The Mom's Choice Gold Award®

# A Wellness Guide for the Digital Age

by Kerry Crofton and twenty-two of the world's leading experts

Yes, you can be tech-savvy, use electronics more safely, and stay connected *and* healthy.

May this comprehensive resource guide bring wisdom and wellness to you, your loved ones and community.

Global Wellbeing Books

Reprinted in July, 2014

Published by Global WellBeing Books

First published as *Radiation Rescue* in 2009
Published as *Wireless Radiation Rescue* in 2010, 2011, 2012



The views expressed in this work are solely those of the author and do not necessarily reflect the views of the publisher, and the publisher hereby disclaims any responsibility for them. This material is not meant to be a substitute for the advice provided by a physician and should not be used for self-diagnosis, or for treatment.

Neither the author nor the contributing experts assume responsibility for how the readers use this information, or for any circumstances arising out of the use, misuse, interpretation or application of any information supplied in this book. The opinions expressed are personal observations, and not intended to malign or defame any industry, agency, individual or product.

Printed in the United States of America

Library of Congress Cataloging-in-Publication Data

Crofton, Kerry

A Wellness Guide for the Digital Age – With Safer-Tech Solutions for All Things Wired & Wireless – All Brains Are Worth Saving

Includes resources and index.

**ISBN: 978-0986473548**

1. Technology – health and safety. 2. Electro-magnetic radiation – Biological effects. 3. Cell phones and cancer risks. 4. Electro-pollution 5. Wireless networks and cell towers – health hazards. 5. Pregnancy and Parenting. 6. Digital Addiction. 7. Digital Detox. 8. Healthy Aging 9. Wellness in The Digital Age I. Title.

Library of Congress Control Number: 2013942411

## A note from the author

WE HUMANS, EACH WONDROUSLY UNIQUE and complex, have an inborn healthiness that is based partially on all the electrical fields – *within and around us* – being in harmony.

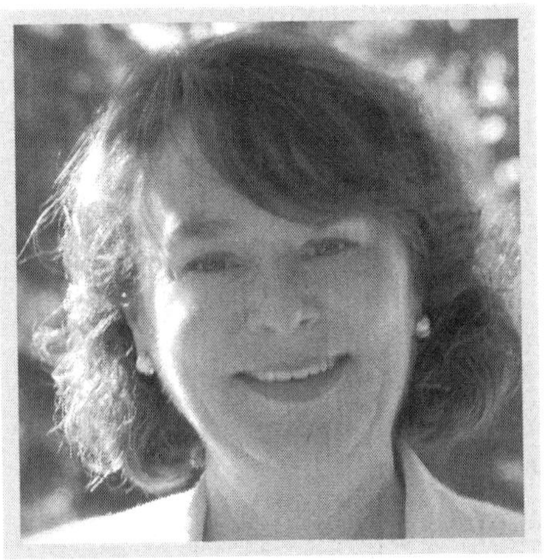

And, our heart and brain cells have their own delicate electrical integrity. Our modus operandi, our wellbeing, so to speak, relies on being attuned in this way.

We are overwhelming this natural state with a new environmental health hazard – the smog of electro-pollution. The waves of microwave radiation – from mobile phones and all WiFi devices – are powerful enough to blast data through concrete. Imagine how easily this radiation travels through us, and our vulnerable children. And, as you may know, this digital generation of inside children is also becoming disconnected – from themselves and the natural world.

Good news: this is a wake-up call with easy-to-implement solutions.

This wellness guide reveals how government-sanctioned levels of radiation, from all things wired and wireless, can be harmful to our health – and how to use all of these electronics more safely.

Our medical team cautions about a range of potential side effects: exposure without symptoms (you don't feel anything but harm is still occurring), mild to moderate symptoms, and electro-sensitivity. And they offer: how to recognize and treat symptoms and how to age well: from conception to college – and beyond. For ourselves, our children, and grandchildren. Not just ours – everyone's.

## Gratitude

In her 1962 ground-breaking exposé, *Silent Spring*, Rachel Carson woke us up to a new environmental concern, "Technology is often so fundamentally at odds with nature that it must be carefully monitored."

I salute the courage of Rachel Carson and other forward-thinking researchers, and especially our stellar team of Contributing Experts – all friends of our future.

Much love, always, to my wonderful husband and children, and my heartfelt thanks for your support.

My gratitude also goes to the media willing to hear this wake-up call. An interviewer once asked me, "Don't you think the train has already left the station?"

I replied, "Yes, and it's a wireless radiation hot spot. However, we can turn this around."

As you read through this book, you will see how. And why.

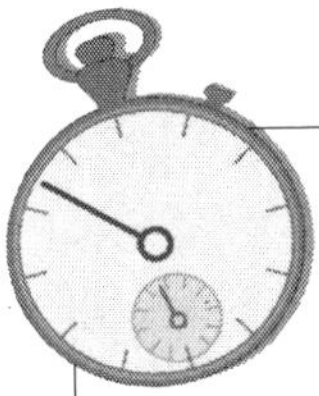

*This is a comprehensive resource guide*

*In a hurry?*

Scan the **Introduction** and **Book Overview** pages 1 - 5

2-minute Quick Read pages begin each section – listed below

The Index begins page 367



- Book website: www.SaferTechSolutions.org

## Safer-tech for the whole family

Some friends are off to see their pregnant daughter and to meet soon their first grandchild.

They welcomed my suggestions to protect this baby:

1. Let the new parents know why the baby should not be within ten feet of any powered-on mobile device – before or after the birth.

2. Buy these new parents landline telephone service and a corded phone. (Like most young people of their digital generation, they are now only using cell phones.) If they insist on a cordless phone, find a second-hand, 900 MHz model – *not* a 2.4, 5.8 or 6.0 GHz digital model.

3. And look for an older analog baby monitor, if they want an electronic monitor. Digital monitors are harmful as they emit microwave radiation.

4. Buy them a wired-only Internet router and a few Ethernet cables and explain why they do not want the baby, or themselves, in a WiFi environment. If they baulk, get them a power bar for turning off the router at bedtime, and make sure it is as far away from baby as possible.

5. If they use a microwave oven, ask them to keep the baby at least twenty-five feet away when it's on.

6. Bluetooth® is not for babies, in the car, or anywhere. And an electric hybrid car has strong electro-magnetic fields.

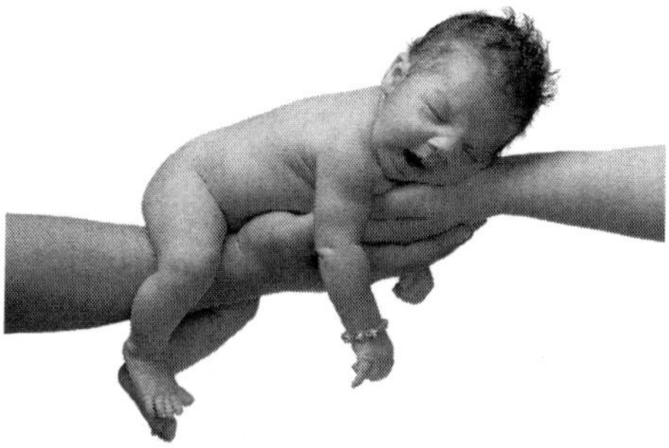

The new parents can use their protective urge to keep their vulnerable child safe, and not let the child play with harmful devices such as phones, tablets or other wirelessly-connected devices. If they read this book, they'll see why.

# Contents

## About the Author

Kerry Crofton is a health educator, children and youth advocate, Medical Commentator on Electro-magnetic Radiation (EMR) for the American Academy of Anti-Aging Medicine, and Founder of the nonprofit Friends of The Future and Doctors For Safer Schools.

She is a member of the International EMF Alliance and The Center for Safer Wireless Medical Advisory Board. Kerry holds a doctorate in psychology, and her 40 years of work include: clinical practice; a newspaper column; co-production of a television program on heart health; and direction of a biofeedback clinic and cardiac programs.

Her first book, *The Healthy Type A* (Macmillan 1998), was based on her program work for the American and Canadian Heart Foundations.

Her clinical background is an asset in working with people who experience electro-sensitivity or digital addiction. She develops wellness programs for pregnant moms and healthy aging programs for all ages.

She also teaches mindfulness meditation and The Mindful EYE contemplative photography with her husband Charles Blackhall.

Kerry worked in aviation with pilots and air traffic controllers and served on the Canadian Aviation Tribunal, enforcing the *Aeronautics Act.* She leads an international coalition of aviation experts concerned about health and safety issues of in-flight WiFi and cell phone use.

In working with experts since 2006, she is well informed in this issue. Her expertise lies in education, coaching people and organizations in effective change, and defending the public's right to know.

Kerry brings together the research and recommendations of many experts in this field, and with their collaboration she developed these Safer-Tech solutions – the basis of this comprehensive resource guide.

# Introduction – Did You Know?

• increasingly powerful electronics, and other radiation exposures, are not properly tested for health safety, and the accumulated doses are not being considered – or monitored – for adverse effects

• radiation from WiFi hot spots and microwave towers (cell towers/ masts) is high enough to have significant impact on human health

• government standards are not accurate, and not protecting us

• there *is* evidence of health risks, especially to our children

• there are safer alternatives – easy and affordable options

**You will find this book useful if:**

- you have heard about wireless radiation health hazards and want an accurate summary of the research and recommendation
- you spend a lot of time on a computer, in a wireless environment, on a mobile phone, live near a Smart Meter, drive a Hybrid, have Bluetooth in your vehicle
- young people you care about use cell phones, iPads/tablets, or WiFi iPods, and you want to know which electronic devices are the safest

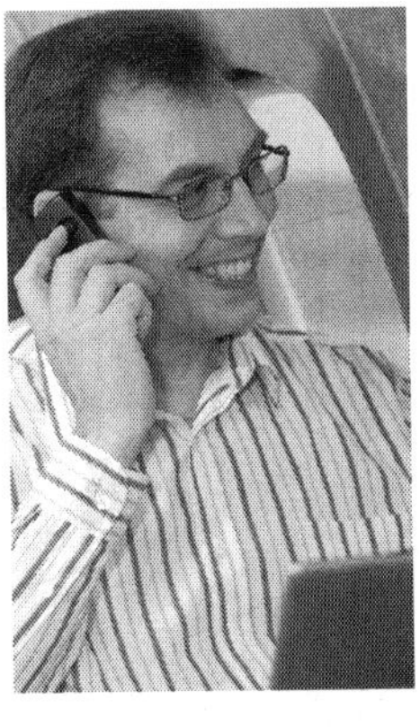

- you travel in high-exposure environments like aircraft and sleep in hotels with WiFi
- you are concerned about the radiation from cell tower antennas, or power lines, near your home, workplace, or your children's school (and the school's wireless Internet)
- you know that you are electro-sensitive and want the best medical and technical advice for this often misdiagnosed condition
- there's a newborn, or one about to be born, in your family and you want to know about baby monitors and other potential hazards

And you will find this book useful if:

- you want the facts on ultrasound, airport security scanners, CT scans, MRI, dental and medical X-rays and other diagnostic imaging
- you are suffering from any of the following conditions:
  - allergies
  - ALS
  - Alzheimer's
  - ADD/ADHD
  - Asperger's Syndrome
  - Autism Spectrum Disorder
  - cancer
  - cardiac conditions - angina, arrhythmia, hypertension, tachycardia
  - cataracts
  - Chronic Fatigue Syndrome
  - depression
  - dizziness/vertigo
  - electro-sensitivity
  - epilepsy
  - headaches and migraine
  - infertility
  - insomnia
  - immune suppression
  - Multiple Chemical Sensitivity
  - tinnitus
  - Parkinson's
  - skin rashes
  - sleep disorders
- you are concerned about aging well. The effects of electro-pollution have been called "rapid aging syndrome," even aging our skin! And there's medical information on how to boost your immune system, and other longevity tips for healthy aging in this new digital age

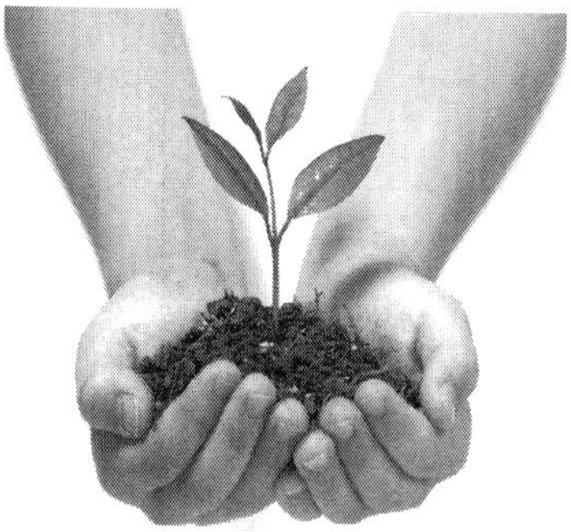

- a healthy balance to your family's need for electronics and screen-free time is a priority. Read about people who are unplugging and being together, outside in nature – tech-free
- you are interested in practical ways to protect our planet, and all life forms, from the environmental impact of electro-pollution and other toxins

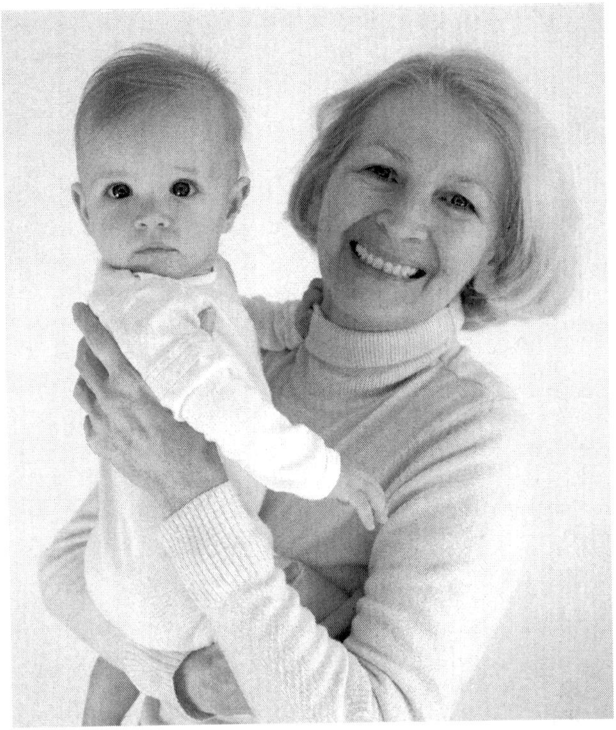

**Overview** – Scan this to reduce being overwhelmed?

**Need to Review the Evidence? Read Strategy 1, page 22**

If you are already well versed in the evidence, the scientists' concerns, the problem with government standards, and the misinformation, you could jump ahead to the second strategy – after you check out our new 4-Day trial on page 49. It will help you recognize and reduce sources of electro-pollution.

However, I encourage you to come back some time to the first strategy so you'll be better equipped to protect your family and educate others. If you find yourself becoming overwhelmed in Strategy 1, please skip ahead to assess your risk (Strategy 2) or to the devices and solutions section (Strategy 3), rather than abandoning this altogether.

## Need to Rate Your Risks? Read Strategy 2, page 96

Here you find a questionnaire to see where you are being exposed to electro-magnetic fields (EMF). Some people refer to this as electro-magnetic radiation, or EMR; this is the term we'll use. We include, in simple terms, what you need to know about EMR – wired and wireless. We also use 'RF' for radio-frequency (wireless radiation, WiFi).

## Need Safer Solutions? Read Strategy 3, 118

This offers information on everything from the lowest radiation dental X-rays, to what you need to know about tucking your child into the back seat of a hybrid car.

Details here include the kinds of cell phone earpieces and headsets to avoid – and the one that is recommended, the safer alternative to cordless phones, what kind of cell phone to buy – and the best way to use it. There's also key information about safer Internet access. You'll discover practical advice about many other devices, and ways to reduce your radiation exposure and related health risks.

## Need Your Action Plan? Read Strategy 4, page 222

Here's how to create a safer environment for you and your family, room by room. Our contributing physicians also offer what you need to know about electro-sensitivity, autism, immune health, dental health and other key factors in your family's wellbeing. They also offer advice on preventing or healing from EMR exposure, and reveal how they protect their own families.

An author on parent-teen communication gives us tips on how to get young people onboard. We look at the Safer-Tech Challenge – this is for families wired on wireless, who take on reconnecting with each other, and with the love of nature.

## Need Hope For the Future? Read page 326

The conclusion brings it all together with inspiration from the families following these guidelines, and from dedicated people making a difference. We hear about hopes for the future – a challenge for some who have been lone voices with their research and warnings ignored.

**Resources** are on page 347

**Index** is on page 367

## You Are The Judge and Jury In This Case

The radiation levels from devices that send and receive have been called "low" but there is enough evidence to cause concern. I am not asking you to jump to this view, but to hear the case and decide for yourself.

You can't see this kind of pollution. However, if the arcs of radiation were visible, you would see the hot zone extends a long way.

These invisible plumes of radiation surround microwave ovens, cell tower antennas, mobile phones, iPads and all wirelessly-connected devices, including video games, cordless phones and baby monitors.

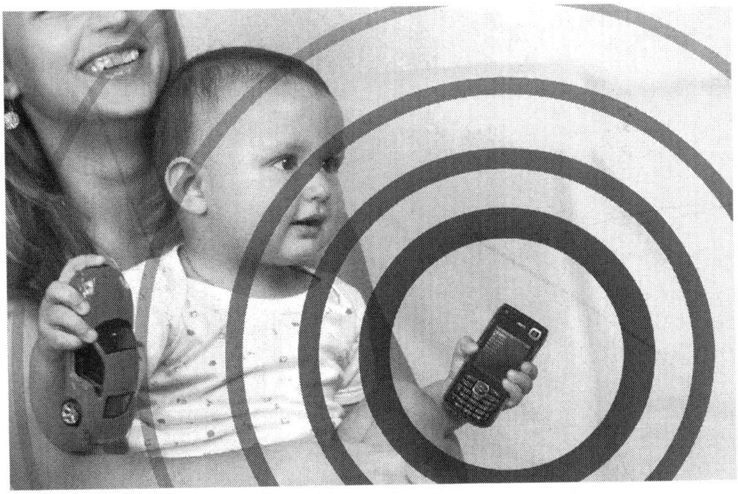

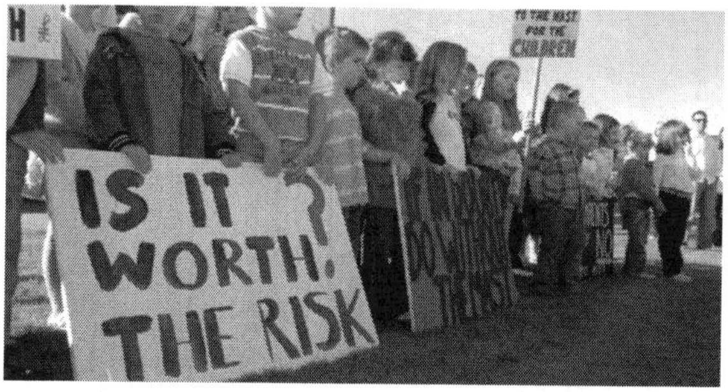


## A Range of Views

Technical expert Grahame Blackwell, PhD, Chartered Engineer and advisor to WiredChild, explains:

> Your body is more sensitive than any wireless device, so if your device can pick up a signal, it means that your body, and your brain cells are also receiving those waves. Unlike natural sources, or radio or TV waves, the harmful frequencies from all digital devices are pulsed and jagged – like a saw tooth.

## Physicians

Many years ago, the surgeon Robert Becker, MD told us:

> Our bodies and brains generate electro-magnetic fields. We live in the Earth's natural magnetic field, and from the beginning we have been dependent on this environment.
>
> However, we have now created a vast global network of man-made electro-magnetic fields – the greatest polluting element in the earth's environment. The human body electric and the Earth's body electric have been damaged.

Cardiologist Stephen Sinatra, MD expresses concern:

> We have seen clinical evidence that electro-pollution affects the normal functioning of the electrically sensitive heart, including the rate and rhythm, and other systems of the body. All forms of pollution impair our health, and the electro-pollution arising from the proliferation of wireless technology has greatly added to this burden. The effects can go unnoticed among even the best health professionals. We need to educate them.

Public health expert, David Carpenter, MD, head of the Institute for Health and Environment at the University of Albany, reported:

> There's enough science to suggest that cell phone radiation can cause cancer, but not enough political will to implement measures to reduce exposure. We're setting ourselves up for an epidemic of cancers in the future that should be preventable based on the knowledge we have now. If you use a cell phone and hold it to your head, the cancers you see elevated are brain cancer, tumors of the auditory nerve, tumors of the parotid gland, the salivary gland and the cheek right by the ear.

Dr. Carpenter also said that the concern is not only about cell phones. He says there is growing evidence that people who live close to radio towers, for example, are at increased risk of cancer:

> If your whole body is exposed, as is the case in people living near towers — there are studies with radio towers in Rome or in Korea — then the cancer that one sees most prominently is leukemia.

Dr. Andrew Weil, Founder and Director of the Arizona Center for Integrative Medicine, offered us this perspective:

> It's vital to focus closely on the most recently published studies, the ones that show the effects of longer-term exposure. The Environmental Working Group (EWG), a Washington, D.C.-based nonprofit organization, reported on key studies that link radiation from long-term cell phone use with increased risks of brain and salivary gland tumors, migraines and vertigo, as well as behavior problems in children, including hyperactivity.

There are many physicians opposing these views. A government health official I know, a physician with many years of medical practice, states firmly, "There is no evidence of harm from wireless technology."

## Scientists

Dr. Devra Davis, epidemiologist and a leading scientist in this field, was involved in other health issues like tobacco. Dr. Davis tells us, "If the cell phone were a drug, it would be banned. And there's concern about other wireless devices including iPads which can be even worse. I am especially concerned about children and teens using mobile devices."

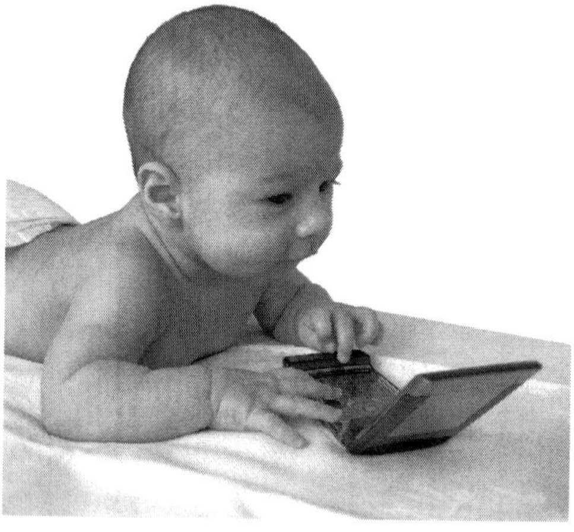

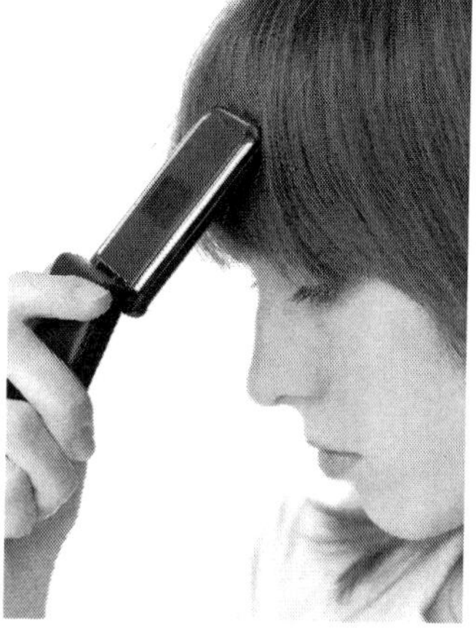

Professor Olle Johansson of the Karolinska Institute in Stockholm:

> There is clear evidence of harm. I am particularly concerned about children and pregnant women, and teens using mobile phones. Existing safety standards are inadequate and do not consider prolonged exposure.

Eminent scientists, including Professor Johansson, issued The Seletun Scientific Statement (*Reviews on Environmental Health* (2010; 25: 307-317) stating there is enough evidence to warrant a new approach to public health with strong preventative actions, especially concerning the growth and development of the fetus and children. They called for biologically-based exposure standards.

## The World Health Organization – Cancer Panel

Their 2011 report changed the WHO/IARC (International Agency for Research on Cancer) long-held "no adverse effects" position on wireless (RF radio-frequency) radiation classifying it as a carcinogen in the same category as DDT and lead. *(Please note this refers to microwave (cell) towers and WiFi as well as cell phone radiation.)* Then they weakened this stance with "the evidence is limited." This equivocation was heralded by the industry. In April 2013, the statement was stronger: "Positive associations have been observed between exposure to radio-frequency radiation from wireless phones and glioma and acoustic neuroma."

## The Industry

> Numerous scientific studies prove wireless technology is safe. This is supported by many health agencies and government standards.

## Your View?

Hopefully, my journey and what I've learned along the way will help you make the best decisions for you and your family in this digital age.

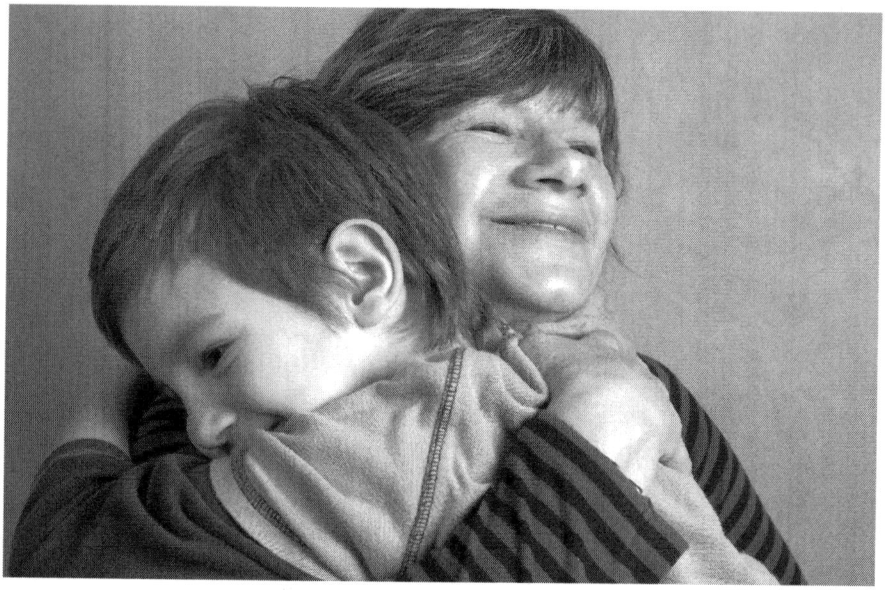

*We don't feel this radiation and we think it's not doing anything, but it's a very potent biological agent and government safety standards are irrelevant.*

Martin Blank, PhD, Columbia University

## My wireless wake-up call and an update

Oh no, you may be thinking, not another dire health warning. Like most people, I often feel fed up with alarming medical news and conflicting studies (one report implicated wine as a risk for breast cancer, and the next day another praised wine as protection from Alzheimer's Disease). What a choice!

Do you remember when it was a pleasure to sit back and read the newspaper – perhaps with a glass of wine? Most have had enough of the 'sky-is-falling' alarms. Yes, it's tempting to hang up on this wake-up call.

But please don't! There are easy and effective solutions in this book.

First, we need to look at how we have become cocooned in convenience, in radiation hot spots, as it turns out. Realizing this hit me hard. I have been a health educator for thirty-five years yet have never faced an issue as challenging, and personally unsettling, as this one.

## Briefly, here's the problem, as I understand it

As the physicians Dr. Robert Becker and Dr. Stephen Sinatra reminded us, we humans are magnificently designed bundles of energy living within the Earth's varied electro-magnetic fields.

The strong forces of the Earth, Sun and Moon affect us, and we have adapted to these. Yes, we can be killed by a bolt of lightning, or develop cancer from too much sun, but overall we have evolved to deal with this natural radiation. However, we're now in a massive soup of human-made radiation, on top of limitless numbers of new chemical toxins.

All the parents I know are concerned about raising children in an environment awash in chemical hazards. We were justly horrified to discover there was lead in toys and baby bibs, toxic Bisphenol A in plastic baby bottles, carcinogens in baby bath products, an array of chemicals in plastics, in just about everything from plastic wrap to shower curtains, and melamine in many pet foods, chocolate bars – and baby formulas!

We hear there can be traces of mercury in high fructose corn syrup, in many processed foods and sugary drinks. Mercury, one of the deadliest heavy metals, is often found in tuna from polluted oceans, in most vaccines, and 'silver' dental fillings. My dentist remarked, "If mercury is such a hazardous material it requires a strict protocol for handling, then how could your patient's mouth be a safe place to put it?" Mercury in dental fillings has been banned in Sweden and Norway.

There's also a seemingly endless list of carcinogens added to color, flavor and preserve our food; toxic chemicals added to our cosmetics, sunscreens, cleaning products, detergents and dryer sheets. Purify and freshen the air with chemically-scented candles, and plug-in, or spray, room deodorizers? What are we thinking?

Whether we're buying children's toys or cell phones, are we assuming that public officials and manufacturers ensure products are rigorously tested for health effects before market? Relying on the fox for the safety of the hen house? It usually takes regulators a long time *after* a marketplace exposure before issuing public health alerts.

Remember asbestos? It took regulators a mere 100 years to take protective action. Tobacco? It was also everywhere. Doctors smoked. Lead? Hear the story that the ancient Romans did themselves in with lead-lined flasks? It's not prudent to wait for government regulators, health authorities, or the industry. Independent scientists are the first to raise the alarm. Rachel Carson, the mother of the environmental movement, took on the chemical industry about DDT and other poisonous pesticides – and won. She was one of the first to warn us that technology can come with a cost to our health.

Toxic sludge and smog are, at least, hazards we can usually see. Imagine how horrified Rachel Carson would be about the environmental impact of electro-pollution, and its connection to the disappearance of the bees. And the birds. Her prediction of a silent spring now seems even more chilling. Yet I am still hopeful that people like you will listen.

The changing landscape, and the World Health Organization stance, are encouraging and I am heartened by medical researchers like Dr. David Carpenter speaking out. He says that the growing mass of evidence that wireless radiation exposes people to increased risk of cancer, explains why the WHO identified it as a 2B carcinogen.

> That 2B classification means the evidence isn't all there but there's reason to be concerned. And a study from the National Institutes of Health demonstrating directly that an active cell phone held to the head resulted in changes in glucose utilization in the brain. So yes, the evidence is getting strong with time.

Yet, many officials still hold the "no evidence of harm" position citing this international agency. They should read the article Dr. Davis and other independent scientists published in *Pathophysiology*, February 2013:

> The WHO determined that cell and cordless phone radiation was a "*possible* human carcinogen" – a category that includes compounds that are subject to serious regulation and control today. Reviewing studies produced since then, this article concludes that this radiation should be re-classified as a *probable* human carcinogen (2A) based on new reports that those who began using cell phones before age 20 have 4 to 8 fold increased risks of brain cancer as well as increases in leukemia.
>
> And, a new study found that cell phones do produce hot spots in living brain tissue, contrary to the assumption used to set all standards today.

This is evidence that cell phone radiation is getting so strong it may heat brain tissue! As you'll see when we look at standards, this news should raise a red flag and provoke serious investigation.

After that WHO report, the industry ramped up its PR campaign and a conference in Brussels reportedly only featured speakers who were directly or indirectly linked to the telecom industry. This is why many people speak out strongly against industry tactics.

In the future, many consumers will wonder why they adhered to the industry's biased views and their spin on the science, and why government complacency was allowed to go on for so long. They may understand why independent scientists, including Dr. Davis, and many advocates, worked so hard to jolt people from their WiFi cocoons.

And, as we've said, it isn't just human health at risk. Our authorities explain how the birds, bees and other life forms, are being adversely affected. Some of this may surprise you. Haven't we had radio and TV waves swirling around our heads, and microwave ovens and portable phones for decades? And aren't we living quite happily with wireless technology without any apparent harm?

Not even the mainstream medical community seems aware of this issue; few recognize related symptoms, conditions and risks. It has taken time, and a lot of research, to discover how to reduce our exposure without unplugging from the power grid and moving to a cabin in the woods. I'll admit, I was resistant to hearing the disturbing evidence and the onslaught of information. I didn't want this bad news.

Have you heard this: Well, everything gives you cancer, so what's the point of worrying? There's nothing we can do so why bother? Feeling overwhelmed and powerless are obstacles that can be overcome. I am hopeful that as this message is being broadcast more clearly, more people will hear not only that there is a problem, but most importantly, that there are solutions. Please remember throughout this book – and when trying to alert others – that we are, at this time, dealing with some areas of scientific uncertainty.

Yes, there is some urgency to this message.

One pioneering researcher told me, "By the time we have scientific consensus, if we ever do, we are going to have lost a lot of people."

Not my children, I protested. Now I am also fighting for yours.

I am often asked how I became so fired up about this issue – my children's wellbeing. In the spring of 2006, I was concerned about the proximity of high voltage power lines – a health hazard I knew about – too close to a new addition at our youngest child's school. Then I discovered the school's wireless Internet, and the cell tower nearby, were also putting the children at risk. Soon I was alarmed by the massive amount of eye-opening research about these health hazards.

Investigating further, I found out that many things in our environment were adding to the problem. Like most people, I carried a cell phone. I seldom used it though – instinctively it seemed that anything that could push a powerful signal through cement might not be good to press against my head. Or my children's. (You may rethink whether arming your children or teens with cell phones is really keeping them safe?) My office contained the usual must-have electronic gadgets: the latest cordless phones, a computer with wireless Internet. So convenient. Being an early adopter I brought the newest conveniences on board. And I took pride in our eco-green home. Then I had a professional electro-magnetic radiation assessment done.

Talk about an electric shock! Our youngest child's canopy bed – so beautifully decorated in pale peach and cream, with luminous stars sprinkled on the blue sky ceiling – was a hazardous hot-spot because of the radiation-reflecting metal frame. I gasped when the radiation detector screamed an alert. Who knew? I whipped that metal frame out of there before we moved on to the next room. I couldn't even bring myself to give it to anyone and thrust it into the recycling bin.

I was also shocked when the cordless portable phone sent the detector off the scale. Doesn't everyone have a cordless phone? Haven't we lived happily with this convenience for years?

The UK physician, Dr. David Dowson, urged caution, "Having a cordless phone is like having a mobile mast [cell tower] in your house." I replaced all cordless phones with safer corded models. Big difference.

Testing a friend's microwave oven was a jolt! Backing up from it, to see how far the radiation extended, I crossed her kitchen floor and almost fell down the stairs. The detector was still blaring at 25 feet (nearly 8 meters). She had known that experts say microwaves can be health risks, so she always stood back when it was on – but not 25 feet away!

Being green at heart we had replaced light bulbs with compact fluorescents. Yes, they are energy-efficient but emit 'dirty electricity' (and then there's the mercury!). My husband protested, "Know how much energy they save?" I waited to tell him about electric hybrid cars. (Occupants are so close to a powerful unshielded electric battery.)

I learned how radiation from the wireless router I'd installed for in-home Internet access was a major problem. Had no idea. As a mother, of course I know the guilt feeling – this time I shuddered, realizing my not knowing put our family in harm's way. (Wired is safer, quicker, and more secure and reliable – and still convenient.)

This is a lot to take in, so I understand if at first you feel overwhelmed. Like me, you may go through flashes (some of us don't need more hot flashes!) of disbelief, outrage, or guilt. However, I did go from being duped to determined and resolved to use my skills as a health educator to alert others. I've worked steadily ever since – sometimes inspired, often discouraged at people's unwillingness to look at this. My heart breaks when I see a pregnant woman or a young child or teen clutching a wireless device, or when a school insists on WiFi and acts as if there's no other way to access Internet. Reading the daily news is rough as reputable organizations are making doubtful decisions: "Apple and the Mayo Clinic are working on mobile health". That's an oxymoron!

Our team addresses a wide range of issues: from healthy aging strategies, how children can become physiologically addicted to gaming and digital devices, to concerns about wireless radiation in aircraft.

Would passengers still demand WiFi if they knew that in 2008 Hans Scheiner, MD cautioned the industry, "Symptoms caused by electro-magnetic radiation: headaches, drowsiness, vertigo, nausea, loss of hearing and vision, loss of consciousness, and a lack of concentration are a concern in transportation safety, including aviation."? A few years ago, two pilots fainted on board WiFi – enabled aircraft. US Senator Jay Rockefeller has called for a closer look at this technology (page 81.)

Here's good news: I met a visionary team at Wisdom 2.0 in San Francisco. Levi Felix caught my attention – typing on his manual typewriter and offering haiku. He and his partner, Brooke Dean lead digital detox retreats. Want to unplug and have tech-free fun? Disconnect to reconnect. Check out: TheDigitalDetox.org and Camp Grounded. This is a radical contrast to the tech giant offering "virtual camp for kids" who never have to leave their laptops, or go outside.

I speak to you as a mother and a health educator. Working together with wisdom and mindfulness, we *can* meet this challenge. You have my commitment to help you and your community as much as I can.

## It's Your Choices That Matter – For Brains Worth Saving

Remember, our goal is for you to have the science-based information, and the effective solutions you need to safeguard your loved ones, maintain your health, and age well in this digital age.

In 2014 Dr. Davis notes, "The case for taking simple precautions to reduce RF exposures is becoming stronger every day, as a number of governments around the world are advising." Are you ready to consider this? Please allow me to introduce our distinguished team.

## Contributing Clinicians, Researchers and Technicians: Experts for The Digital Age and Friends of The Future

**Martin Blank, PhD** – Dept. of Physiology and Cellular Biophysics, Columbia University, author of *Overpowered* (Seven Stories Press, 2014);

**Carolyn Dean, MD, ND** – physician and naturopathic doctor specializing in complementary medicine and environmental health;

**Professor Devra Davis, PhD**–epidemiologist, Founder and President of Environmental Health Trust, a Lead Author with Nobel-prize winning group, author of *Disconnect* (Dutton, 2010);

**Lawrence Gust** – electrical engineer and Institute for Bau-Biologie® (IBE) certified Building Biologist;

**Katharina Gustavs** – Building Biology environmental consultant specializing in electro-magnetic field testing and environmental health;

**Stan Hartman** – environmental health consultant with Radsafe in Boulder, CO specializing in EMF/EMR issues;

**Magda Havas, PhD** – Associate Professor of Environmental and Resource Studies at Trent University;

**Olle Johansson, PhD** – Associate Professor at the Department of Neuroscience, Karolinska Institute, Stockholm, Sweden;

**Vini Khurana, MD** – Neurosurgeon at Canberra Hospital, and Associate Professor of Neurosurgery at Australian National University;

**Dietrich Klinghardt, MD, PhD** – founder of the Klinghardt Academy of Neurobiology offering training programs for health practitioners;

**Henry Lai, PhD** – Research Professor, School of Medicine and College of Engineering, University of Washington;

**Heather McKinney, PhD** – researcher who specializes in strategic planning within individuals, organizations and communities;

**Rob Metzinger** – Electronics Engineering Technologist and instructor with the International Institute for Bau-Biologie® (IBE);

**Joel Moskowitz, PhD** – Director, Center for Family and Community Health, School of Public Health, University of California, Berkeley; disseminates information on EMR at saferemr.com;

**Alasdair Philips** – the Director of Powerwatch (UK), qualified in Electrical and Electronic Engineering;

**William Rea, MD** – former surgeon, Founder the Environmental Health Center in Dallas, Texas, and a leader in environmental medicine;

**Hans Scheiner, MD** – was a physician practicing complementary medicine, who treated thousands of electro-sensitive patients;

**Peter Sierck** – industrial hygienist with IBE and IBN certification performing professional EMF and RF measurements;

**Stephen Sinatra, MD, FACC** – board-certified cardiologist, Fellow in the American College of Cardiology, founder of Heart MD Institute, and writes a newsletter entitled *Heart, Health & Nutrition*;

**Louis Slesin, PhD** – founder and publisher of Microwave News, a reliable source of scientific information and news updates;

**Sarah Starkey, PhD** – neuroscientist in the UK with a specific concern about wireless systems in the school environment;

**Jacob Teitelbaum, MD** – author of *From Fatigued to Fantastic* and a leading physician in the field of complementary medicine.

All of these experts have generously offered their quotes and expertise; none are responsible for any other material included here.

## Update: Microwave Madness in The Marketplace

Just when we thought awareness of WiFi health hazards was growing:

• Baby seats by Fisher-Price with iPad holders so close to the infant

• Pendant mobile phones to hang between women's breasts (Dr. Devra Davis' report about the potential breast cancer link is on page 40)

• Google™ Glass – more radiation than a cell phone, close to the brain

• Google™ Driverless Cars, "Our software and sensors do all the work"

• Smart Conductive Clothing and Wearable Gear, Hearing Aids with Bluetooth™ for WiFi connectivity – microwaves up close and personal

**Product Disclaimer?** Suppose a product came with the following warnings. Even if it were cool and everywhere, would you buy it?

– Not tested for long-term [or short] impact on human health, and in tiny print in the manual: keep this ___ [distance] away from your body

– Thousands of physicians and scientists, and some countries, are raising a medical alert about its use and inaccurate regulation standards

– The World Health Organization has labelled its microwave radiation emissions a possible carcinogen [along with DDT, lead and car exhaust]

– People report reaction symptoms when exposed to this product: heart problems, sleep disruption, vertigo, headaches, cognitive impairment, skin rashes, bloodshot eyes, tingling hands, ringing in the ears. Scientists warn of brain cancer and other health risks.

– Evidence of pre-natal exposure causing harm to offspring

– There are class action lawsuits based on health claims

**Consumer Beware 'Smart' WiFi technology**:

Diapers, Clothing, Medical devices, Classrooms, Watches, Wearables, Guns, Meters, Appliances, Heart Monitors, Hospital beds, Home Security, 'Smart' Cities with sensors in every house and on every street, and 'talking' cars with WiFi signals emitting from car to car – for safety! Please hear what our experts have to say and decide for yourself.

## Safeguard The Children

Meet another friend of the future using the precautionary principle.

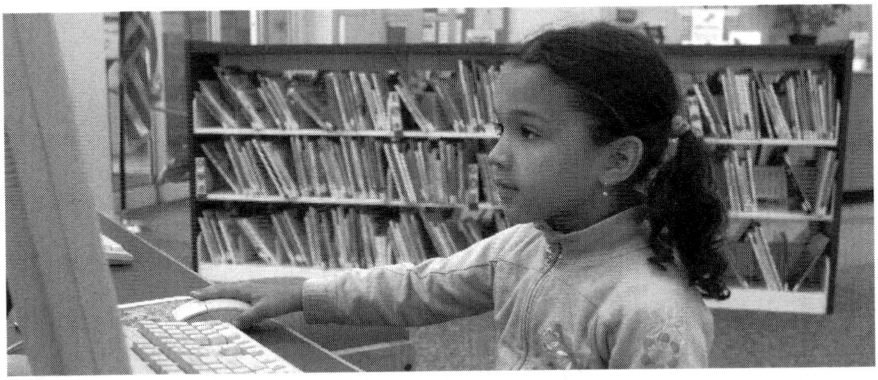

> As a school principal, I see the health and safety of our children as a non-negotiable responsibility. Although there is far from universal agreement as to the dangers of wireless technology, and there are many with vested interests in its continued use, evidence of harm is extensive. The default position must be on the side of safety. I have removed all wireless technology from our school and banned the use of cell phones within our building. In our older classes, every child has a laptop, connected to the internet through a hard-wired cable. We have advanced technology without the dangers of wireless radiation.
>
> Kristin Cassie, Principal, Roots & Wings Montessori, British Columbia

Many other educators and public officials throughout the world have removed WiFi citing health concerns, including the school of a 10-year-old boy in New Zealand who died recently of a brain tumor.

**Our question: why expose students (and staff) to a known health hazard when there are safer, more efficient, options available?**

Are your children and/or grandchildren among those facing this risk?

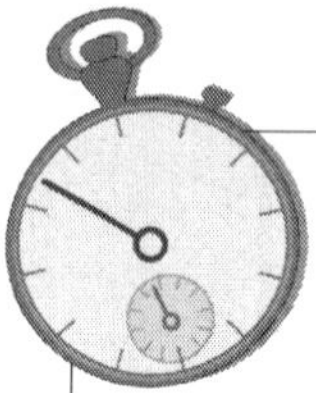

*2 Minute Quick Read Summary*

## Strategy 1. Know the Evidence

WE ARE ADAPTIVE BEINGS who have adjusted well to the other electrical fields in our environment. Until now.

Electro-magnetic radiation exposure from massive man-made wireless and wired sources has been shown to cause harmful effects, especially to children.

Some of the adverse biological effects:

- damage to our DNA
- suppression of the immune system
- leakage of the blood-brain protective barrier
- thickening of the blood

There are also other harmful effects to the cardiovascular, neurological and endocrine systems.

Why bother with yet another health concern? 30 minutes per day on your cell phone, over 10 years, can increase your risk of brain cancer by 40% (Interphone study) or as much as 140% (Professor Hardell). Then Hardell reported a 300% increase with 25 years of cell phone use – some motivation to keep it away from your body.

How many minutes per day do you spend on a cell phone, or a new high-powered multi-media device? And having wireless Internet and cordless phones in your home could be the reason you are not sleeping well. Or those dizzy spells?

**See Strategy 1 for more details.**

*The voluntary exposure of the brain to microwaves from hand-held mobile phones is the largest human biological experiment ever.*

Professor Salford, MD, Lund University, Sweden

The digital-age generation is un-knowingly, and un-necessarily, at risk.

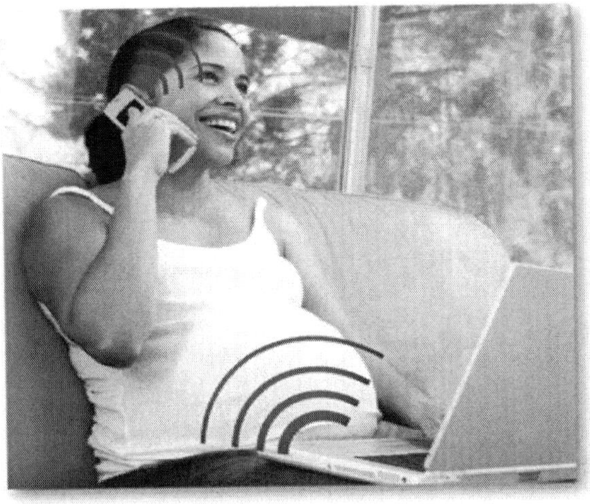

## Strategy 1. Know the Evidence

- the levels of electro-magnetic radiation that we are exposed to today are billions of times higher than for our ancestors (yes, *billions*, and this is a conservative estimate);
- this technology was never pre-market tested for safety;
- the current government standards we assume are protecting us are, evidently, just plain wrong;
- **fortunately, there is good news** - this is not an insurmountable problem; there are safer solutions and hope on the horizon.

*Facts do not cease to exist because they are ignored.* Aldous Huxley

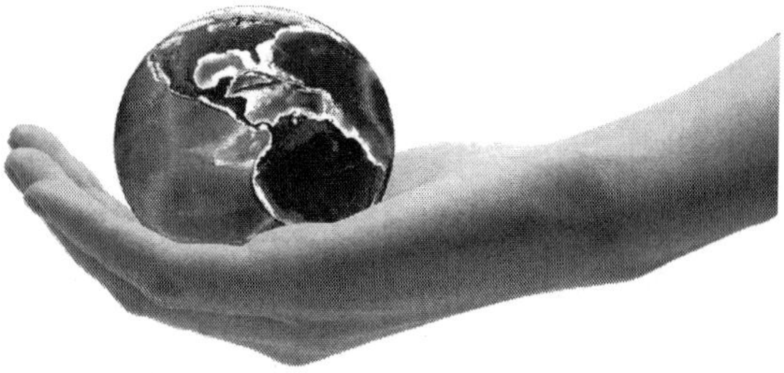

## Microwaving this Blue Planet

As if satellites hovering over us in space, city-wide canopy wireless systems, and powerful electrical grids weren't enough, Mt. Everest – "the roof of the world" – has become another radiation hot spot. You may be wondering if many scientists report evidence of harm, then why haven't our governments done something to protect us? And, how did untested wireless devices make it to market in the first place?

## Why Government Regulations Are Not Protecting You

Guess what? Safety standards are IRRELEVANT to WiFi, cell phone radiation, and other wired and wireless devices, as the standards were only based on thermal damage. Thermal means the energy is strong enough to warm human tissue (non-thermal means it is not.) Unbelievably, regulators only considered thermal effects and ignored less powerful (non-thermal) frequencies – the lower parts of the spectrum. Tell that to the officials trying to reassure you that the WiFi levels in your child's school, "fall well within safety standards," as if that means they are safe. In Canada a government scientist, Dr. James McNamee, admitted their standards (Safety Code 6) are only based on thermal levels – preventing damage from heating, like electrical burns.

Because short-term exposure from cell phones did *not* heat the tissue of a 200 lb adult male, the industry argued wireless devices were safe and should be excluded from pre-market testing. Potential damage to smaller, more vulnerable, beings was *not* tested, or considered. Professor Gandhi – his graphic of the skulls is on the book cover – worries about this, "All the standards used for cell phones apply only to the 'big guy' brain." How is this oversight affecting your children?

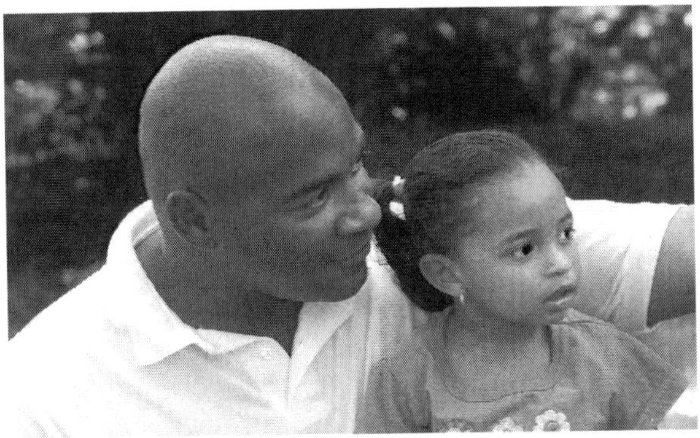

This is still the only thing that government regulations are based on, and still govern the marketplace. And you should know that the standards for radiation emitted from your cell phone, wireless network, cordless phone, baby monitor, or nearby cell tower antenna are not a little bit off; they are *thousands to millions* of times apart from what many eminent scientists consider safe.

So why are our schools installing WiFi? And hospitals. And parks. And planes. No government agencies seem to be monitoring the impact on human health – on us – or considering the affect in five years. In two?

Professor Johansson cautions:

> People should know about the difference between acute (immediate) and long-term health effects. The current standards only look at acute effects.

As you see, we need to take a course of action to safeguard our families, and not wait for regulators and public health officials to wake up.

## Government Regulators are "just plain wrong"

The environmental health physician, Dr. David Carpenter, made that hard-hitting statement. Remember this when you have concerns about the wireless at your children's school, question the cell tower antenna, or ask about cell phone safety. You may get: "The radiation levels fall well within government standards." Public health officials may insist, "There is no clear evidence of harm." The industry also holds to these positions. Here are some questions you could ask.

### 7 Key Questions

1. Are those standards up to date?

2. Have these levels been proven safe for women, children, pregnant women, or the fetus? (RF exposure tests were only based on short-term, thermal – heating – effects, only considering adult males.)

3. Did they investigate long-term, and/or non-thermal effects? (No, and brain cancer can take 10-30 years to develop; 3 years for leukaemia in children. While DNA damage, leakage of the blood-brain barrier, cognitive impairment, sperm damage and cardiac effects can occur within a short time at those 'low' government-sanctioned levels.)

4. Have you, as an official/expert, taken steps, like many European countries, to re-evaluate standards and use a safer-tech system? (See page 167.) Why not adopt this precautionary principle?

5. Will you, as an official/expert, give us your personal assurance that the standards you are upholding are safe, and tell us if there are any published, or unpublished, exposure restrictions? We assert our right to know why you are defending this position if you refuse to sign. (See Statement of Accountability on page 330.)

6. What agency is monitoring any adverse health effects, including wireless Internet access in aircraft, or other modes of transportation?

7. What agency is measuring the cumulative dose we are being subjected to, and the potential impact, even if we don't use a cell phone, or have removed wireless exposures from our homes?

**See this news headline? Use your mobile all you want – It's safe!**

"Why haven't we heard about this hazard before?" Good question when headline-making research [studies funded by?] often gives the all clear, including a Danish study several years ago. Then two more Danish studies reported, "No increase in brain tumors from cell phones." However, scientists not working for the industry found serious study flaws. How are we to know the truth, even if we are willing to hear it?

Our team of scientists explains that some studies don't ask what side of the head the person uses the phone on – a key variable in assessing risk – and subjects are included even if they only had rare or occasional exposure. Also it can take more than 10 years for a cancerous tumor to develop. In our WiFi world, with more mobile devices than people, the data will be hard to ignore; Norway and Finland, where mobile devices have been in use longer, are already seeing an increase. How many decades did it take before it was accepted that smoking caused cancer?

There are numerous peer-reviewed studies, published in reputable journals, that should raise medical alerts, including pre-natal exposure and damage to the fetal brain. In March 2014, an animal study on maternal exposure to cell phone radiation reported structural damage to the neurons in the offspring. (Razavinasab M, Moazzami K, Shabani M. *Toxicol Ind Health.* 2014 Mar 6.) See it in the daily news? Did obstetricians alert their pregnant patients about a possible risk, as they surely do about alcohol and tobacco exposure? *See page 41 for more studies and "Pregnancy" in the Index.*

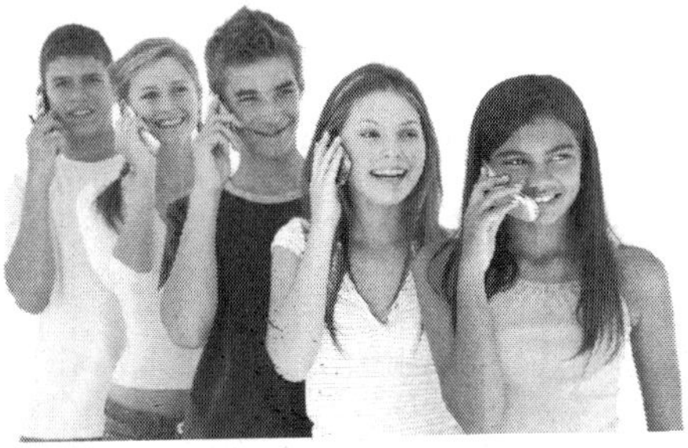

## Evidence is Building

Damage can be immediate, or it can take years to become evident. What fate for a generation using mobiles, and WiFi, day and night? And virtually all pregnant women?

Those saying there's no problem, or who do not take precautionary action – in the face of growing signs of harm – may have a lot to answer for, one doctor confided to me. Educating doctors is crucial.

Dr. David Servan-Schreiber, was Professor of Psychiatry at the University of Pittsburgh, and Dr. Annie Sasco who worked with the World Health Organization agreed about cell phone health concerns:

> What we have now are highly suggestive results from a number of different studies…that point to a non-negligible long-term risk for a brain tumor.

Dr. Magda Havas, from the Environmental and Resource Studies Program, Trent University, confirms other risks:

> Headaches, numbness and tingling sensations in their fingers and face, and difficulty with cognitive functions either when using, or being in the presence of, cell phones and/or cordless phones. Also, people who live within 400 meters (437 yards) of the antennas are experiencing adverse health symptoms. Studies show an increase in cancers and symptoms of what is being called electro-hypersensitivity or EHS.

## Biased Evidence in Industry-Funded Studies?

Dr. Henry Lai is one of a number of credible scientists who have faced attempts to discredit their findings. The trouble started when Dr. Lai's work at the University of Washington showed that radiation at frequencies similar to those emitted by cell phones broke the DNA in rats' brain cells after just two hours of exposure (Lai & Singh 2004).

In "The Cellphone Game," an excellent article published in the September 2008 edition of *The Walrus* magazine, Dr. Lai reports:

> Industry-funded studies are roughly twice as likely as government-funded ones to conclude that cell phones are harmless.

Follow the funding, read the study yourself and/or a trusted review.

### The Controversial Interphone Study

This massive study began in the late 1990s with researchers from 13 countries investigating the possible tumor risks with mobile phones – a good example of misleading headlines: "Interphone Study Inconclusive, Cell Phones Safe, After All." I wish that were true. Check out the Interphone's 'heavy user.' If you had been on your cell phone only *30 minutes a day* over a 10-year period, then you'd qualify as their *'heavy user'*, with a 40 percent increased risk of a brain tumor. If your usage was only *4 minutes a day* (the amount the average person in that study used a cell phone) then you'd fall into their 'no conclusive link' category – as long as you are not exposed to other sources of radiation.

### Cell Phone/Wireless Radiation Update

Joel Moskowitz PhD, Director, Center for Family and Community Health, School of Public Health, UofC Berkeley has conducted research on chronic disease prevention and health promotion for more than 30 years, and has authored dozens of peer-reviewed health publications. Dr. Moskowitz offers this update with some compelling evidence:

• 25 or more years of cell phone and cordless phone use was found to be associated with a tripled risk of brain cancer.

• Women who used cell phones for ten or more years were two-and-a-half times more likely to develop acoustic neuroma, a tumor on the nerve from the ear to the brain.

• Only 30 minutes of exposure to LTE, 4th generation cell phone radiation, was found to alter activity on both sides of the human brain.

• Children with slightly elevated lead levels in their blood who used cell phones were found to be at greater risk of developing Attention Deficit Hyperactivity Disorder (ADHD).

• The American Academy of Pediatrics (with its 62,000 physicians) urged the adoption of standards: that protect children's health and well-being from radiation emitted by cell phones and other wireless devices; that reflect how people actually use their cell phones; and that provide sufficient information to enable consumers to make informed decisions Visit Dr. Moskowitz's excellent site for the report with scientific references and to request email updates: www.saferemr.com.

What is the daily usage for your family? You may have a great savings plan but consider the cost to you and your family's health.

**No one yet knows the risk of several hours a day of exposure?**

What is the risk for today's 'heavy user'? People of all ages chat and text, catch the news, watch online movies and locate a restaurant. Note: whenever you are online with your mobile device: cell phone, tablet, iPad, laptop or desktop computer, in its sending/receiving mode, you are absorbing microwaves. Does it seem wise to hold one, with its hot-spot plume of radiation, against your head? Your heart? Your unborn baby? Your child? Is it prudent to entertain/educate your kids with mobile apps? Tips: only have a device in the sending/receiving mode when necessary; disable that function (put in airplane mode) whenever you can; hold away from your body, and far away from children.

The Interphone study scientists and the US report from The President's Cancer Panel called for more research. Do you think we already have enough evidence to take some precautions? Or should we wait?

Let's take a look at the various systems of the body that are affected. You will see why so many symptoms and medical conditions can be related. The good news: there are many health benefits when you reduce your exposure with our safer-tech solutions.

This section gives you a detailed list of potential effects. Why are we still standing and not crashing under all this wireless radiation? A good question. Noticeable harm can be immediate, or take many years.

## Biological Effects – Evidence of Damage

Yes, there *are* numerous peer-reviewed and published studies that strongly suggest harmful effects. Here we go ...

### Functioning of Our Cells

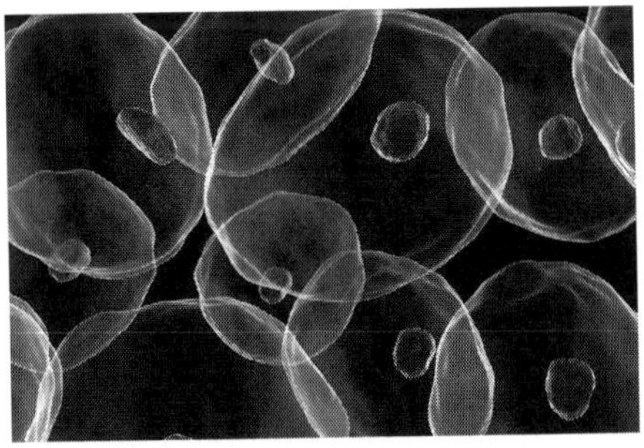

Scientists now have far more sensitive measures of how human cells respond to EMR than they did in the 1990s.

As the research of Dr. Blank demonstrates, these fields can affect our cells even when present at very low intensities – low enough that our senses can't detect them, let alone feel any heat. (Could this be the crux of the problem?)

Along with Dr. Reba Goodman, Dr. Blank has been studying these biological effects on the stress response in cells. He explains for us how the cells interpret this stimulus.

> The cells react as if this energy is harmful! They make stress proteins only when they sense they're in a bad situation, such as when they are exposed to heat, toxins or the wrong pH. The research is showing that when

> exposed to low frequency they're responding in this way, even without thermal stressors. When the cell starts making stress proteins, it's trying to tell you something!

There are other troubling signs of reactivity. In 2011 Drs. Blank and Goodman published a new paper on DNA in the *International Journal of Radiation Biology* 87(4): 409-15, 2011. This review of the responses of DNA to electro-magnetic fields, in different frequency ranges, shows that the DNA in cells can react as a fractal antenna, able to pick up many frequencies. This property of DNA is probably due to its structure. This DNA damage could account for increases in cancer.

## Our Immune and Other Systems

Another scientist, Dr. Ted Litovitz, who was Emeritus Professor of Physics and Bioelectro-magnetics, Catholic University of America, Washington, DC, found that when a cell is subjected to too much stress, this fundamental protective response itself becomes stressed and stops making proteins. (Litovitz 2002) In other words, the cell becomes less able to protect itself and this impairs our immune system strength and affects every system in the body.

## Our Cells' Ability to Communicate

The pioneer in the field of environmental health, Dr. Neil Cherry of New Zealand, described this mechanism in detail. Sadly, this highly respected scientist died in 2003 after suffering from Motor Neuron disease (ALS). Professor Cherry wrote:

> Nature has developed many advanced and complex biological processes in, and between, cells for cell-to-cell communication, intra-cellular communication and regulation, and brain and CNS systems. Dr. Ross Adey's

description of cells 'whispering to each other' in this cell-to-cell caring society, checking on the health of their neighbours and suggesting subtle changes to keep them healthy are part of biological homeostasis.

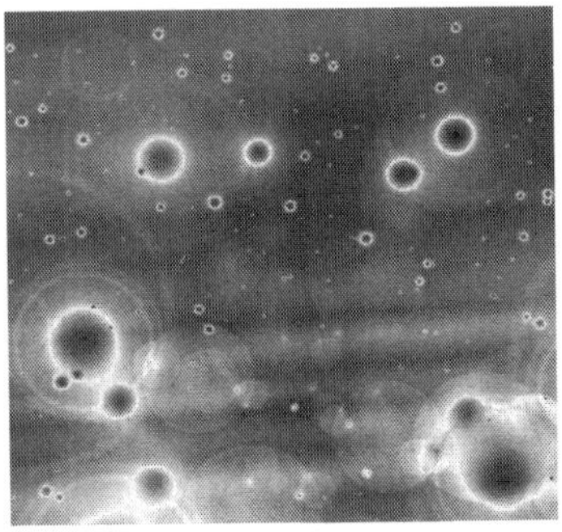

Our brains and cells primarily use calcium ions for these processes and Dr. Adey's laboratory, followed by Dr. Carl Blackman's monumental work, confirms that the natural and vital processes for cellular health are interfered with ... at the cell membrane level, by the oscillating signals from mobile phone base stations.

These waves of radiation confuse and damage the cell's signal system while the strong emissions of a cell phone next to your head almost drown out the signals.

This alters the EEG and hormones, damaging the cells and producing acute symptoms such as headache, concentration problems, memory loss, dizziness and nausea, and long-term problems including brain tumors, Alzheimer's Disease, depression and suicide.

The cardiologist Dr. Stephen Sinatra told me about this hypothesis:

Receptor sites on the cell membrane do not recognize the chaotic electrical disturbances from mobile phones and other wireless exposures, and interpret this as a foreign invader, sending the cell membranes into a protective 'lock down' mode.

One theory is that electro-magnetic radiation (EMR) impedes the active transport channels that should allow nutrients into the cell, and waste products to get out, as well as the cells' ability to communicate and work well with each other. Waste products can build up inside the cell causing a high concentration of molecules called free radicals.

## Our DNA

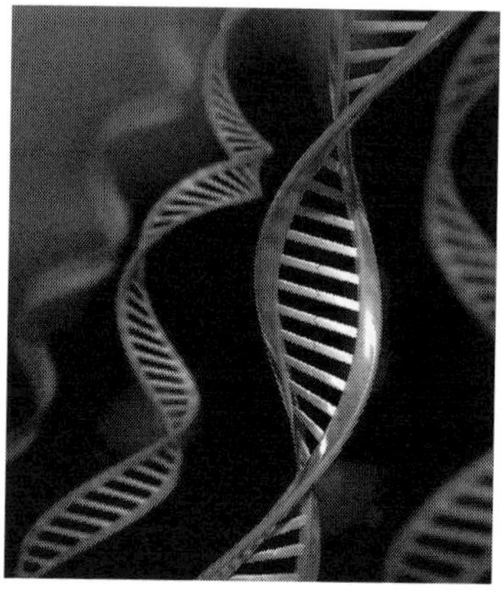

Free radicals interfere with DNA repair and alter future DNA. Damaged DNA is passed along to the next generation of cells. This is worrying, because, as Adey explains, the cells can no longer 'whisper' with each other, they can no longer call in the immune system to remove dead cells and damaged DNA.

The researchers Drs. Henry Lai and Narendra Singh have been studying DNA for many years, and their results are strong evidence. Even with brief exposures, at very low levels of EMR, there are signs of significant damage to DNA, and they report this can lead to changes in cellular functions and cell death. (This study, with J.L. Philips, was published in *Pathophysiology* 16 (2009) 79–88.) I asked Dr. Lai and Dr. Singh about security scanners and our DNA -- more on that later.

This disruption to the normal functioning of cells affects all life forms, not just us wireless-crazed humans. Dr. Carrie Hyman voiced her concern:

> This radiation affects every living cell in ways we are only beginning to understand. Because of the genotoxic effect of radio frequencies in particular, we may be altering the genetic expression of all life on earth.

## Our Cardiovascular System – Your Heart At Risk

Having worked for many years in the field of heart health education, I welcomed Dr. Sinatra's contribution and peppered him with questions about the possible connection between EMR and cardiac symptoms.

> The heart is electrical in nature so it is vulnerable to all electro-magnetic fields as well as the microwaves from wireless technologies. The non-harmonious, jagged waveform of wireless radiation impairs the normal functioning of the heart, including the rate and rhythm.
>
> Some people can feel discomfort in the chest area when around mobile phones or wireless hot spots.
>
> People are usually unaware of the cause of these 'unexplained' cardiac symptoms, and unknowingly, their doctors may not offer the appropriate diagnosis, or treatment. Even if you are not aware of any effects, it does not mean that you are safe from harm.
>
> Cardiac effects may include: variability of heart rate and rhythm (tachycardia and arrhythmia), palpitations, chest discomfort/pain (angina), high blood pressure (hypertension – this is now better understood: oxidative stress/free radical damage from toxins, environmental pollution, emotional stress etc. impairs the delicate lining of small blood vessels, causing constriction and an increase in blood pressure), blood clumping (this thickening of the blood also happens with the stress response, as you can imagine, thicker, more viscous blood is not a healthy condition).

## Our Blood-Brain Barrier – Vital For Brains Worth Saving

The blood-brain barrier is a vital filtering system in the blood vessels in the brain to keep toxins out and cerebrospinal fluids in, so that the environment of the brain is kept clean and the brain itself is cushioned against any contact with the skull. Published, peer-reviewed research by Leif Salford, MD, the neurology professor at Lund University, shows that EMR is capable of causing leakage of the blood-brain barrier. (Salford et al. 1992, 1993, 1994, 1997b, 2001.) See the graphic below.

Dr. Salford's research team reported rat brain cross-sections showed first ever evidence of brain damage from cell phone radiation. While the controls (top) appeared healthy, the test subjects (below) – exposed to a 2-hour dose of cell phone radiation of varying intensities – were heavily spotted with proteins leaked from the surrounding blood vessels, and show signs of significant neuronal (brain) damage.

Think that what applies to rat brains doesn't apply to humans? Sorry. Professor Salford says that the blood-brain barrier is anatomically the same in both species and some years ago stated, "It is my sincere belief that non-thermal electro-magnetic fields from mobile phones do have effects upon the human brain." Now there is even more scientific evidence to support this concern – a good reason not to hold a mobile against your head, or your baby.

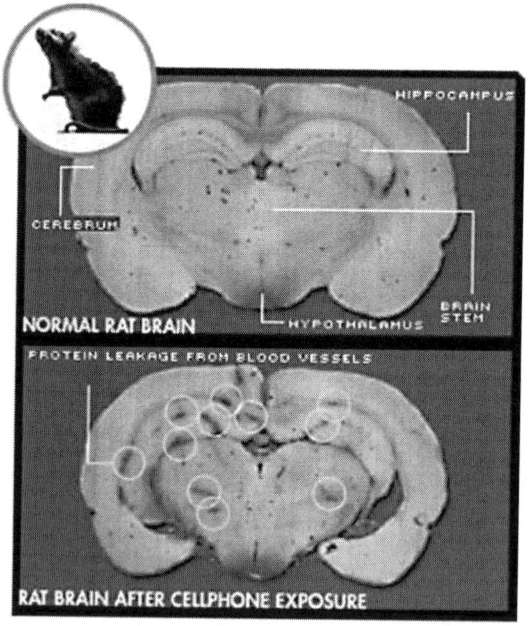

## Medical Researchers Raise The Alert About Brains At Risk

Wireless microwave radiation impairs the blood-brain barrier leaving us vulnerable to an increasing number of toxic chemicals – chemicals doubled in the last seven years! In March 2014, *The Lancet Neurology* published a review by Philip Landrigan, MD, of Mount Sinai School of Medicine and Philippe Grandjean, MD, of Harvard School of Public Health. They say this is so troubling they are calling for a worldwide overhaul of the regulatory process in order to protect children's brains.

> Neurodevelopmental disabilities, including autism, attention-deficit hyperactivity disorder, dyslexia, and other cognitive impairments, affect millions of children worldwide, and seem to be increasing in frequency. We know from clinical information on poisoned adult patients that these chemicals can enter the brain through the blood brain barrier and cause neurological symptoms. When this happens in children or during pregnancy, those chemicals are extremely toxic, because we now know that the developing brain is a uniquely vulnerable organ. Also, the effects are permanent.

## Our Cognitive Abilities – Evidence of Impairment

Researchers in Israel confirmed cognitive functions of human subjects exposed to wireless radiation were impaired, including slower response times to a memory task (Luria, Eliyahu, Hareuveny, Margaliot, Meiran). Professor Wilhelm Mosgoeller, MD, University of Vienna, reports: "When healthy human subjects were exposed to RF, certain brain waves changed – faster response times during exposure which seem to occur at the expense of the quality of the response. *Wrong responses were given within shorter time periods.*" (Not good in transportation or education!)

## So why are we flooding our schools with WiFi?

I challenged one Principal, "If the safety of the school's playground equipment was being questioned by scientists and medical associations, there were reports of children being harmed by this equipment, many schools were removing it, and several countries advising against it, how long would it take you to remove this equipment from your school?"

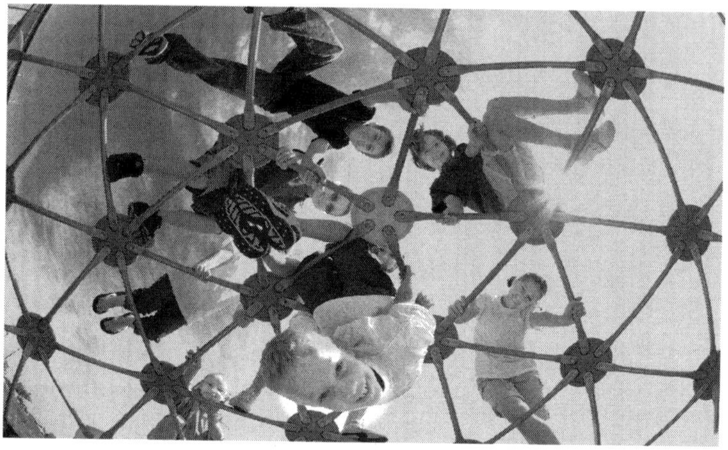

## Neurological Conditions, Including ADHD and Autism

There are many symptoms reported with EMR exposure including difficulty sleeping, headaches, dizziness, eye pain, cardiovascular reactions, and many more. Sadly, medical researchers also suggest an extensive range of brain and nervous system-related conditions.

These include: learning disabilities, ADD and ADHD, Asperger's Syndrome and the Autism Spectrum Disorders, MS, ALS, Parkinson's and Alzheimer's Disease. A 2003 published study by Professor Salford suggests an EMR and Alzheimer's link; with 4 billion cell phone users, if microwave radiation turns out to be a causative factor what will we do? Studies have reported a link between electrical occupations and neuro-degenerative disease including ALS (Suavity et al, 1998). I know otherwise healthy men who worked in the computer industry and now in their 60's are afflicted with ALS, and with Parkinson's. A connection?

## Rapidly Rising Incidence of Autism

A few decades ago autism struck 1 in 10,000 children. In 2002 it affected 1 in 150, then 1 in 110 in 2006, then 1 in 88 in 2008. In 2014 it's 1 in 68 [according to the CDC (Center for Disease Control)]. Dietrich Klinghardt, MD who works with these families, made a chilling prediction, "With this rapid increase, in 10 to 15 years we may have no neuro-typical (neurologically-healthy) children born. Implausible? Show me a pregnant woman who is not around mobile devices, WiFi or strong electro-magnetic fields."

Pediatrician Toril H. Jelter, MD, FAAP, raises a medical alert, "In addition to the pain and suffering these children with autism and their families experience, this problem alone threatens to bankrupt whole school systems. When I, as a physician, need to perform a potentially dangerous procedure on a child, such as a spinal tap, I need to explain why it is necessary and the risks, and obtain written consent from the parents who have the right to refuse. Currently, we are performing large-scale experiments on children without informing them or their parents of the risk, nor have they been given an option to opt out."

Dr. Jelter and a technical consultant report families with autism can improve significantly in a low EMR environment (see pages 278, 279).

## Our Memory

This function dims as we age, but there's an EMR factor, says Prof. Olle Johansson, "If you look in the literature, you have a large number of various adverse effects like chromosome damage, impact on the concentration capacity, and decrease in short-term memory."

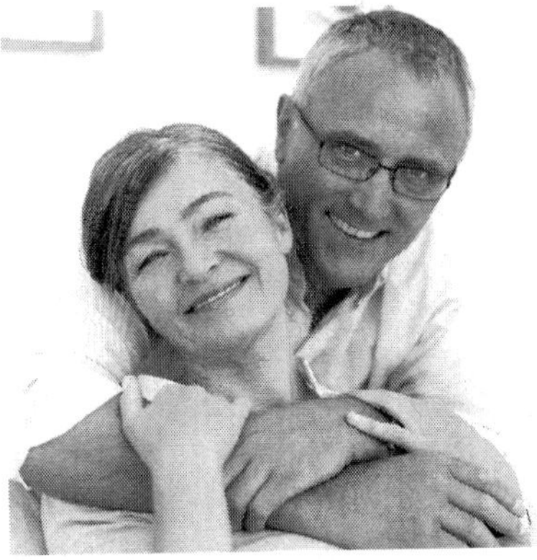

Memory loss and concentration problems may occur as radiation affects the ability of the brain to process and remember information (part of distracted driving?), and can damage and kill brain cells, most of which do not re-grow. This could be a factor in dementia.

## Our Skin

We have just heard about free radical damage to our DNA; there's more. Dr. Benetti, at the French company, Clarins Laboratories, exposed skin cells to EMR and found it damaged the quality of the skin, accelerating the aging process by causing a production of free radicals and a loss of cellular renewal. The skin became dehydrated, more sensitive, and less radiant. They are developing plant-based protective formulas.

## Our Breasts

Research indicates damage from wireless communication – time spent in WiFi, on cordless, or cell, phones – can include risk of breast cancer. There's evidence that breast tissue absorbs electro-magnetic radiation. Awful news. All of us have lost loved ones – wonderful women. This is a good reason to avoid carrying a powered-on cell phone on your body, and to limit its use. (I've seen mobile phones as pendants!) Dr. Davis, cancer epidemiologist and veteran breast cancer researcher warned, "A cellphone's microwave radiation seeps directly into soft fatty tissue of the breast – not a good thing." In 2013, a small study published in *Case Reports in Medicine* found carrying a cell phone in a bra may have led to cancerous tumors in the breast – tumor sites outlined the shape of the women's cell phones.

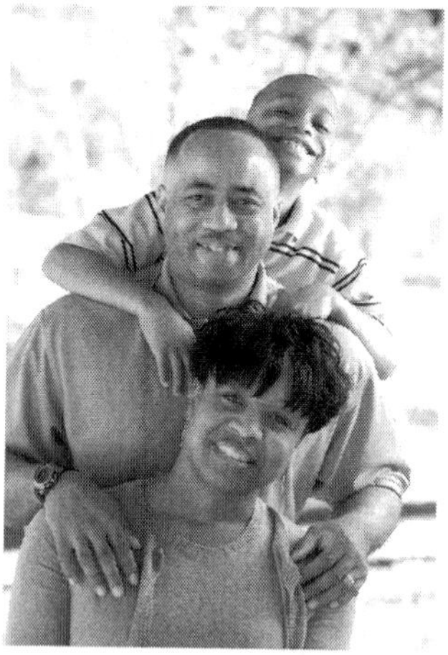

## All this evidence is too scary?

If you are feeling overwhelmed, maybe it's time to put down this book and go for a brisk walk in the fresh air?

## Pre-natal Exposure

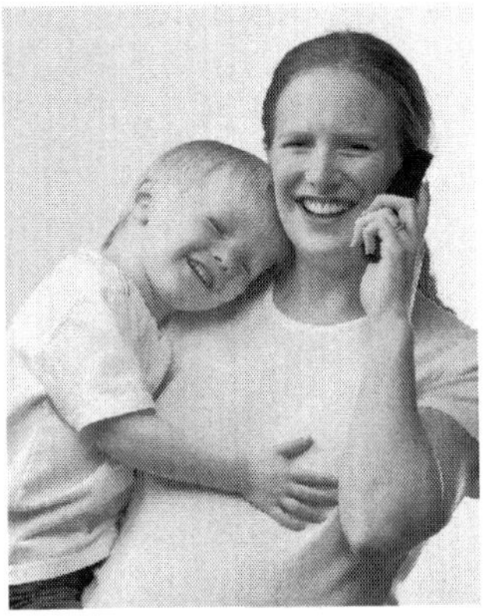

Did you see a recent study on page 27? Here are others: [Lowenthal et al. 2007; Infante-Rivard and Deadman, 2003] report that a fetus and young children are at greater risk than adults from exposure to environmental toxins, such as electro-pollution. This is consistent with evidence that the fetus and young child are more vulnerable than older persons are to chemicals [Makri A, et al. 2004] and ionizing radiation [Preston, 2004].

• Birth defects linked to proximity to high voltage power lines. *Reprod Toxicol.* 1993 May-Jun; 7(3) 283-7. Childhood leukemia is also linked.

• RF exposure (from wireless radiation) and adverse effects on the developing fetal brain. Nakamichi N, Ishioka Y, Hirai T, Ozawa S, Tachibana M, Nakamura N, Takarada T, Yoneda Y. *Journal Neuroscience Research*, August 2009, Volume 87, Issue 11, Pages 2399–2614.

• Bellieni et al [2012] assessed the RF exposure of the 26-week fetus of a pregnant woman using a laptop computer, and found the fetus was adversely affected, as these fields pass directly through the mother's tissues to the fetus.

• RF exposure and possible promotion of neuronal differentiation in fetal rat brain neural progenitor cells. Nakamichi N, et al. *Journal Neuroscience Research* 2009, Aug 15;87(11):2406-17.

• Rabbits and rats – with RF exposure – evidence of damage to the fetal brain, eyes, liver and skin. A. Tomruk, Gazi University, Ankara.

• And abnormal changes in different types of fetal brain cells and structure. Prof. Sulleyman Kaplan, Ondokuz Mayis University, Samsun.

• Also biomarkers of genetic and other damage to fetal cells and organs. Prof. Nesrin Seyhan et al., Gazi University.

How much evidence do you need in order to protect your baby?

## Childhood Cancers

In Australia, the UK and Italy, studies found that the closer people live to broadcast towers (radio and/or tv transmitters) the higher their incidence of leukemia (Michelozzi 2001, 2002, Hocking et al 1996). Other studies looked at people living near power lines – with a small increase in the number of power lines, there was a doubling of childhood leukemia by age 3 or 4 (Draper et al 2005).

For 30 years experts have investigated how EMR could increase the risk of childhood leukemia. In 2008, medical researchers in Shanghai, led by Xiaoming Shen, reported a ground-breaking theory: children who carry a defective gene that normally helps repair damaged DNA and also live near power lines or transformers are up to 4 times more likely to develop leukemia than neighboring children who have a fully-functioning gene. They report that children who have this faulty gene cannot repair DNA that's damaged by EMR, even low-frequency fields. This impairment could increase their risk of cancer.

A mother's exposure in her work environment during pregnancy, or just before she conceives, may also put her child at greater risk of developing certain types of brain cancer. In 2009, researchers at Canada's McGill University raised this concern after following the pregnancies of women working on electric sewing machines. And there are new reports that pre-natal exposure to cell phone radiation may increase the risk of glioma in the offspring, and a range of electro-magnetic fields may be factors in infertility and miscarriages.

Seeing a pregnant woman chat on her cell phone or rest a cell phone, tablet or laptop on her abdomen will soon be as shocking as if she is smoking or drinking alcohol. The new warning: refrain from drugs, alcohol, tobacco, prolonged proximity to electric devices, and avoid mobile technology. See page 137 for obstetricians' BabySafe warnings.

As with tobacco, asbestos, and other health issues, it's a long time between people getting sick and governments taking action. Not only are most not funding research and providing precautions, most are still defending existing 'safe' levels which respected scientists warn are not protecting us. Meanwhile, reports from the European Union alert us that childhood brain cancers are on the rise.

British neurosurgeon Kevin O'Neill, MD reported in 2009:

> Brain tumours are on the increase, reportedly in the region of 2% per year. But in my unit we have seen **the number of cases nearly double in the last year**.

In 2014, a cancer breakthrough – an experimental treatment known as immuno-oncology (IO) harnesses the body's natural defences to fight off tumours by undermining the evasion tactics used by tumours, which can "hide" from the body's immune system by disguising themselves as normal cells. This is good news as many scientists predict a global pandemic of brain and other cancers. We feel harrowed seeing the bright face, and shiny bald head, of one child with cancer. How would we cope with many? Around the world, dedicated researchers and children's advocates like me are fighting hard to prevent this. We need your help. Start by safeguarding your family.

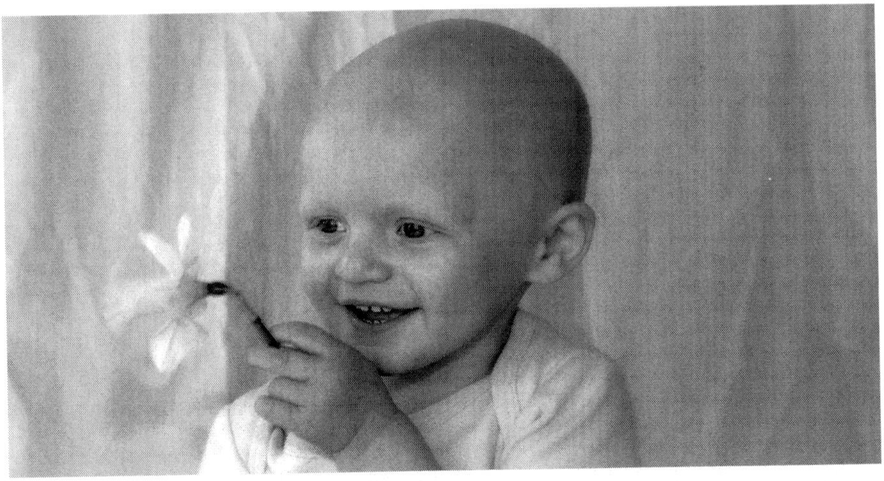

Epidemiologist Dr. Davis is concerned about our children's future:

> When it comes to proof of human harm, we've kind of been led down a garden path that says the only proof that really counts is enough sick or dead people. I think that approach has got to change, and particularly with respect to something like brain cancer. Brain cancer can take 10, 20 or 30 years to develop. Our children are using cell phones in growing numbers. Companies are marketing cell phones now to five-year-olds. Should we wait until we have proof of sick, or dead, kids before acting?

## Life Expectancy for This Digital Generation?

In our WiFi world, at what age should we start healthy aging strategies, and see that reducing EMR exposure is essential to longevity? We hear predictions of children born today living way past 100. I wonder. With more than four billion people using mobiles, the global fallout could be that young people, and the rest of us, will face related adverse health effects: cancer, cardiac symptoms, neurological and other diseases. Already some countries are reporting an increase in brain tumors and clusters of childhood cancers in close proximity to power lines and cell towers. What will happen when we are all living in close proximity? What kind of world will it be for our grandchildren? What kind of nature-deprived children are we leaving for our world?

I'd like to ask Dan Buettner, author of *The Blue Zones,* and his globe-wandering team, to consider reducing EMR exposure as the new longevity factor and one of their 'lessons for living longer.' In his book it was obvious, to me at least, that while not all the long-living 'Blue Zone' people were off-the-grid, none of them were living under power lines or near cell towers, nor did they use cell phones, or have much exposure to the wireless radiation that surrounds us all these days.

## A Partial Summary of EMR Biological Effects

"No clear evidence of harm," some claim. However, even at low exposures (a fraction of government-sanctioned levels) EMR is bio-active, every part of the body is affected and published evidence includes:

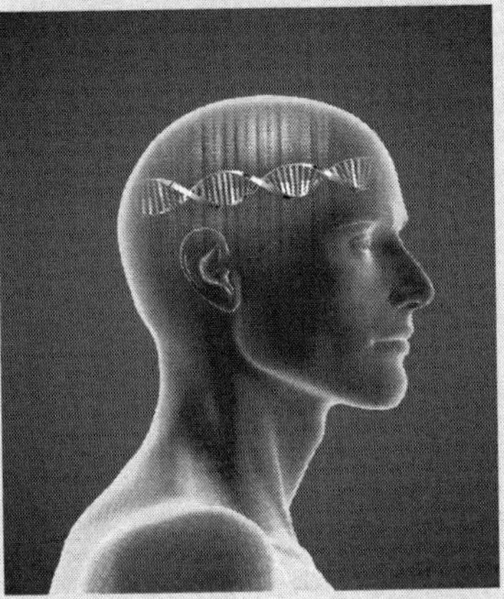

- DNA damage and disruption of DNA repair (Lai, Singh, Philips)
- Suppression of the immune system (Johansson, Nakamura, Litovitz, Veyret, Hocking, Draper)
- Disruption to normal functioning of neurological, cardiovascular and endocrine systems (Lai, Salford, Becker, Cherry, Hurtado, Johansson, Karasek, Schilowsky)
- Leakage of the brain's protective blood-brain barrier (Salford, Persson)
- Impaired cognitive functions, including reaction time (Mosgoeller, Scheiner, Lai, Becker, Cherry, Luria, Eliyahu, Hareuveny, Margaliot, Meiran)
- Increased agitation, sleep disruptions and food, chemical and electro-sensitivities (Becker, Holt, Rea)
- Stress protein synthesis (body's reaction when stressed at the cellular level) (Blank, Goodman, Mosgoeller)
- Inter- and intra-cellular functions (cell membrane permeability and the cells ability to communicate with each other) (Cherry, Adey, Blackman)

## More Evidence of Harm

Building Biology consultant and Industrial Hygienist, Peter Sierck, with his colleague Thomas Haumann PhD, offer this summary of non-thermal biological effects from wireless technologies. (Nonstop Pulsed 2.4 GHz Radiation Inside US Homes) You can show this to your friend (or government agency, or industry spokesperson) who protests, 'there is no real evidence of harm'.

"Much experimental evidence of non-thermal influences of microwave radiation on living systems has been published in the scientific literature during the last 30 years – relating both to in vitro and in vivo studies.

- Changes in the electrical activity in the human brain,
- Increase in DNA single and double strand breaks from HF exposure to 2.45 GHz,
- Increased lymphoma rates (2 fold) in transgenic mice exposed twice a day to 30 minutes of cell phone (GSM) signals over 18 months,
- Increased permeability of the blood-brain barrier in rats,
- Observation of an increase in resting blood pressure during exposure,
- Increased permeability of the erythrocyte membrane,
- Effects on brain electrochemistry (calcium efflux),
- Increase of chromosome aberrations and micronuclei in human blood lymphocytes,
- Synergistic effects with cancer promoting and certain psychoactive drugs,
- Depression of chicken immune systems,
- Increase in chicken embryo mortality,
- Effects on brain dopamine/opiate electrochemistry,
- Increases in DNA single and double strand breaks in rat brain,
- Stressful effects in healthy and tumor bearing mice,
- Neurogenetic effects and micronuclei formation in peritoneal macrophage."

## Brain Cancer and More Medical Warnings

As I mentioned, no one seems to be measuring, or monitoring, the combined daily dose of radiation we receive from wired and wireless exposures. Even if we don't use a cell phone; we are not escaping.

David Carpenter MD, Director, Institute for Health and the Environment at the University of Albany and co-author of The BioInitiative Report warns:

> **This report stands as a wake-up call that long-term exposure to some kinds of EMF may cause serious health effects.** Good public health planning is needed now to prevent cancers and neurological diseases linked to exposure to power lines and other sources of EMF.

Several years ago, Dr. Carpenter testified at a US Congressional hearing along with Dr. Ronald Herberman, an internationally recognized tumor immunologist. They stated that according to the government's own statistics, the incidence of brain cancer has been increasing over the last ten years, particularly among 20-29 year-olds.

If it takes more than ten years for brain tumors to grow, and if these are, in fact, being caused by cell phones, cancer rates might not peak for at least another five years in Dr. Herberman's opinion. Then what?

You see why I jumped in to safeguard my family without waiting for the cancer rates to peak, and why I am urging you to protect yours.

Julius Knapp, from the Federal Communications Commission (FCC), also testified at those hearings, revealing "**nobody at the agency is competent to evaluate the biology**." The FCC's job is to implement regulations. The industry's trade group declined to testify, and issued a statement assuring us that there's no scientific basis for any concern.

Dr. Herberman reported an alarming rise of brain cancer in Scandinavian countries with longer cell phone use:

> Based on the laboratory and epidemiological evidence to date, the grounds for taking precautionary actions to reduce direct exposure to the brain and body from cell phone radiation are stronger than ever.

The American Academy of Environmental Medicine issued this medical alert, "Adverse health effects from RF radiation – learning disabilities, altered immune responses, and headaches – are well documented in the scientific literature. It is better to exercise caution and substitute with a safe wired connection."

Our international Advisory Board Doctors for Safer Schools focuses on a range of issues and what has been called 'nature-deficit disorder.'

Surgeon and DFSS board member John Barnhill MD warns, "The medical, psychological and social effects of wireless (RF) radiation are quite concerning. Evidence that exists in medical literature is in keeping with our understanding of the physiology and carcinogenic capability of radiation. And this radiation exposure is against any consent."

Yet, most health officials and regulatory agencies still insist there's no clear evidence of biological effects that could lead to illness or disease.

Not so, according to Dr. Magda Havas, who says there are "literally thousands of studies showing serious adverse health effects, studies reporting a range of symptoms and illness from RF exposure go back a long way, and adverse effects occur at a fraction of government standards." *(See page 61.)* The width of the gap is astounding.

In the US and Canada those allowable levels are a whopping 2 to 10 million units. Yes, that is millions, while for many people sleep can be disrupted at levels below 5 – that is 5 single units, not 5 million units.

## Your symptoms EMR related? The 4-day Safer-Tech Challenge

Are you not sleeping well, feeling dizzy, having cardiac problems or other symptoms? Wired and/or wireless radiation exposures could be one reason. Electro-pollution can make a healthy person feel unwell, and worsen symptoms in someone with compromised health.

Here's how to try our test.

- Unplug all 2.4, 5.8, or 6.0 GHz cordless phones. Replace them with older 900 MHz cordless phones, or even better switch to landlines – phones with a corded handset. If you have done away with landline service and use mobile phones, you may really benefit from this test, and will need to power them off, especially at night.
- For safe Internet access: use a wired router and Ethernet cable, or power off your wireless router when not in use, and at night. Disable your computers' sending and receiving functions – Airport (MAC) – and use airplane mode on all digital devices, including iPads, iPods.
- Avoid or limit use of all mobile communication devices, talking and texting. See our safer use guidelines.
- Unplug wired devices in your bedroom: magnetic biomats, grounding sheets, heating pads, electric heaters, charging stations, electric clocks.
- An RF meter will test the wireless radiation levels. Test the electrical, wired devices with a Gauss meter. You need the right meter (available at www.slt.co). Test the levels, then reduce exposures – unplug devices and/or replace them as suggested above – then retest.
- Other home sources to disable/unplug: baby monitors, wireless security systems, wireless speaker/entertainment systems, Bluetooth devices, microwave ovens.
- At night you can turn off the non-essential circuits in the fuse box

You may have not be able to reduce the external sources, such as your neighbor's Smart Meter, WiFi and cordless phones, or the nearby cell tower antennas and power lines, but you can control the closest sources: what is in your home. After 4 days, how are you feeling?

## The jury is still out? Or not?

In a 2013 episode of "The Doctor Oz Show," cardiologist Mehmet Oz, MD and his guest Sanjay Gupta, MD, a neurosurgeon and chief medical correspondent for CNN, discussed the research about cell phone radiation health effects. Based on the research, Dr. Gupta issued important precautionary warnings about cell phone use.

CNN's Larry King was one of the first to take this issue seriously. He asked neurosurgeon, Vini Khurana, MD about his view that this could have far broader health ramifications than asbestos or smoking.

Dr. Khurana's reply:

> I base my [2008] statement on the fact that at this point in time, there's just over three billion users of cell phones worldwide – half of the population. [In 2014 there are now more mobile phones than people.] And the concern is not just brain tumors, but other health effects including behavioral disturbances, salivary gland tumors, male infertility and microwave sickness syndrome.

Flash forward to Larry King's program when the Interphone study was big news in 2010. One of his guests, Ms. Ellie Marks, became a fierce campaigner when her husband Alan was diagnosed with brain cancer.

Alan writes:

> Doctors determined that my brain tumor was directly attributable to my long term use of my cellular phone. I know of other brain tumor patients much younger, and many no longer alive. I am in real estate and used a cell phone for over 20 years for about 10,000 lifetime hours. I held my phone to my right ear and the tumor was on

> the right side of my brain, by my right ear. The very thing that was an integral part of my business to enhance my productivity will kill me.

Ellie Marks was Director of Government & Public Affairs for Environmental Health Trust (founded by Dr. Davis.) Ms. Marks is Director of the California Brain Tumor Association and works with brain cancer victims and their families. Her concern is not just Alan:

> My husband is just the tip of the iceberg of a pandemic of brain tumors as he used one longer than many people. These tumors have a lengthy latency period. What has happened to my husband could easily happen to you, your children, or grandchildren. There is strong evidence.

Dr. Johansson, "I have been studying this issue for 30 years and have seen enough evidence of harm, first hand, and in the literature, to allow me to say with high scientific certainty that even low levels of this radiation – well within government safety standards – are harmful to human health. To those who deny this I say, this means that all the thousands of papers that have published very serious effects of electromagnetic fields in fully approved peer review-based scientific journals must all be wrong?

**Your family's screen time?**

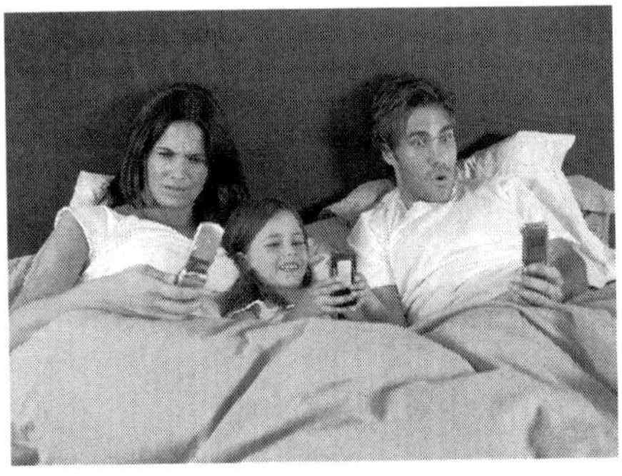

One of our readers wrote:

"We spent lots of time on our digital devices. My husband had headaches, dizzy spells, a skin rash, and was having trouble sleeping. Your plan has been very helpful. His symptoms have greatly improved and all of us are sleeping much better – now without any medications."

## Concerns: mobile devices in education, for safety, as games for activity. And digital addiction at all ages.

A teacher shares the changes he has seen over 35 years, "Increasingly, there is a marked decline in handwriting and the ability to spell and to read. Give students several pages of written text – on paper – and they're overwhelmed. They are distracted by, and addicted to, mobiles and some use them to cheat. I won't have these devices in my classroom. This generation is so used to fast-paced images (and violence) that their attention spans are minimal, and there is a disturbing empathetic disconnect: Looking at images of the collapse of the Twin Towers, some enthused, 'Hey, that's cool'. We must wake up to the violence and/or isolation in some young people, and to the disconnect in most."

## How many minutes (or hours) per day do your children spend gaming? Teens online and texting? Are they addicted?

Many parents feel safer knowing their children carry mobiles: you know where they are, and they can call in an emergency. The kids text, surf, and play video games. The games that get them up off the couch and firing away at the screen are great exercise, some believe. Most parents don't realize kids are getting a lot more from this rapid-fire obsession – many are becoming addicted. They often sleep with the

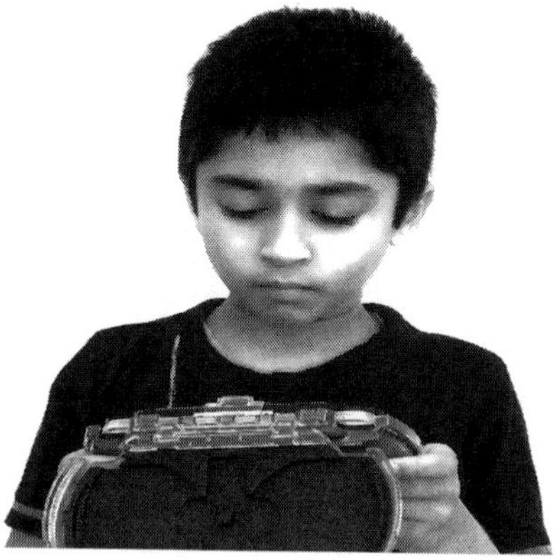

mobile under the pillow to catch every text message. Maybe this is why many have trouble sleeping. Who wants to sleep when you can tweet?

Dr. Scheiner explained the physiology of digital addiction:

> People of all ages can become physiologically addicted to wireless radiation exposure. So excessive cell phone use and wireless computer games are not just an addictive habit, or a behavioral issue. **This radiation opens the blood-brain barrier in the same way as alcohol and drugs** giving a feeling of euphoria, and when you take away the device they'll experience withdrawal symptoms, as you may know if you've tried to reduce your child's tablet/computer/gaming time and cell phone use.

In 2013, British newspapers reported on toddlers so obsessed with the dazzling screens of their iPads/tablets that they needed psychological treatment. Due to significant health concerns and the vulnerability of the young, it's time for a digital detox. These radiation-emitting and addictive devices are not benign. They are harmful – they are not toys.

Scientist Dr. Johansson offers us this concise summary:

> The radiation emitted by wireless communication devices has been shown to damage DNA leading to possible mutations and cancer development, and is linked to impairments to immune function and neurological diseases and functions including cognition and behaviour, as well as affecting fertility and reproduction.

**Overload alert?** Step away from the machines and get outside in fresh air. We created this situation and can change it. The next section details the challenges. Then we focus on strategies – how to take effective steps with our safer tech solutions to reduce the risks, for all of us.

## Children and Teens on Mobile Devices: Cell Phones, iPads, iPods, Cordless Phones

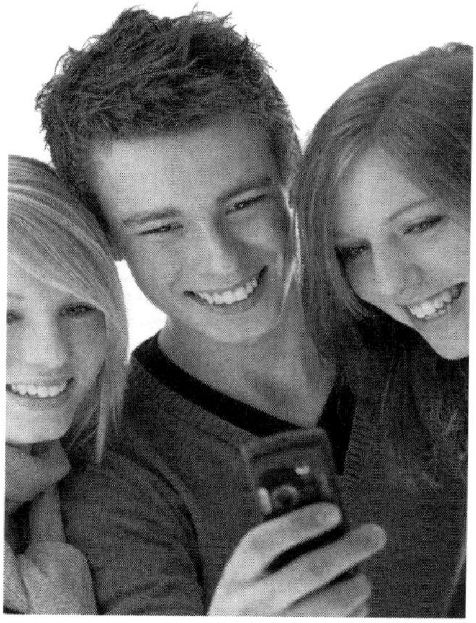

Swedish oncologist Professor Lennart Hardell, MD offered an analysis from one of the biggest cancer risk studies: children and teenagers are five times more likely to get a certain kind of brain cancer – glioma – if they begin using cell phones before the age of 20. The extra risk from cordless phones was almost as high.

In 2013 Dr. Hardell updated the research in the peer-reviewed journal, *International Journal of Oncology*: people who used mobiles for more than 25 years were at greatest risk – **300% greater risk of brain cancer** – than those who used them for a year or less. Dr. Hardell et al published "Mobile Phones and Cancer: Next Steps," *Epidemiology* 2014 Jul;25(4):617-618 (At: www.saferemr.com)

In a 2013 television program, Dr Mehmet Oz and breast cancer surgeon Dr. John West warned about keeping mobile phones in bras, especially young women with their developing breasts. Dr. Oz's 21-year-old guest said she carried her mobile phone in her bra for four years prior to her diagnosis. The audience gasped when she added a large tumor was found exactly where she'd kept her cell phone. Her mother said they've heard from women of all ages who say they carried a mobile device in their bra before their breast cancer diagnosis. Alert your loved ones.

How many women are at risk? Un-knowingly and un-necessarily. On page 40, Dr. Davis discussed the potential of this new breast cancer risk; this is also in her excellent newsletter. (At: www.ehtrust.org)

After the WHO reversed its position on cell phones and related radiation, Health Canada issued a cautionary note about those under age 18 using mobile phones. Yet few people are making the connection with WiFi and other devices like iPads which have four embedded transmitters emitting harmful radiation. So why are some schools providing iPads for young people, children with autism and those with special needs – the most vulnerable to the harmful effects. We can give them tech advantages in a much safer way – see page 167.

## iPods – Another Invisible Source of Microwave Radiation

Music is good for the soul and the brain, and children should be exposed to its many benefits. That iPod glued to your child/teen may look harmless, entertaining and kid-friendly, however they will be exposed to harmful radiation if the iPod goes online – to send/receive messages. If it can, consider replacing it with one that cannot, as young people should not be relied upon to keep it on the safe, airplane, mode.

If you still believe mobile devices are safe because they are everywhere, consider the strengthening of the WHO position: in 2011 the radiation emission is labelled a carcinogen and in 2013, a stronger statement, "there is a positive association" between cell phone radiation and a certain type of brain cancer. Hardell's research shows risks also increased with the number of hours of use, the intensity of the phone's power, and the younger the child was when starting to use cell phones.

Studies from two other European labs, published in *Physics in Medicine and Biology* (June 7, 2008) showed that young children's brains absorb twice as much radiation from a cell phone as the brains of adults. Children also have thinner skulls and smaller heads than adults, so radiation can penetrate more deeply into the brain as you see on the book cover that shows an estimation of the absorption of cell phone radiation based on age.

Dr. Davis explains:

> Few parents know that radio-frequency signals reach much more deeply into children's thinner and smaller brains than ours – a fact established through the pioneering work of Professor Om P. Gandhi, head of the University of Utah's electrical engineering department. In 2004 standards became looser, because industry modelers decided to use a new approach – basically doubling the amount of radio-frequency that could reach the brain of an adult and quadrupling that reaching a child's. The brain of a child doubles in the first two years of life and keeps on developing until their early 20s. Professor Gandhi no longer works with the cell phone industry and none of his grandchildren uses a cell phone.
>
> Radio-frequency energy is another word for microwave radiation. If people understood that they (or their children) were holding a two-way microwave-radiating device next to their brain, or their reproductive organs, they might think differently about it. The fine print warning with the Android says, 'Keep it 2.54 centimeters from the pregnant abdomen or the abdomen of a teenager.' The iPhone 4S also has fine print warnings.

Scientists in Europe and the USA endorsing the BioInitiative Report called for following precautionary actions were proposed:

- **children under 16 should only use cordless and mobile phones in emergencies**
- **no WiFi, Wi-MAX, or other wireless networking, be placed in homes, schools, or public areas**

- **conduct independent, widely publicized, frequent audits to ensure base stations do not exceed newly warranted, biologically based standards**

(Professor Johansson. The London Resolution. *Pathophysiology*.)

## How can we limit our teens' risky behaviors?

This generation is hard-wired to wireless gadgets. And most of their age group has never been prone to accepting adult advice.

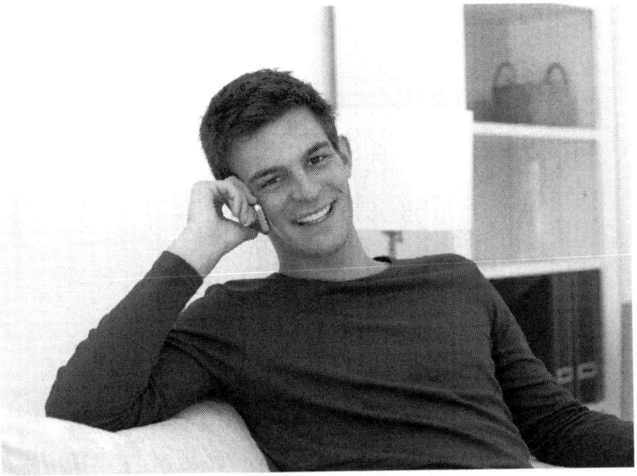

When I was buying a pair of shoes the other day, the young sales person was working his cell phone every few minutes. I felt compelled to ask him if he had heard about health hazards. The look he gave me wasn't quite the adolescent eye-roll I get from my own children, but it was certainly an expression of disbelief.

"Not interested," he shrugged, "I use this cell phone for everything." Let's hope someone who loves him will tell him about safer-tech tips.

Professor Johansson offers some sobering science:

> Children/teens are vulnerable due to the skull's permeability. The risk may turn out to be equally large for all ages, but the effect on children is much more serious for mankind. As our knowledge stands now, interaction with fertility, the immune system capacity, shattering of the DNA, or impaired learning and intelligence, will be much more dangerous than the extra cases of cancer. Of course, anyone with cancer, or being a relative to a cancer victim, will suffer tremendously. But, just considering mankind, as a species, we can lose a few, but not everyone.

In 2009, Joel Moskowitz PhD, with his UofC Berkeley colleagues and researchers at the National Cancer Center in South Korea, synthesized data from case-control studies published in the peer-reviewed literature, and found a 32% increased risk of tumors across eight high quality studies that examined mobile phone use of 10 years or longer.

In 2014 Dr. Moskowitz reports, "We have growing evidence that long-term cell phone use is associated with increased risk of head and neck cancer, sperm damage and male infertility, and health effects on children from pre- and post-natal exposure (e.g., attention deficit hyperactivity disorder). And a recent study showed four women developed breast tumors proximal to where they kept their cell phones."

A 2014 study led by the University of Exeter strongly suggests that being exposed to radiation from carrying mobiles in trouser pockets negatively affects sperm quality – the motility and viability. *Environment International.* 80 (2014):106-112. DOI: 10.1016/j.envint.2014.04.015 Imagine the ramifications of this to our species? And to others?

Researchers have warned that with ten years of cell phone use, the brain cancer risk increases between 30% – 140%. Then we have Dr. Hardell's chilling 25 years and 300% increase in risk! If you also have a mobile device powered on while sleeping or on your body, and/or digital cordless phones, 'Smart" technology or WiFi in your home, office and/or car, the health risks will be even higher. As concerned as we are about the young digital generation, we must remember the increase in adult brain cancers, as Ellie Marks tells us. As with most potential calamities, we assure ourselves, "Not me, not my family."

I attended the standing-room only 'Celebration of Life' of a truly marvelous man and witnessed the tragedy that can strike any family. Michael inspired everyone who met him with his humour, modesty and grace – before and after his diagnosis. Even with a scar on the side of his bald head; even when he could no longer walk, he greeted each person, and each situation, with an ear-to-ear smile, radiating kindness. He accepted each day with joyful zest, and always put others first, even toward the end of his journey when he was utterly dependent on them. His wife with such courage, and his two young children with such promise, brought tears to our eyes and somehow hope to our hearts, as they remembered the love and laughter that he brought to them.

Michael was 42. He was a wonderful teacher who inspired his students.

I am sure he and his wife never thought this could happen to their family. We seldom do. And this is what keeps us from taking the proactive steps that could protect us. People often tell me, "Yes, but, my son (husband, daughter) would never give up the convenience of wireless mobile devices that are essential these days."

A positive biopsy wakes you up quickly. I know from working with cardiac patients how motivating 'a bolt from the blue' like a heart attack can be. I have talked personally with most of these experts, made a lot of changes in my life, and experienced a lot of benefits. And I have had time to try and come to terms with this, and still find it hard to swallow and digest, so I empathize if you are choking on it.

## Safe levels and levels allowed by existing standards

**Why is this chart relevant?** To see the massive disparity between the levels considered biologically safe, and the government safety standards that govern the marketplace: A. electrical; B. RF/wireless.

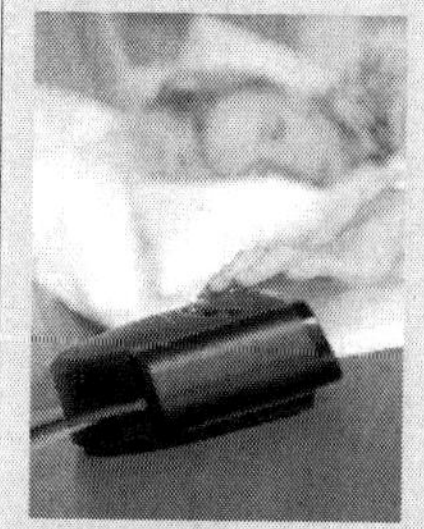

### A. ELECTRICAL SOURCES

AC MAGNETIC FIELDS from plugged in devices, household appliances, power lines, ground current issues. Test with a Gauss meter (mG = milligauss).

1. **Daytime exposure levels** are preferably kept below **1**
2. **Nighttime exposure levels** are preferably kept below **0.2**
   Building Biology Guidelines for sleeping areas (SBM 2008)

| all measures on this page are in milligauss mG | No concern | Slight concern | Severe concern | Extreme concern |
|---|---|---|---|---|
| | **< 0.2** | **0.2 - 1** | **1 - 5** | **> 5** |

**North American Standards:**

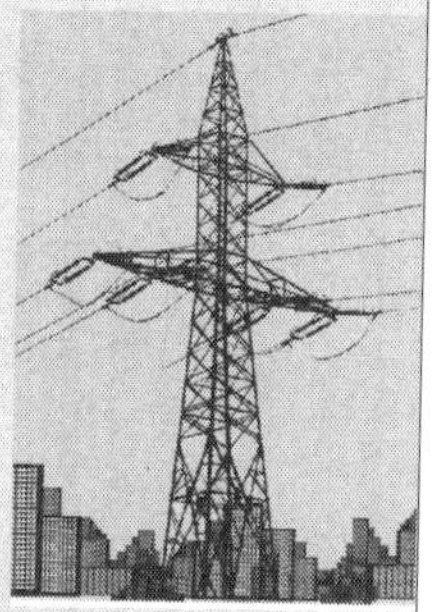

**833** for the general public

**4,166** for occupational exposure

**European:** Levels are the same – appear lower as they are based on a different frequency

**1,000** for the general public

**5,000** for occupational exposure

Source: ICNIRP, 1998.

Take into consideration the duration, proximity and intensity of all exposures.

## B. RADIO-FREQUENCY (RF)/WIRELESS RADIATION

Cell tower antennas (masts), Wi-MAX, wireless networks, cell and cordless phones, tablets, laptops, and other wireless devices.

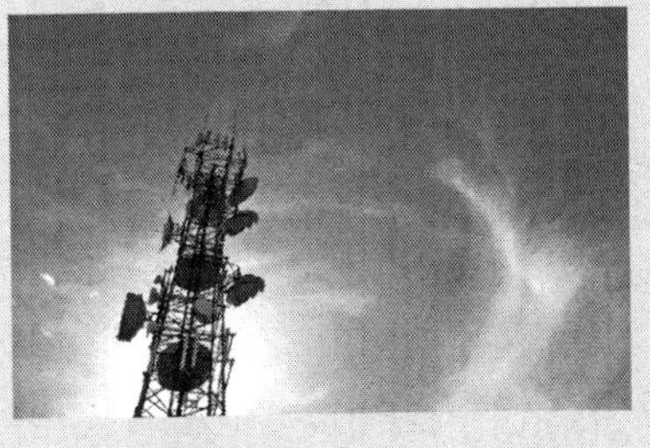

Test with an RF meter. Make sure your meter's frequency range is high enough. Many meters don't have a high enough range to test newer cordless phones, for example, so you may get a false low reading.

1. **Daytime exposure** levels are preferably kept below **10**

2. **Nighttime exposure** levels are preferably kept below **0.1**

Building Biology Guidelines for sleeping areas (SBM 2008)

| measures in microwatts per square meter µW/m² | No concern | Slight concern | Severe concern | Extreme concern |
|---|---|---|---|---|
| | **< 0.1** | **0.1 - 10** | **10 - 1000** | **> 1000** |

**What levels are allowed in government standards?**

**2 - 10 million** Source: ICNIRP, 1998.

Yes, the government standards are MILLIONS of times higher exposure than what is biologically safe. They are based only on thermal levels – the ability to warm human tissue. Wireless radiations emitted by a mobile phone, tablet, Smart Meter, Bluetooth and the cell antenna beside your child's school are deemed non-thermal.

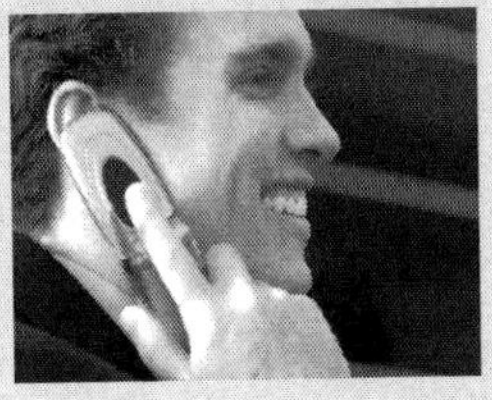

This is why these standards are irrelevant. Assurances such as, "These levels fall well within government safety standards," should be questioned, and standards re-evaluated.

In a few pages you will see the RF Guidelines table that shows international levels of this radio-frequency radiation (also known as microwave radiation) from broadcast antennas, cell towers (masts), radar, satellites – wireless communications that now encircle all parts of our planet.

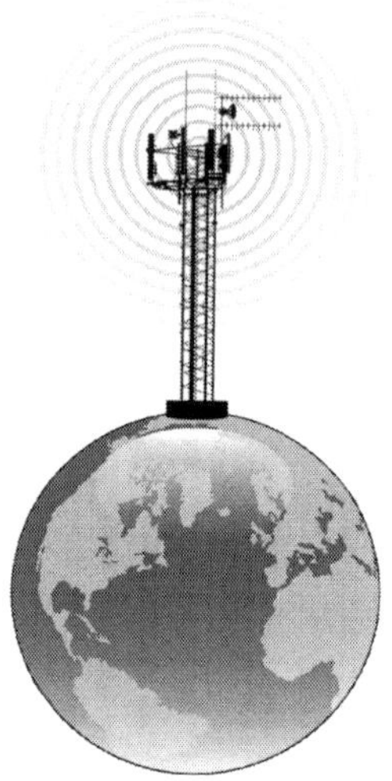

Remember what you just learned about thermal and non-thermal? Some of these international standards are based on the view that as long as the radiation is not powerful enough to cook tissue, then we're just fine. (Or, so their thinking goes.)

I asked the Building Biology environmental consultant, Katharina Gustavs, "just how high are those so-called 'safe' thermal levels?"

Ready for an astronomical number to stretch your comprehension? She answered, "At exposure levels of around 1,000,000,000 (microwatts per sq. meter in the frequency range of 400 MHz to 3 GHz), the eye lens starts to turn opaque; this is referred to as the thermal level."

Yes, that is one billion! So you see why some occupational exposures, including the military in many countries, allow 100,000,000 – why, it's only 1/10th of the allowable thermal level.

If you don't recognize the evidence of biological effects that have been shown to occur at a minuscule 0.1, it can seem that there's 'no problem'. This is the core of the issue, as I see it.

To put this into perspective, I also asked Peter Schlegel, a Swiss civil engineer, "What was the natural background of RF radiation for our ancestors?" I had to pause and count the zeros when he replied, "0.000001 is the estimate."

How's that for an indication of how far we've come in a century of technological development? Schlegel goes on to explain, "this is the cosmic background radiation arriving on earth (source H.-P. Neitzke, ECOLOG Institute, Germany) and it is also a level that living cells respond to."

Knowing this is useful, he tells us, for raising the awareness of the harm we have caused to our environment. However, this low natural level does not exist anymore because it is overpowered by the emissions of our human-made technology.

From 0.000001 to 100,000,000 – anyone have a calculator? One presumes the various species living on this planet had millions of years with the natural background. You can see why so many experts are alarmed at the dramatically increased levels of radiation exposure we're forced to endure now.

I find the recommendation of maximum levels of exposure below 10 for daytime, and below 5 for sleeping, to be very helpful. You need a reliable RF meter to determine these levels – see our Resources section.

The gap between what many scientists consider safe (0.1) and what some organizations/regulations allow (100,000,000) is the same difference in magnitude between the length of a few football fields and the distance from the earth to the sun. Isn't that unbelievable? (See the next page.)

## RF Exposure from Cell Towers

**Worldwide Limits and Standards** in μW/m² (microwatt per square meter)

| | |
|---|---|
| 100,000,000 | U.S. Standard C95.1-1966.<br>The first standard limiting exposure to microwaves in the Western world. |
| 10,000,000<br>to<br>4,000,000 | ICNIRP Guidelines (1998) are based on biological effects of short-term, high-level exposures that cause a rise in temperature, also referred to as thermal effects. Germany (1996), USA (1997), Japan (1997), Switzerland (2000), Australia (2002), Finland (2002), Sweden (2002), UK (2004), Austria (2006), Canada (2009) and many others. Exposure limit depends on frequency of carrier wave (800 MHz to 10 GHz). |
| 2,500,000<br>to<br>1,000,000 | Belgium law (2001). In 2009 a ruling of the constitutional court concluded that the setting of exposure levels for cell towers lies with the regional not the federal government. Exposure limit depends on frequency of carrier wave (800 MHz to 10 GHz). |
| 100,000 | Russia law (2003), China law (1987) |
| 100,000 | Italy law (2003): attention level not to be exceeded in sensitive areas. |
| 95,500<br>to<br>42,500 | Switzerland law (2000): precautionary exposure limit for sensitive areas. Based on the carrier wave frequency of the respective antennas (900 MHz, 1800 MHz, or both), the limit applies to a single transmitter site, including all antennas located on the same cell tower or building. |
| 24,000 | Ukraine Health & Safety Guideline (1996) |
| 1,000 | France: 16 cities chosen by Environment Ministry for pilot project (2010) |
| 1,000 | Parliamentary Assembly of Council of Europe(2011)<br>Precautionary recommendation for indoor environments |
| 1,000 | Salzburg Resolution for sum total of GSM (2000) |
| 100 | BUND (Friends of the Earth Germany) recommendation for hazard protection (2008) |
| 3 - 6 | BioInitiative Working Group precautionary recommendation (2012) |
| 1 | BUND (Friends of the Earth Germany) recommendation for precautionary protection (2008) |
| 1 | Health Department, Federal State of Salzburg, Austria precautionary recommendation for indoor environment of sum total of GSM (2002) |
| < 0.1<br>No concern | **Building Biology Evaluation Guidelines** (SBM 2008) specifically designed for sleeping areas and empirically established on the basis of many thousands of individual cases, including EHS sufferers. |

**0.000001 Natural background** – mostly this low natural level does not exist anymore.

Prepared by Katharina Gustavs, 2014. Printed here with permission.

How is this massive safety margin gap affecting our families? Do we even know? I have a cousin in a navy radar unit; it is chilling to realize the extreme levels he is being exposed to onboard ship. Now that you know about this measurement of RF radiation let's take a look at some of the levels we may be exposed to.

Katharina Gustavs reports on this RF (radio-frequency):

> For the sum total of the background RF radiation level in urban areas, you can find in the literature levels ranging from one hundred (microwatts per sq. meter) all the way up to a few thousand, or even into the ten thousands, depending on how close the next base station is located.

## Risks from Cell Tower Antennas / Masts In Your Community?

A German study reported that living within 400 meters (1300 ft) of two antennas over 10 years increased rates of cancer three fold. Living closer than that, they warned, the risk could be 100 fold. In Israel, a Tel Aviv University study also showed an increased cancer risk with proximity to antennas. Researchers in Australia, the UK and Italy found significant increase in leukemia. Many advocacy groups are fighting the installations of cell towers/masts in their communities. You can find a group in your area, or start your own. (Check out page 330 for our Statement of Accountability – a useful tool in this fight.)

In the US, the proliferation at www.antennasearch.com will alarm you, as will the rate at which transmitters are installed close to your home, child's school or hospital. Why are we allowing these so close? Outdated safety standards. Regulatory inertia. Talk to your school, other parents, and local representatives. At www.electromagnetichealth.org there is an important report "The BRAG™ Antenna Ranking of Schools" by Dr. Magda Havas who is working tirelessly, and effectively, for us all.

## Proximity to cell tower antennas/masts/base stations

Many experts report that harmful biological effects occur at so called "safe" levels. The neuroscientist Dr. Sarah Starkey sent us this update:

> In 2010 Dr. Khurana reported in the *International Journal of Occupational and Environmental Health* that 8 out of 10 published epidemiological studies reported increased adverse neurobehavioral symptoms or cancer in populations living **within 500 meters (1640 feet)** of cell tower antennas (mobile phone base stations). Also in 2010, Balmori found developmental abnormalities and 90% mortality of tadpoles (compared to 4.2% mortality for those screened from the radiation) after two months of living near a cell tower antenna. In the journal *Pathophysiology* (2009), Otitoloju reported developmental sperm abnormalities from mice living near an antenna for six months and many associations between this proximity and damage to wildlife. The Stewart Report, commissioned by the UK Government in 2000, recommended that the beam of greatest intensity of this radiation should not fall on a school's grounds or buildings.

In 2011 a Brazilian study led by engineer Adilza Dode, PhD also linked cell tower radiation with cancer deaths among people living within the same distance – 500 meters (1640 feet). Dr. Dode warns that emission limits are not based on health criteria, but upon industrial, economic and technological criteria. A study by Dr. Henry Lai and Blake Levitt, published by the National Research Council Press, recommended **"keep cell towers far from people"** and cautioned that proximity to WiFi, Wi-MAX, and SmartGrids also increases people's cancer risks.

It's not just cancer; a long-term study from Rimbach Germany, published in 2011, showed harmful effects on neurotransmitters – electric impulses in our brain. This is a concern for us, at every age!

## Risks at your school?

A mom wrote that her school principal reassured her that, "The levels in the school were well within the government safety standards." I told her about the research and suggested she show it to the school, and other parents. Who better to fight for our children than us, the parents?

## Some RF risks in your own home?

While it is essential that we have some comprehension of the exposures in our external environment, and that we make our voices heard, we should also be mindful of our exposures inside. Building Biology consultant, Peter Sierck, comments:

> We see many people fighting the installation of cell towers (masts) and going home where they have wireless routers and cordless phones which constantly radiate without being in use, microwave ovens, and often mobile phones.

**Common Exposure Levels** (all in microwatts per sq. meter)

Let's take a look at some measures taken by Gustavs and others.

**Wireless Internet access** An average-powered home wireless router within one foot (30 cm) – 30,000, within 10 ft (3 meters) – 3,000

**A cordless phone** (5.8 or DECT 6.0) within one foot (30 cm) – 200,000, within 10 ft (3 meters) – 2,000

**A microwave oven in use** (new, not defective) within one foot (30 cm) – 10,000-1,000,000, within 10 ft (3 meters) – 1,500

**In an average 2-3 bedroom home** that has a wireless router and at least one cordless phone: (KG) "If the cordless phone is in the bedroom, the person in bed may be exposed to 20,000 all night long, and in the kitchen maybe only 200. Again, the router at the desk may expose the computer user to 20,000, while in the living room next door you may have 1,000 and in the bedroom further away – 100."

## Cognitive Impairment, Cardiac Effects and Cancer Risks?

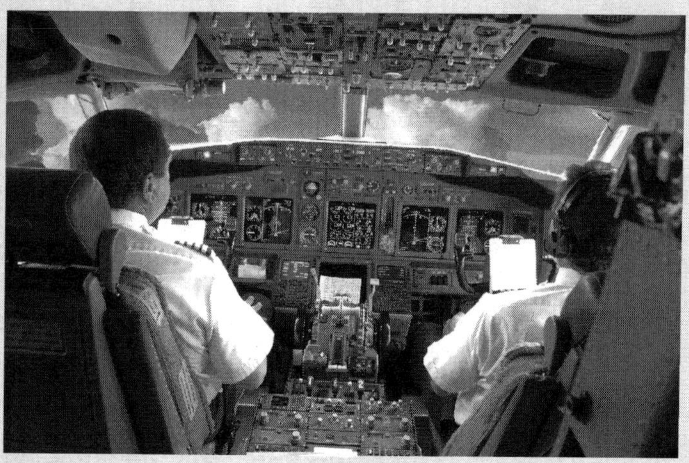

After the memorial service for her husband – her high school sweetheart – who died of a brain tumor, the widow was consumed with grief. Now she is getting angry. He was a commercial pilot who used a cell phone for many years. One year she gave him one of those in-the-ear wireless bluetooth headsets, hoping it would help.

She discovers that air crews' EMR exposure, including cosmic radiation, has caused cancer concerns for many years; and that now there is more exposure in the skies. She reads that a group of European physicians have issued an urgent medical alert about cell phones and wireless Internet onboard. Evidently, it was ignored.

The physicians had warned that this radiation can affect cognitive function and reduce reaction time – crucial factors in aviation – and put the crew at greater cancer risk. She used to assume that the strictly controlled aviation industry, and other regulatory agencies, were being vigilant about the health and safety of the flight crews and passengers. Now she is not so sure.

## Smart Meters, Smart Grids and Smart Appliances

Are you suspicious yet of technologies labelled "smart"? The health concerns are *not* just about one Smart Meter, but hubs of them in high-density dwellings, the prospect of billions of them around the world, and their powerful wireless Smart Grid/Wi-MAX networks. Smart Meters send out frequent bursts of data (energy consumption readings) from your house to your neighbor's, then to the power company. Electro-sensitive people, and others, could suffer from this involuntary exposure. The emission levels "meet government standards and are too low to cause harm," officials declare. Let's ask some hard questions: Where is the evidence that this radiation, re-classified in 2011 by the WHO as "possibly carcinogenic," will not be harmful? What agency is monitoring our accumulated dose of exposure? Why are you forging ahead, when some utilities are removing Smart Meters? (Due to health concerns, in the fall of 2011, California's PG&E was 'quietly' replacing wireless Smart Meters with analog/wired ones – the safe option.) And is your agency/company insured for health claims?

**Fiber optics** is the best choice for data communication, according to many technical and health experts. This system has many benefits. The data are sent along fiber optic cables, using pulses of light – safe – and also secure as this is a closed system. There are no radiation emissions blasting through space and all living creatures. Fiber optics can deliver Internet access and other communication data. Initially, this may be more expensive, but consider the health savings – see page 333.

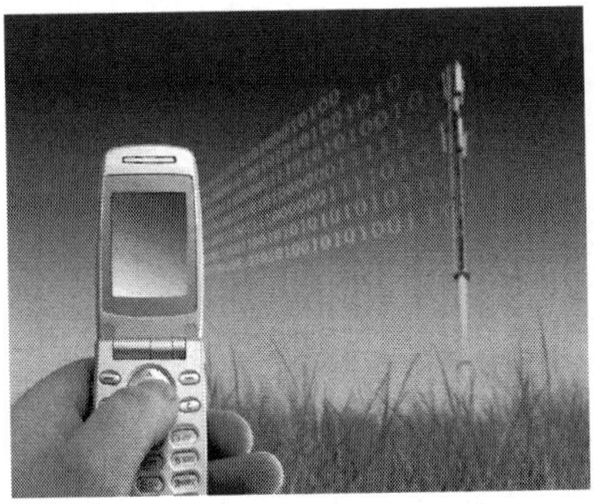

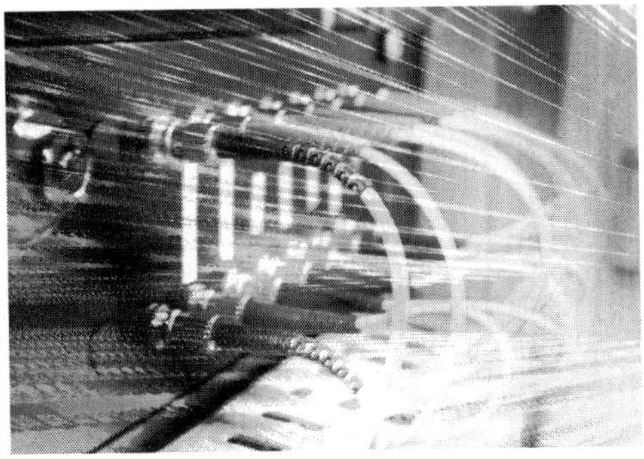

## Natural World at Risk – Where are all the bees?

As we mentioned, electro-pollution affects all life forms, not just us.

With mounting concern, a beekeeper notices bees have disappeared again this year. As he inspects empty hives, he glares at the cell tower on the nearby hill. Half a world away, a church custodian is unaware of the new cell antenna embedded in the metal cross on the church tower.

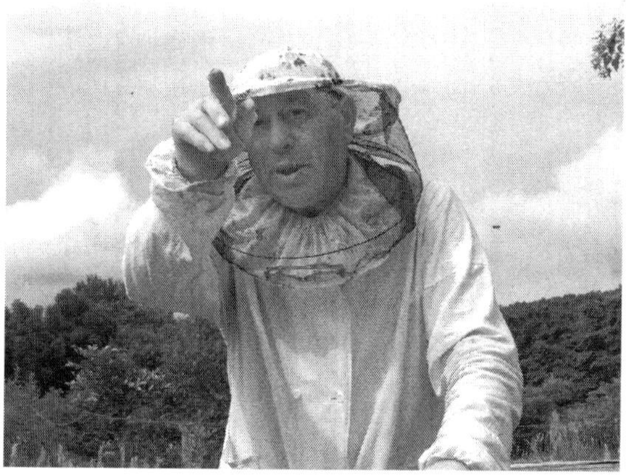

He has been watching for the return of the barn swallows. Here is a possible connection: The adverse effects of disrupting the intra-cellular whispering that Dr. Ross Adey (formerly of the Brain Research Center at the University of Southern California) described are not limited to inside the human body. Leading researchers caution that wireless radiation from cell tower antennas, mobile phones, 'smart' grids, etc. is disrupting the essential natural navigation abilities of whales, birds, and bees. It is biologically plausible that exposed bees become disoriented, cannot find their way back to the hive, and starve.

(Someone warn the determined Outernet developers who want to engulf our entire planet. Alert parks departments to halt plans for WiFi in the wilderness. Innovations can bring unintended consequences.)

## Colony Collapse Disorder – Disappearance of The Honey Bees

You might not give much thought to the wellbeing of bees, or be aware of their crucial role in ours: Much of the food we eat – some say one-third – depends on crops being pollinated. The health of bees is vital to human survival. Colony Collapse is just that: something affects the bees so that after they leave the hives they don't return. Around the world bees are dying in record high numbers. Why? Theories include: parasites, viruses, bacteria, GMO crops, pesticides and/or climate change. Is there another factor? The US Department of Agriculture weighed in, "Despite a great deal of attention having been paid to the idea, neither cell phones, nor cell phone towers, have been shown to have any connection to colony collapse or poor honey bee health." However, researchers in India conducted a study on this. In groups of bees periodically exposed to cell phone radiation, there was a significant decrease in the number returning to the hive. By the end of the study's three months, "there was neither honey, nor pollen or brood and bees in the colony". This was not the case with the control group. "The present study suggests that colony collapse does occur as a result of exposure to cellphone radiations," the researchers concluded. *Current Science*, Vol. 98, No. 10, 25 May 2010.

**Albert Einstein, "No more bees, no more pollination ... no more humans!"**

## Agriculture and All Things Green at Risk

In May of 2013, Jean Savedge (author of green parenting blogs about raising eco-aware children) wrote about a student science project in Denmark, "The girls noticed that if they slept with their mobile phones near their heads at night, they often had difficulty concentrating at school the next day. They wanted to test the effect of a cell phone's radiation on humans, but their school did not have the equipment to handle such an experiment. So the girls designed an experiment that would test the effect of cell phone radiation on a plant instead.

Over the next 12 days, the girls observed, measured, weighed, and photographed their results. By the end of the experiment the results were blatantly obvious — the cress seeds placed near the router had not grown. Many of them were completely dead. While the cress seeds planted in the other room, away from the routers, thrived."

## It's Not Just the Bees

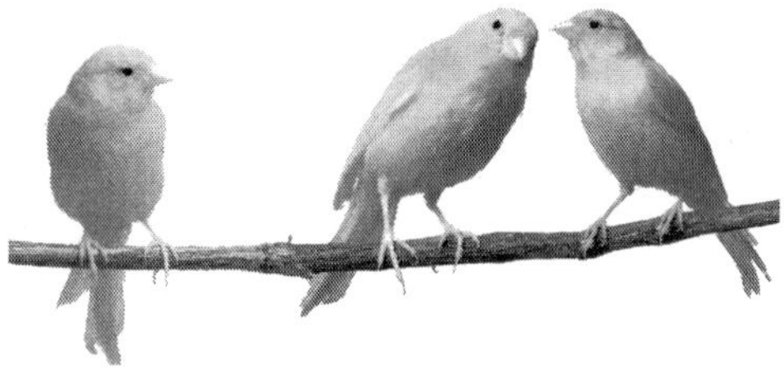

In 1971, William Kenton of Cornell University studied the effect of electro-magnetic fields on birds' ability to migrate:

> ...with 1-gauss (electrically-charged) magnets attached to their heads the birds couldn't find their way home. Each bird without magnets faultlessly navigated the 150 miles ...and fluttered in like a helicopter to a perfect landing.

Arthur Firstenberg wrote in *The Ecologist* in June 2004:

> Canadian researchers working with parakeets, chickens, pigeons and seagulls reported that these birds avoided microwave fields (EMR) if they could, and collapsed within seconds if they couldn't. Many years later, Alfonso Martínez carefully documented the decline and disappearance of white storks, house sparrows, and free-tailed bats from the vicinity of cellular phone base stations.

More than 45 years ago, Rachel Carson wrote:

> Over increasingly large areas of the US, spring now comes unheralded by the return of the birds, and the early mornings are strangely silent where they were once filled with the beauty of bird song.

As a species we take much for granted; we cannot imagine the effects of drastic climate change, and losing the natural world as we know it.

More than 100 years ago, Anton Chekhov warned:

> Human beings have been endowed with reason and creative power. But they have been more destructive than creative. Forests are disappearing, rivers are drying up, and wildlife is becoming extinct.

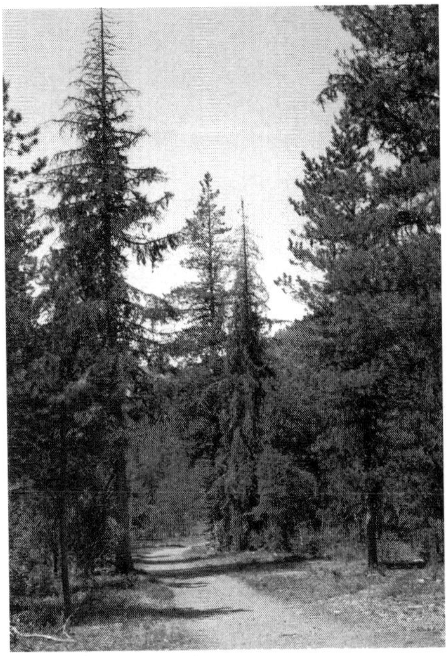

Before a radar station in Latvia was shut down at the end of the Cold War, a co-ordinated effort was made to determine whether the station had any environmental impact. Even at extremely low levels of exposure, researchers found these effects: smaller growth rings in trees, premature ageing in pine needles (a factor in raging wildfires in heavily populated high-EMR areas), and they found chromosome damage in cows.

Wolfgang Volkrodt linked forest die-back to microwave radiation rather than acid rain. Also in Germany, Löscher and Käs documented illness in dairy cows caused by cell towers. You don't have to be a dairy farmer to realize the serious implications of this.

In 2014, the Director of the Office of Environmental Policy of the US Department of the Interior sent a letter to the National Telecommunications and Information Administration with a concern that cell tower radiation has had negative impacts on the health of migratory birds and other wildlife.

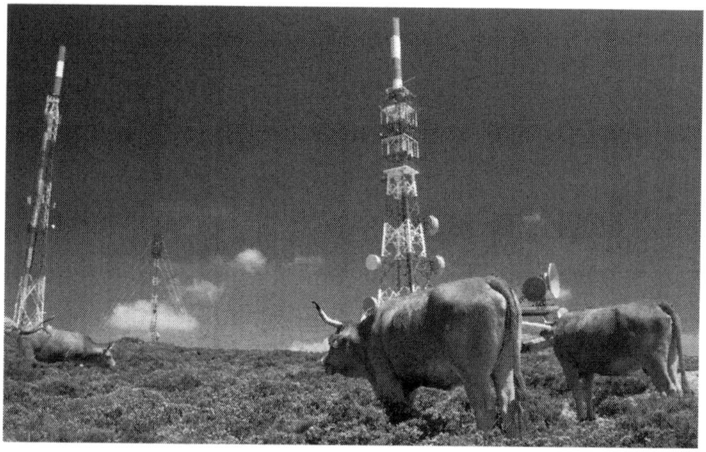

## Wildlife and Domestic Animals at Risk

Wildlife biologist Alfonso Balmori, PhD reported:

> **Electromagnetic radiation is a form of environmental pollution which may hurt wildlife.** Phone masts (cell towers) located nearby are irradiating continuously some species that could suffer long-term effects, like reduction of their natural defenses, deterioration of their health, problems in reproduction and reduction of their useful territory through habitat deterioration. Therefore microwave and radio-frequency pollution constitutes a potential cause for the decline of animal populations and deterioration of health of plants living near phone masts.

## Your Pets at Risk

If radiation harms wildlife, our pets are also at risk. When I reviewed stories of people with electro-sensitivity, it was sad to read how these families, including their pets, suffered. Many reported symptoms when they were near cell towers or WiFi signals. One story was heartbreaking: soon after a Smart Meter went in next door, the family watched helplessly as their healthy dog had a seizure, for the first time.

## Nature at Risk

Dr. Ulrich Warnke of the University of Saarland, in Germany cautioned a recent conference organized by Radiation Research in the UK that electro-smog was "disrupting nature on a massive scale."

Dr. Warnke went on to say:

> Today, unprecedented exposure levels from numerous wireless technologies interfere with the natural information system and functioning of humans, animals, and plants. The consequences of this development, which have already been predicted by critics for many decades, cannot be ignored anymore. Bees and other insects vanish; birds avoid certain places, and become disorientated at others.
>
> Humans suffer from functional impairments and diseases. And insofar as the latter are hereditary, they will be passed on to next generations as pre-existing defects.

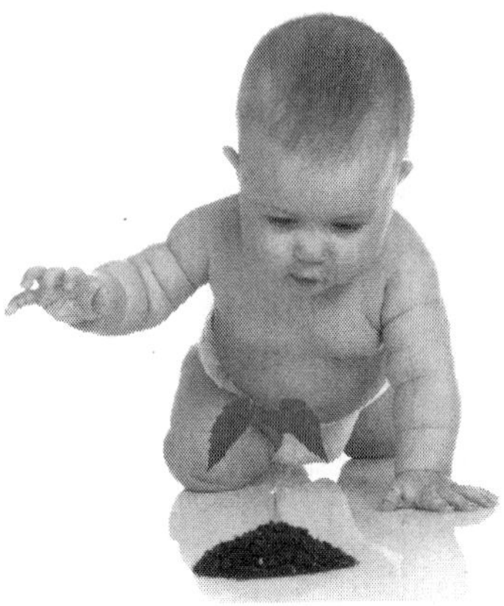

Now that we have investigated some of the evidence of harm from the electro-pollution which surrounds us, I must pose these questions: How much more evidence do we need before taking a course of action? And where are those who are charged with public health safety?

## Agencies Passing the Buck?

Alasdair Philips, the Director of Powerwatch, is realistic:

> I am a practising engineer and scientist who did amateur radio transmitter work. I thought wireless was brilliant. I now believe that the mistake we are making will have much more serious long-term effects than either smoking tobacco, or asbestos. Wireless is one of the few boom industries today, and one that brings governments massive tax revenues. So neither governments, nor the wireless industries, want any official word of precaution to be issued – however gently it is worded.
>
> There is good evidence of some harm (at least) and we should be warning people not to use such technologies when other, less invasive, ones are available that often (like Ethernet wired networks v.s. wLAN/WiFi) actually perform better, and do not expose people to radio-frequency radiation. Why can't we warn people about the dangers of excessive exposures to relatively low levels of radio-frequency radiation. To use caution.

## Economics Over Public Health?

Relying on government and public health officials to safeguard our wellbeing has seldom been prudent. Whenever I hear an official proclaim, "there is no conclusive evidence," I vow to find more brave souls like the feisty Canadian physician Dr. Francis Kelsey. She was working in the US and prevented the use of thalidomide by pregnant women. Canada and many other countries didn't heed her wise use of the precautionary principle. We know the tragic cost of their negligence: thousands of babies born with birth defects.

Unfortunately, the dispute about the regulations controlled by ICNIRP, the World Health Organization, and various federal government agencies, continues. This controversy is not very helpful when you're wondering about that powerful multi-purpose mobile device.

I heard one expert warn that these powerful new multi-task phones are getting close to thermal levels. Is some government agency monitoring this? Or monitoring the people getting sick, or those who are dying? I discovered that the European Union's main environmental watchdog, the EEA, and the BioInitiative Working Group – an international team of scientists, researchers and public health policy professionals – were both warning that government standards are woefully inadequate. Truth is, they're irrelevant, according to the BioInitiative Report.

(Check out www.healthandenvironment.org for information, and for the BioInitiative Report go to www.bioinitiative.org.)

A few years ago, Dr. Louis Slesin commented on these regulations:

> The Finnish Radiation and Nuclear Safety Authority recommended that parents limit children's use of mobile phones and, on the same day, the French government announced a series of environmental health proposals, which include a ban on advertising that promotes the use of cell phones among those under 12. In contrast to all this activity, the lackadaisical approach of the International Commission on Non-Ionizing Radiation Protection (ICNIRP) is striking. Some 40 countries, many of which have only limited expertise in RF radiation health effects, look to the Commission for advice. **Yet, ICNIRP has been silent for ten long years. Their last standards on RF exposures were published in 1998.** How long could it take to write a simple statement urging caution?

Dr. Slesin explains the WHO 2B classification:

> It's not easy to reach unanimous agreement on anything to do with cell phone radiation, but IARC (the International Agency for Research on Cancer – part of the World Health Organization) nearly pulled it off. In May 2011, a group the WHO/IARC Director called 'the world's leading experts' – issued a joint statement that cell phone and other types of radiofrequency (RF) and microwave radiation might cause cancer.

In 2013 the same World Health Organization group increased the caution in a 471 page report concluding that there is now "limited evidence" in both humans and laboratory animals that wireless radiation, especially from cell phones, causes cancer. Did the media and marketplace take notice? Did the industry?

At a 2009 gathering, The Mobile Manufacturers Forum (a lobby organization) said why it believed its members are sufficiently protected from potential litigation – because products (i.e. mobile phones and other wireless devices) comply for the most part with ICNIRP, the international regulators' safety standards. Is the wireless industry even insured against health claims?

David Gee, one of the authors of the BioInitiative Report, warned:

> The mobile industry will not be able to claim immunity if, in ten years or so, it is determined that use of mobile phones causes brain cancer or other illness. They are forewarned now, and simply saying 'but we were in compliance with ICNIRP safety limits' will not be sufficient reason for ignoring the growing evidence.

## US Federal Regulations – Protecting Americans?

Dr. Davis, "The U.S. agency that offers recommendations on cell-phone emissions – the Federal Communications Commission – doesn't employ a single health expert. The standards the FCC adopts are based on advice given by outside experts, many of whom work directly for the cell-phone industry. And the Food and Drug Administration lacks the authority to set standards for cell phones and can only act if a phone is shown to release hazardous signals."

In 2013 the FCC requested public input on its 17-year-old regulatory limits on cell phone radiation. Pediatrician Toril Jelter, MD, wrote to them, "I am writing to request that you reevaluate current FCC safety standards for wireless technologies. Current research, and what I see in my clinical practice, indicate a revision is long overdue. Children are suffering disability and disease in much higher numbers than 30 years ago. Their EMF exposure is clearly a significant contributing factor. Children have a right to live and play and learn where their DNA will not be damaged; their immune systems, neurology or behavior not adversely affected; and where they are not at risk of developing cancer at an early age. They need to be adequately protected from (wireless) non-ionizing radiation. This is not the case today."

In Canada, also in 2013, there was a public hearing on Safety Code 6. Their panel decided to opt for the status quo. Sad but not unexpected.

Scientists including Dr. Davis and Dr. Blank, and dedicated advocates including the publisher Dr. Louis Slesin, are highly effective in educating people about this issue, and media coverage is increasing.

## Your Assessment So Far?

As you can see, I have formed mine and sincerely believe that we are putting ourselves and our loved ones at risk. I have taken steps to protect my family. But it is *your* view that is most relevant here.

**Are the wireless or insurance industries alerting customers?**

Did you read the fine print on your cell phone contract to see if you agreed not to participate in any class action lawsuits, or to review their safety precautions? An industry defence if/when they are sued?

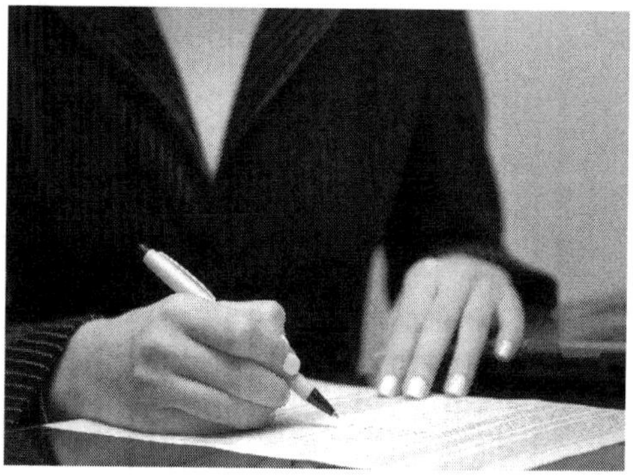

Evidently, after 2002 the insurance industry began refusing to insure the wireless industry against health-related claims. What science did those insurance executives see? And when did they see it? And why were we consumers not made aware? Think we know that.

Took only a few class actions to strike fatal blows to the asbestos and breast implant industries. Since as much as 30% of retirement fund shares are invested in telecom stocks, a global tsunami of class action suits could be disastrous to retirees, world economies and the industry

If you use a magnifying glass to read your mobile phone/device user manual, you may see the recommended distance from your body [does that include your hands?]. If pressed against the head or touching the body, emissions may exceed government standards. Warning: It is in tiny print.

In 2014, Australia's largest telecom warned its customers with a "reminder msg" to visit their website for information on "electromagnetic energy and tips to reduce exposure" with advice from the World Health Organisation and points such as, "Use hands-free devices to keep mobile phones away from the head and body during phone calls. Limit the number and length of calls".

So we've been fairly warned. Or have we?

## So Who is Taking Action?

There are some encouraging signs that people are listening to the independent scientists urging them to bring the safety regulations in line with the science. Many parent and consumer advocate groups are demanding product safety and accountability – the wellbeing of people over profit. Proactive people all over the world are deciding *not* to wait for the indisputable smoking gun before taking precautions, especially with young, developing brains. And while most governments are lagging behind, others are opting for the precautionary principle.

## In the US – Transportation Hazards and More

Fortunately, some legislators show the leadership we need. In December 2013, U.S. Senator Jay Rockefeller (D-WV), chairman of the U.S. Senate Committee on Commerce, Science and Transportation, sent a letter to FCC Chairman Thomas Wheeler and U.S. Department of Transportation Secretary Anthony Foxx. Senator Rockefeller wrote,

> The ability to make a call on one's cell phone is not worth compromising the safety of a flight. I encourage you to carefully consider the possibility of banning in-flight mobile calls and to fully examine all safety issues that the use of cellular voice services on aircraft may create.

Yes, many want the convenience of receiving and making calls on their mobile in flight. Do you? If you only knew the potential hazards: not just the proven damage to your DNA, or long-term brain cancer risk; we are talking now about the potential of more immediate danger. Our team is briefing transportation officials on cardiac problems and cognitive impairment, including Professor Mosgoeller's work on the adverse effects on human performance, and neurological symptoms (dizziness, loss of consciousness) – want this for your pilot? More evidence from top aviation health and safety experts is on page 209.

I attended a 2009 conference on cell phones and health, organized by Dr. Devra Davis in Washington, DC. We attended a US Senate Hearing, requested by Senator Arlen Specter of Pennsylvania and chaired by Sen. Tom Harkin of Iowa. Sen. Mark Prior of Arkansas also attended. A scientist (speaking for the wireless industry?) caused a stir in the gallery with the claim, "The current scientific evidence does not demonstrate that wireless causes cancer, or other adverse health effects." (Flashback: one after the other, a line up of Big Tobacco executives assures a Senate hearing, "Senator, nicotine is *not* addictive.")

It was captivating to witness the eminent scientists Drs. Henry Lai, Om Gandhi, Martin Blank and Leif Salford in attendance. During a discussion between the panel of presenters and the senators about Dr. Lai's seminal work on DNA damage, I wanted to leap up and shout, "Dr. Lai is here. Let's ask him about the evidence."

At the closing, Senator Harkin commented, "I found this really very interesting and very challenging, and I can assure you we are going to do some follow-up on this." I am grateful to Dr. Davis for her clear and compelling testimony at this Senate hearing, and for her book, *Disconnect – The Truth About Cell Phone Radiation* (Plume, 2011).

Other US legislators are responding. Christiane Tourtet, BA, Founder of International MCS/EMS Awareness, brought this issue to Connecticut Governor M. Jodi Rell and Colorado Governor Bill Ritter, Jr.

In 2010, Maine Rep. Andrea Boland presented a bill that would have required cell phones to carry warning labels, like tobacco. It was voted down. In 2014 the bill was finally passed and then it was 'killed'. Industry influence? San Francisco Mayor Gavin Newsom had passed a bill which requires retailers to post cell phone radiation levels. "This will protect the consumers' right to know," said Mayor Newsom, "and encourage the redesign of devices to function at lower radiation levels."

In 2010 California Senator Mark Leno introduced a similar state bill that would require disclosure of cell phone radiation levels.

Congressman Dennis Kucinich (D-OH) held a Congressional hearing on this issue in 2008 in which Ellie Marks testified and he promised Marks that he would see this through. Then four years later he introduced a bill to create a new national research program to study cell phone risks and to grant a consumer's right to know by providing warning labels. He declared, "Obviously, cell phone companies should not be the ones making decisions for us."

Please contact your representatives and ask what they know about this issue. Without overwhelming them, offer the evidence about wireless radiation and human health, with references, and ask for a response. Best to avoid an angry, alarmist tone, even if you are feeling that way.

Also in 2010, the President's Cancer Panel, which had received extensive information from Eileen O'Connor of EM Radiation Research Trust, issued its report, "Reducing Environmental Cancer Risk."

In Microwave News, Dr. Slesin summarizes that report:

> The Panel's #1 recommendation is: 'A precautionary, prevention-oriented approach should replace current reactionary approaches to environmental contaminants in which human harm must be proven before action is taken to reduce or eliminate exposure. It is vitally important to recognize that children are far more susceptible to damage from environmental carcinogens.' Martha Linet, the head of the Radiation Epidemiology Branch at the National Cancer Institute says: 'The most urgent issue that we need to address is whether children or adolescents using cell phones are at increased risk.'

## In Canada

Keith Martin, MD – a physician and retired Member of Parliament, "Canada needs an independent assessment of EMR and human health."

Carol Hughes, MP, has spoken out, "Health Canada must tell Canadians the full story about the microwave irradiation of children. Exposing them to WiFi in school is a big experiment, with unknowing volunteers."

Elizabeth May, MP, leader of the Green Party of Canada,"It's disturbing how quickly WiFi has moved into schools as children are the most vulnerable." The Green Party is also up to date on climate change.

## In the UK

The Leader of the UK Green Party, Caroline Lucas, MEP, "In keeping with the precautionary principle, we need a moratorium on masts (cell towers) until there is sufficient evidence to guarantee their safety."

Dr. David Dowson is a physician who advises the House of Commons and the House of Lords. They need to hear this as electro-sensitivity (ES) is increasing in that country as Dr. Dowson explains, "The incidence of ES in Switzerland, with its very strict and low levels of allowed exposure, will have a very low incidence compared to the UK."

In May 2014, the UK launched the largest study of mobile phone effects on children's brains: "The Study of Cognition, Adolescents and Mobile Phones". An estimated 70% of 11– to 12-year-olds in the UK now own a mobile phone, rising to 90% by age 14. Remember Dr. Hardell's research on page 54? This does not bode well for the future.

## In Europe

After an extensive study, The European Environment Agency called to reduce exposure from cell towers, "Delay may result in a crisis more serious than AIDS, smoking, pesticides, asbestos and leaded gasoline".

In its report this agency advised us about standards around the world:

> Safety limits set for radiation are thousands of times too lenient. We will increase pressure on governments and public health bodies to take precautionary action over the radiation from rapidly expanding new technologies. The German government is advising its citizens to use wired Internet connections instead of WiFi, and corded landlines instead of mobile phones.

In 2013 the EEA called on governments to reduce exposure to cell phone radiation, especially children and young adults who are at greatest risk for brain and salivary gland tumors. The report recommended texting, use of hands-free sets, and improved cell phone design; governments should reconsider exposure standards; cell phones should be required to have labeling and warnings; and funding should be provided for "urgently needed research into the health effects of phones" and base stations.

In 2008 the European Parliament had voted by 522 to 16 to urge ministers across Europe to bring in stricter limits for exposure stating: "The limits on exposure to electro-magnetic fields which have been set for the general public are obsolete." In 2009 these same parliamentarians passed a major resolution that antennas, mobile phone towers and other EMR-emitting devices should be placed a specific distance away from schools, retirement homes, health institutions, and consumers, especially children.

At a 2009 Andrzej Rys, MD, Director of Public Health for the European Commission, spoke of the need for continuing progress on new, biologically-based exposure standards, and implementing precautionary strategies. In 2011 the Parliamentary Assembly Council of Europe recommended that "for children in general, and particularly in schools and classrooms, preference should be given to wired Internet connections -and the use of mobile phones by schoolchildren on school premises- should be strictly regulated." Some European member states have taken action. Wireless Internet has already been banned in public schools in Frankfurt, Germany, and Austria's Medical Association is pressing for a similar ban.

Also in 2013, Belgium banned children's cell phones and requires the specific absorption rate (SAR) be listed on every cell phone at the point of sale and a warning provided to customers to choose a lower SAR phone, use it moderately, and wear an earpiece.

The French Agency for Food, Environmental and Occupational Health warned the public to reduce their exposure to cell phone radiation.

Several libraries in Paris removed their wireless Internet networks due to health concerns. In 2009 the French government moved to prohibit cell phone use in elementary schools, and 2013, citing the precautionary principle, the National Assembly passed a bill to promote the use of wired Ethernet in schools and to reduce the use of WiFi systems.

Herouville-St.Clair, France was the world's first municipality to remove wireless from schools and public buildings. Mayor Rudolphe Thomas,"Our job is to protect people's health. We are *not* willing to gamble with our children's health." They are also investing in a WiFi-free fiber optics network – the wave of the future!

The Mayor of Oullins decreed that new mobile phone masts could not be built within 100 meters of schools or day care centers. Also in France, the Senate moved toward banning cell phone use in schools, by children up to about age 14, and telecom companies would be required to make sure emissions, within this protected zone, do not exceed the low levels recommended in the 2012 BioInitiative Report.

Health agencies in Switzerland, Germany, Israel, France, the United Kingdom, and Finland have issued warnings to limit cell phone use, particularly by children. A district court cited the precautionary principle when in an injunction stopping a French company from installing cell phone antennas on a hotel, 15 meters from an apartment building in Paris. The plaintiffs argued that the antenna would beam radiation directly into their bedroom. The judgment said, "Even if present scientific knowledge does not enable us to determine precisely the impact of electro-magnetic radiation when it penetrates the communal parts of the building, there exists a risk that cannot be ignored of repercussions on the state of health of the residents."

It's not all success stories. Industry pressure is strong. In Salzburg, Austria, with the guidance of renowned physician, Dr. Gerd Oberfeld, had set limits based on biological effects. However, only one of the operators observed the agreement, for a short time, then withdrew. And the Liechtenstein Parliament intended to restrict exposure from base stations to the BioInitiative Report's recommended levels, by 2013, in sensitive areas such as homes, workplaces, schools, hospitals and public buildings. The wireless companies threatened to pull out, saying this would not be financially viable. In a referendum, initiated by industry, the voters rejected the reduction of the safety standard value.

## Scientists are Also Taking Action

Many researchers are calling for nations to adopt biologically-based standards. The BioInitiative 2012 Report (bioinitiative.org) was prepared by 29 authors from ten countries: ten holding medical degrees (MDs) and 21 PhDs. And Elizabeth Kelley, MA directs the International Commission for Electromagnetic Safety (ICEMS) composed of many concerned scientists. Another excellent resource is the Seletun Scientific Statement (*Reviews on Environmental Health* (2010; 25: 307-317) where leading experts provide their research and recommendations.

The International EMF Alliance (IEMFA), a global consortium whose members cover a diversity of medical, scientific and related disciplines, provides health-oriented information and advice.

## Citizens are Taking Action

### USA

The EMR Policy Institute – led by Janet Newton and Diana Warren – focuses its activities on the recommendations to protect human health set forth in the BioInitiative Report.

The Environmental Working Group is a nonprofit organization based in Washington, DC to protect children, babies, and infants in the womb from toxic contaminants, including electro-pollution, as well as federal policies.

Center for Safer Wireless is an expanding national non-profit group, founded by health advocate Christine Hoch, to enhance the public's understanding of the safety concerns about wireless products.

Another effective voice is the dedicated Camilla Rees, the founder of ElectromagneticHealth.org and co-author with Dr. Havas of *Public Health SOS: The Shadow Side of the Wireless Revolution.*

Here is an inspiring grandmother: when her grandsons became ill by EMR exposure, Joanne Mueller started Guinea Pigs "R" Us.

### Canada

Martin Weatherall and the Canadian Initiative to Stop Wireless, Electric, and Electromagnetic Pollution (WEEP) educate the public, and provide help for electro-sensitive people.

In British Columbia Sharon Noble, founder of CAUSE, was a leading force in getting Colwood to adopt the Porto Alegre Resolution.

Frank Clegg, former President of Microsoft Canada, is the CEO of Canadians For Safe Technology (C4ST). It is a not-for-profit volunteer-based coalition whose mission is to educate and inform citizens and policy makers about EMR issues and solutions, and to work with all levels of government to create healthier communities for children and families. C4ST provides information for people with electro-sensitivity.

Una St Clair-Moniz is founder of Citizens For Safe Technology. They focus on a range of issues; their mission is to empower the public to protect children and nature from unsafe wireless technologies.

## The UK

Alasdair Philips (Powerwatch), an electrical engineer, has advised the British government and is a Contributing Expert for this book.

Eileen O'Connor, Director of EM Radiation Research Trust is an effective voice informing the EU, British Parliament and WHO.

Sarah Dacre (ES-UK.info), and others, are educating the public, and providing information and support for those with electro-sensitivity.

Safe Schools Information Technology Alliance (SSITA) is a new group focusing on the need for safe environments for students of all ages.

WiredChild raises awareness of risks from wireless technology. And Mast Sanity campaigns against the unsafe placement of masts.

## Europe

HESE (Human Ecological Social Economical Project) is an international group of researchers and advocates, many with ES/EHS.

## France

PRIARTéM helps citizens fight for protection of their health. Next-Up is another effective French non-governmental group.

### Sweden

Sweden has support for people with electro-sensitivity. Several of the world's leading researchers are Swedish. In Gothenburg, Anne-Li Karlsson and Jennie Öberg, with others, built a radiation-blocking Faraday cage, in the shape of a house, to show sources of radiation.

### Norway

Citizens' Radiation Protection is a group founded by Sissel Halmøy, MS. She is also Founder and Chair of the International EMF Alliance.

### Australia

EMFacts Consultancy, founded in 1994 by Don Maisch, PhD, has published a range of reports and papers. And three neurosurgeons, Drs. Vini Khurana, Charles Teo, and Richard Bittar, are speaking out with their concerns about brain tumours and mobile phone use. The Australasian College of Nutritional and Environmental Medicine has published a number of papers. And EMR Australia is a consumer advocacy group alerting people about the growing concerns.

### New Zealand

Oururah NZ provides information to people on the adverse health effects of antennas and mobile phones with an extensive website. Another active group in New Zealand is Ban The Tower.

These are just some of the citizens' groups who are taking action. The Resources section has the websites of these groups and Microwave News has a detailed list of organizations around the globe.

### We can turn this around

With any wake-up call we can just go back to sleep. We are fighting against the tide (and waves!) But please don't despair. There's progress and safer-tech solutions. Let's 'keep calm and keep going.' We won't save everyone; we can make a difference for our families and communities.

## Mindfulness For The Digital Age

Never underestimate the impact of dedicated experts, informed consumers, and protective instincts of parents and grandparents. We *will* make regulations based on biological effects. We will get safer technology. We will live closer to nature in saner and less materialistic ways. We'll find more friends of the future, as in *For The Next 7 Generations: 13 Indigenous Grandmothers Weaving A World That Works.*

Here are three other excellent documentaries raising public awareness:

*Mobilize* is a 2014 documentary film directed by Kevin Kunze featuring scientists, doctors, and politicians, with telecom executives Apple's co-founder Steve Wozniak and Virgin Mobile's Sir Richard Branson. *Mobilize* explains why many experts say brain tumors, infertility, and breast cancer are related to cell phone radiation and explores potential long-term health effects. The film also features personal narratives of cancer patients who believe cell phone radiation caused their disease. (www.mobilizemovie.com)

*All The Time In The World,* by Suzanne Crocker, MD and her family, explores the theme of disconnecting from technology-laden lives to reconnect with each other, ourselves, and our natural environment.

*Full Signal* is an award-winning film by veteran journalist and director Talal Jabari, and it includes several of our experts.(www.amazon.com)

We are here to support you, in supporting your loved ones.

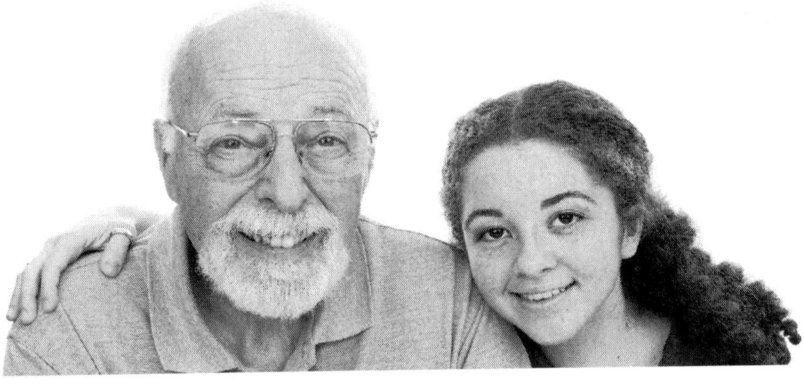

Some days I wish I could walk away from this. Then I see a child pressing a hot pink cell phone against her head, a baby in the arms of someone on a cordless phone, or a person lying on a heating pad.

As you know, many people will have to mull this over; others act quickly.

A take-action kind of mom got the message about wireless networks right away, "That's it, I'm ripping that router out of our house and going back to our Ethernet connection. It worked fine."

I did point out that the risk is not yet a scientific certainty. She shot back, "With my children, I don't wait for that."

A grandmother also woke up on the spot, "My son put this wireless thing in my house so he could get his email in the living room. What about their home and my grandchildren? Their bedrooms are full of electrical things. I'm calling him right now."

Another parent, whose child has autism symptoms, spontaneously hugged me when I told her that many of these children were thriving in a low-EMR environment, and about a new study with promising results, which we will discuss later on.

Let's not fall into the extremes of ignoring this, or becoming anxious. We have a plan that works, and we must not forget that there are many health-enhancing electro-magnetic fields. Some are known as life force, chi – the healing energy in us, and around us. We generate our own bio-electrical field, which is inherently in harmony with the energies that surround us in the natural world. To reconnect with these natural energies is another good reason to push back from the computer and step outside. Acupuncturists, and many other practitioners of energy medicine, work with our inner energetic flow to encourage our innate self-healing mechanisms.

In later strategies, we will look at these natural energies and the healing benefits of these traditions. The key, as in many things, is balance. We can withstand a certain amount of EMR and other toxicity, as long as our innate wellbeing is not overwhelmed. Our basic healthiness and ability to heal are miraculous beyond measure, and can be supported in ways we will discuss. Every contributor to this book is supporting you.

We industrious human beings created this electro-pollution, and we can reverse it. We will meet this Safer-Tech Challenge, for all of our children.

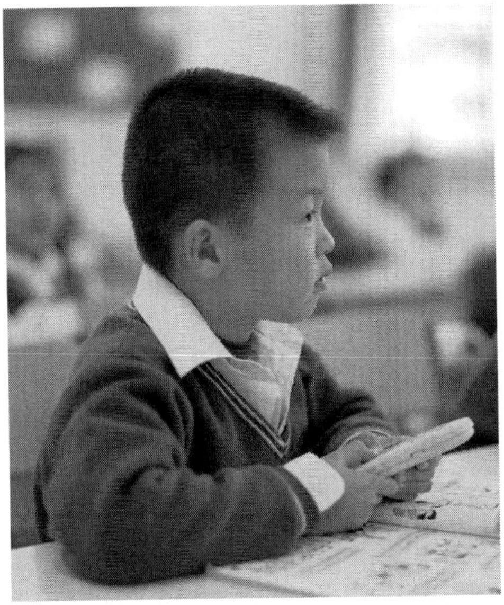

In the next section we turn to the crucial strategy of taking stock.

The benefits of this include knowing how much EMR exposure you, and your family, are dealing with on a daily basis; how this may be affecting you, and symptoms and medical conditions. Then we look at safer options for your living, working and travelling environments.

First, I'd like you to read about a teen with electro-sensitivity and understand why we are fighting for him, and for all the others.

**Is your child being affected by wireless radiation? A mom's story:**

> Our 17 year old son was complaining of headaches; an inability to focus; exhaustion even after a long sleep; stomach pains and nausea; clumsiness, and weak legs. Many specialists, from allergists to neurologists, found nothing. Running with his gym class, he'd get sudden pains in his head and nausea – at the same place on the run. (Close to two cell towers, as it turns out.) He always felt really good in remote and unpopulated mountains. No symptoms there.
>
> About a year ago, a building biologist did some testing in our home and suggested he might be electro-sensitive. We had WiFi and cordless 6.0 phones, including one by his bed. His symptoms worsened about a month after we got these 'conveniences'. Was there a connection I wondered?
>
> One evening he was on the computer, near the WiFi router, slouched over his work and struggling with homework. Without his knowing, I unplugged the router. He sat up straight – like a puppet being pulled up on strings. After 15 minutes, secretly, I plugged the router back in. He slumped back down. This was enough proof for me. We removed every radiating device. (Amazingly, my heart palpitations, and my husband's arthritis symptoms, also improved.)At the end of this summer, our son was full of energy. Now he is back at school and has gone from a clear-thinking, sociable, happy teenager into a foggy-brained zombie. He says he feels isolated. There are WiFi routers at his school – for staff use only – one is in his English class. In that class he can only do a few questions in an hour. While at home, he can easily complete 23 questions in half an hour. I have asked the school administration if cabled options could replace the WiFi. They defer to School District policy, which defers to government exposure standards.

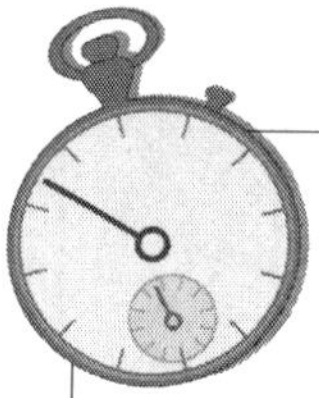

*2 Minute Quick Read Summary*

## Strategy 2 Know Your Risks

THIS SELF-ASSESSMENT QUESTIONNAIRE will help you identify:

- the sources of radiation from wireless and wired devices
- the symptoms and conditions that may be related

Remember, just because there are no symptoms it does *not* mean there are no adverse effects.

Do you know where you are on this spectrum, and what to do?

- exposure without symptoms
- mild to moderate symptoms
- electro-sensitivity
- electro-hypersensitivity
- electro-allergy
- other serious medical conditions

And in this step you learn the basics of electro-magnetic radiation – a simple and accurate primer including the difference between wired and wireless radiation. This will help you understand how to take steps that will decrease – not increase – your risk.

**See Strategy 2 for more details.**

*Difficulty sleeping, headaches, increased stress, trouble concentrating, dizziness, impaired immune systems, food allergies and chemical sensitivities can all be connected with EMR exposure.* Hans Scheiner, MD

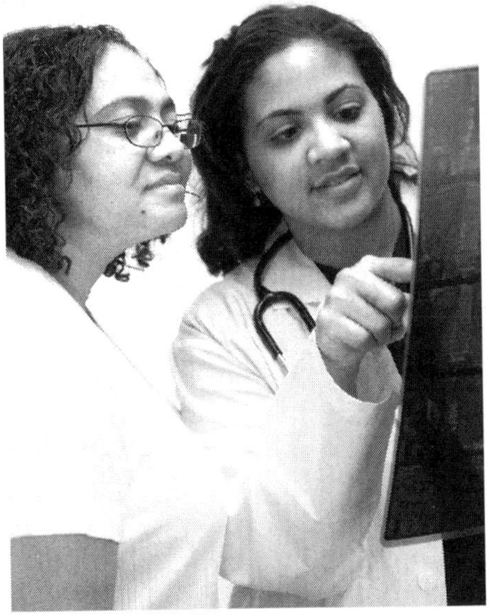

## Strategy 2. Know Your Risks

- throughout each day, we are exposed to artificial EMR;
- these levels have been shown to have adverse biological effects;
- this exposure now begins in utero;
- there is a range of related symptoms and health conditions;
- many medical tests and treatments expose us to EMR;
- millions of people around the world are affected by new conditions: electro-sensitivity or electro-pollution syndrome;
- knowing your risks is essential to reducing them.

## A Family Like Yours?

Before we get to the questionnaire, let me introduce you to a mother, perhaps much like you, or someone you know. I met this woman and her family at our local library.

After discussing books, including this one, she asked if she could read it. It was still in process so I sent her sections to read, inviting her feedback.

Here's an excerpt of what she wrote:

> Sorry that it's taken me so long to get back to you about the second chapter. I think that I had some fear around what I might learn – after all the evidence in part one. So there was some resistance for me to overcome before I could read it properly!
>
> I was definitely intimidated by the checklists in Strategy 2. I have so many of the symptoms.
>
> I think also, that it might be useful to suggest to the reader that they do a cost/benefit analysis ie. what is the potential long term risk of EMR exposure vs. what is the potential loss that they will incur by restricting their EMR exposure.
>
> They will probably find that many of the lifestyle changes required to restrict EMR are not life-threatening--but are actually life enhancing.

As you'll see in the questionnaire that follows, there's a surprisingly long list of symptoms and conditions that may be linked to EMR exposure; this is because every cell and system in the body is adversely affected. It can be challenging to figure out whether EMR is a factor in an individual's case. More about this in Strategies 3 and 4.

## The Safer-Tech Questionnaire©

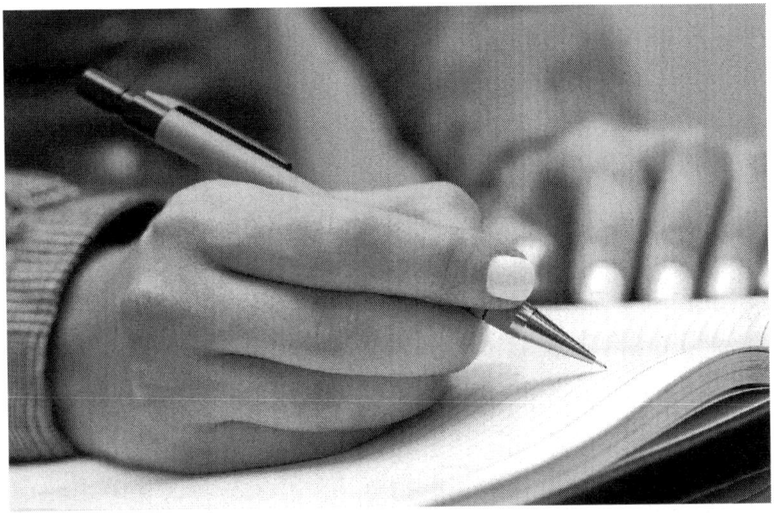

The information contained within the questionnaire does not provide medical advice and is not intended for use in medical diagnosis or treatment.

In the case of any disease, you should always consult your health care practitioner.

You'll notice this survey is not scored; that's because there is no way at this time to weight the effects of the various exposures. While the power of your mobile phone makes a big difference so does the usage.

For example, **Professor Hardell's early research indicated that 500 minutes per month (less than 30 minutes per day) of cell phone use significantly increases brain cancer risk – as much as 140%.**

Other studies show up to a 300 per cent increase when using the cell phone between 500 and 1000 minutes per month.

Source: Wire Technology Research, Second State of the Science Colloquium Book; January 2001 *Journal of the American Medical Association*; Early Hardell studies.

We need to find out how much the risk increases when combined with exposure to wireless radiation, cordless phones and/or overhead power lines. As Professor Johansson cautions, we are part of that experiment. I created this questionnaire by extensive research and input from many experts and documents compiled by others. I had the editing assistance of Dr. Heather McKinney.

If you wish to use this questionnaire in any form, please contact me via our website: SaferTechSolutions.org.

**Can you connect the dots?**

This is one of the objectives of our risk reduction plan.

Is the radiation from your cell phone, and/or cordless phone, one of the reasons you can't sleep? Maybe it's not just the worry.

Is the wireless router in your home, and in their schools, why your children need new glasses again, and are having trouble concentrating?

Is the mobile device – always powered on – in your husband's pocket the reason he is having cardiac symptoms? Maybe it's not just the stress.

As you answer the questions in Sections III and IV, you will see your exposures. Then you may see a connection with the Symptoms and Conditions that you answered in I and II. Reduce your exposures with our action plan and see if your symptoms improve.

## Section I – Symptoms:

If the length of this list seems to diminish its impact (as there can be many causes), consider that these symptoms are commonly reported by people with electro-sensitivity and are recognized by doctors. Check those that may affect you when exposed to electro-magnetic radiation from wired and wireless devices.

- ☐ Anxiety or depressive disorders
- ☐ Dry, painful or bloodshot eyes
- ☐ Erratic blood pressure
- ☐ Excessive sweating at night
- ☐ Headaches
- ☐ Heart palpitations/irregular heartbeat
- ☐ Inability to focus
- ☐ Light-headedness/dizziness
- ☐ Nausea
- ☐ Pain/discomfort in the heart area
- ☐ Pain in the head, a feeling of pressure
- ☐ Panic attacks
- ☐ Ringing of the ears
- ☐ Sensitivity to noise and/or light
- ☐ Sleep problems
- ☐ Skin rashes
- ☐ Tingling and/or numbness – in the hands and/or feet
- ☐ Vision problems

Do any of these symptoms worsen when you are exposed to wired and/or wireless devices or environments?

☐ No

Yes
- ☐ Mildly
- ☐ Moderately
- ☐ Severely

☐ I don't know

### Section II – Conditions:

If the length of this list seems to diminish its impact (as there can be many causes), consider that there is evidence that these conditions can be related to, and/or exacerbated by, EMR exposure.

Check the items that apply only to your personal health history.

- ☐ Allergies
- ☐ ALS/Motor Neuron Diseases
- ☐ Alzheimer's Disease
- ☐ Autism Spectrum Disorder
- ☐ Brain aneurism
- ☐ Cancer
  - ☐ Eye
  - ☐ Ear
  - ☐ Brain (adult or child)
  - ☐ Breast
  - ☐ Testicular
  - ☐ Other
- ☐ Leukemia (adult or child)
- ☐ Candidiasis
- ☐ Cataracts
- ☐ Cardiovascular disease
  - ☐ arrhythmia
  - ☐ heart attack
  - ☐ hypertension
  - ☐ stroke
  - ☐ tachycardia
  - ☐ TIA (Transient Ischemic Attack)

- ☐ Cold or flu (persistent)
- ☐ Heavy metal toxicity
- ☐ Infertility
- ☐ Insomnia
- ☐ Learning Disorder
  - ☐ ADD
  - ☐ ADHD
- ☐ Lupus
- ☐ Lyme Disease
- ☐ Migraine and/or other severe headaches
- ☐ Multiple Chemical Sensitivities (MCS)
- ☐ Parkinson's Disease
- ☐ Sleep disorder
- ☐ Thyroid gland disorders
- ☐ Tinnitus
- ☐ Vertigo

Do any of these conditions worsen when you are exposed to wired and/or wireless devices?

- ☐ No
- Yes
  - ☐ Mildly
  - ☐ Moderately
  - ☐ Severely
- ☐ I don't know

**Section III – Sources of EMR Exposure – Wireless Devices:** Please check 'Yes' or 'I don't know' in the columns, as appropriate. Leave an item blank to signify 'No'.

| | Yes | I don't know. |
|---|---|---|
| Do you regularly use a cell/mobile phone? | ☐ | |
| **If Yes:** | | |
| Less than 4 minutes daily? | ☐ | |
| More than 30 minutes daily? | ☐ | |
| More than 60 minutes daily? | ☐ | |
| In your car? | ☐ | |
| For 10 years or more? | ☐ | |
| Do you experience Symptoms with use? | ☐ | ☐ |
| **If No:** | | |
| Do you experience any Symptoms around cell/mobile phones? | ☐ | ☐ |
| Do you use a wireless in-your-ear cell phone? | ☐ | |
| Do you use a tablet or other mobile device? | ☐ | |
| **If Yes:** | | |
| Less than 4 minutes daily? | ☐ | |
| More than 30 minutes daily? | ☐ | |
| More than 60 minutes daily? | ☐ | |
| In your car? | ☐ | |
| For 10 years or more? | ☐ | |
| Do you experience Symptoms with use? | ☐ | ☐ |
| **If No:** | | |
| Do you experience Symptoms when you are around mobile devices? | ☐ | ☐ |

| | Yes | I don't know. |
|---|---|---|
| Have you ever checked the SAR (radiation absorption level) of your cell phone/mobile device? | ☐ | |
| **Do you...** | | |
| Have your cell phone and/or other mobile device powered on at night? | ☐ | |
| Use your cell phone and/or other mobile device as an alarm clock? | ☐ | |
| Use a headset or ear piece with your mobile? | ☐ | |
| **If Yes:** Check the type you use | | |
| ☐ Wireless ☐ Wired | | |
| Use a wireless game station, or wireless video box? | ☐ | |
| Use a wireless device with Internet access, or that downloads music, movies or other wireless transmitted data? | ☐ | |
| Use a portable satellite, or wireless broadband, radio? | ☐ | |
| Have a GPS, satellite radio or wireless system in your car? | ☐ | |
| Drive a commercial vehicle with a satellite/GPS locator? | ☐ | |
| Use a personal computer connected to wireless Internet? | ☐ | |
| Have wireless Internet access.... | | |
| a) in your home? | ☐ | |
| b) in your workplace and/or school? | ☐ | ☐ |
| c) in your neighborhood? | ☐ | ☐ |
| d) in your city? | ☐ | ☐ |

| | Yes | I don't know. |
|---|---|---|
| Live or work near a cell tower, or mast? | ☐ | ☐ |
| **If Yes:** | | |
| a) Within 100 metres? (110 yards) | ☐ | ☐ |
| b) Within 200 metres? (220 yards) | ☐ | ☐ |
| Work with or live near,radar devices/systems? | ☐ | ☐ |
| Use an amateur radio, 2-way or CB radio? | ☐ | |
| Have a cordless/portable phone? | ☐ | |
| **If Yes:** | | |
| a) In your home/office/school? | ☐ | |
| b) In your bedroom? | ☐ | |
| c) Your total number of cordless/portable phones and/or baby monitors is: | | |
| 1____ 2 ____ 3____ 4_____ | | |
| Are your cordless/portable phones | | |
| 900 MHz | ☐ | ☐ |
| 2.4 GHz | ☐ | ☐ |
| 5.8 GHz | ☐ | ☐ |
| DECT 6.0 | ☐ | ☐ |
| Have a wireless SmartMeter installed by your utility company at your home/apartment? | ☐ | ☐ |
| Live near a wireless SmartMeter hub and/or SmartGrid network? | ☐ | ☐ |
| Around wireless "hot spots," or devices, do you experience Symptoms from Section I? | ☐ | ☐ |

## Other exposures:

| | Yes | I don't know. |
|---|---|---|
| Are you an airplane pilot or flight attendant? | ☐ | |
| Do you travel often, and go through security X-ray scanners? | ☐ | |
| Are you going through *whole body* X-ray scanners? | ☐ | ☐ |
| Do you work at a supermarket checkout or library near scanners, or go through security X-ray scanners at your workplace? | ☐ | |
| Have you had a CT scan? | ☐ | |
| Have you had an MRI? | ☐ | |
| Have you had medical diagnostic X-rays (chest etc.) | ☐ | |
| Have you had dental X-rays? | ☐ | |
| Have you had a long-term hospital stay – more than one week? | ☐ | |

**Section IV – Sources of EMR Exposure – Electric Devices:** Please check 'Yes' or 'I don't know', as appropriate. Leave an item blank to signify 'No'.

| | Yes | I don't know. |
|---|---|---|
| **Do you...** | | |
| Use an electric blanket, and/or heating pad? | ☐ | |
| Sleep on a/an: | | |
| a) Electric adjustable bed? | ☐ | |
| b) Metal bed frame? | ☐ | |
| c) Coiled mattress/box springs? | ☐ | |
| d) Electrically-heated mattress or water bed? | ☐ | |
| Sleep within 2 metres (2.2 yards) of electric devices: a clock, a radio, compact fluorescent or low voltage halogen lights, or plugged in transformer? | ☐ | |
| Sleep within 6 metres (6.5 yards) of an electrical panel (fuses or circuit breakers)? | ☐ | |
| Stay in a hotel more than 5 nights per month? | ☐ | |
| Regularly use a hair dryer and/or electric shaver? | ☐ | |
| Use a microwave oven? | ☐ | |
| Are you often near the front burners of an electric stove while they are operational? | ☐ | |
| Are you often near electric heaters or "off-peak" or "overnight" electric storage heaters? | ☐ | |
| **Do you...** | | |
| Live/work/school near overhead power lines? | ☐ | ☐ |
| Live in a densely populated urban area? | ☐ | |

| | Yes | I don't know. |
|---|---|---|
| Work/live near electrical transformers? | ☐ | ☐ |
| Work/live near a electricity sub-station? | ☐ | ☐ |
| Live/work near an airport? | ☐ | ☐ |
| **If Yes:** | | |
| a) Within 0-5 km? (0-3 Miles) | ☐ | ☐ |
| b) Within 5-15 km? (3-9 miles) | ☐ | ☐ |
| Work/live in a brightly lit room more than 5 hours daily? | ☐ | |
| Work with power tools? | ☐ | |
| Work with other electrical or high frequency equipment? | ☐ | |
| Does your home/work have dimmer switches on any lights? | ☐ | |
| Do you have low voltage halogen, tube or compact fluorescent lights at work and/or at home and/or at school? | ☐ | |
| Do you live/work in an area with high radon gas? | ☐ | ☐ |
| Do you drive/ride in a hybrid car (gas/electric), or a car with wireless Internet and other high-tech electronics? | ☐ | |
| Do you experience Symptoms from Section I around electric devices? | ☐ | ☐ |

As you know, when artificial electricity was introduced it was a whole new kind of energy that created many obvious advantages and some great gadgets. Obviously, there's harm if you put your finger in a live socket, but generally, we have come to view electronics as benign; this may explain why many people sleep with a cell phone close by their heads without concern. I'm hoping that by now you are viewing our electrified conveniences in a more cautious light.

You may well be thinking, "Okay, I've got it. What can I do about this problem?" So, let's get on with it.

To begin, we need a quick crash course.

## Why do we need to know the EMR basics?

You don't really need to be an expert in the various kinds of radiation to reduce your exposure. However, you want to be sure that you are decreasing, not increasing, your electro-magnetic load. (This is an important reminder for the get-on-with-it types who dive into assembling something without reading the instructions.)

Here's an example of a little knowledge being a less-than-safe thing. I visited a friend who has a few testing meters. I was surprised to see she was standing close to her microwave oven when it was on. I asked gently if she felt this was safe. She said, "It's okay, no problem. I tested it and it's fine at this distance." She was using her Gauss meter, which tests the magnetic field around this plugged in appliance. She didn't, however, test the microwave radiation with the instrument which measures that – the RF meter. Not only did she test the wrong exposure, she missed the most harmful one. More on this in a few pages…

## **The Electro-magnetic Spectrum** – what you need to know.

**An electric field** is the energy surrounding wiring in the walls, or a plugged-in electric device or power cord – even it's when turned off.

**A magnetic field** is the energy surrounding the same wires or appliances when an electrical current is flowing – for example, a lamp is turned on.

**Radio-frequency (RF) radiation** – these wireless waves (fields) are also called microwave radiation. Here the frequency is so high that small packets of energy are released from the antenna – as in mobile devices. With a microwave oven, you can cook with these waves.

**Electro-magnetic radiation (EMR)** – also known as **electro-magnetic fields (EMF)** – is the overall term for most of the spectrum – see the next page. Technically, EMR/EMF includes everything (the highest frequencies are termed ionizing radiation – X-rays etc).

## Energy Consumption In The Digital Age – a personal rant

The power demand of electronics is surging. If you're concerned about energy conservation, and all of us should be, read a 2014 report by the International Energy Agency that says billions of plugged-in devices and Smart Appliances, even when on standby, are a huge energy drain in our energy-challenged world. A July 2014 TIME Magazine cover story offers "The Smarter Home: The dwellings of the future will make you calmer, safer, richer and healthier – and they already exist". There's some good energy-saving ideas but, overall, is 'Smart' healthier?

Where is Rachel Carson when we need her? How about Ralph Nader? Our ever-increasing energy consumption, rampant consumerism and mindless digital addictions could hurry us to a place we don't want to be. Lemmings R us?

## The Three Windows

| A. Lower Frequencies | B. Higher Frequencies | C. Highest Frequencies |
|---|---|---|
| *Electricity* | **Microwaves/Radio-frequency** | |
| | All wireless communication devices except microwave ovens | Nuclear material |
| Power lines | | The Sun |
| Transformers | | Cosmic Rays |
| Electrical wiring | Microwave ovens | Gamma Rays |
| Plug-in appliances | Fluorescent lights | CT Scans |
| Electric blankets | Satellite uplinks | Medical X-rays |
| Electric heaters | Cell tower antennas | Dental X-rays |
| Electric shavers | WiFi, wLAN, Wi-MAX | Airport security scanners |
| Hair dryers | Cell phones, Tablets, Mobile devices | Ultraviolet (fluorescent lights) |
| Power tools | Cordless phones | |
| Office equipment | Wireless: devices/games/speakers/ headsets/earpieces/keyboards/ printers/mouse/small appliances/ TV with Bluetooth | TEST WITH instruments that measure X and gamma rays, like a GEIGER COUNTER or a SCINTILLATION COUNTER. |
| Lamps, light fixtures | RF identification tags | |
| Dimmer switches | Baby monitors | |
| Electric clocks | Security systems | |
| Power cords | Dimmer switches | |
| Extension cords | Police and other radar devices | |
| Power bars | Pagers, Walkie-talkies | |
| Computers | Radio-frequency sealers | |
| TVs - Video Display Terminals | Radio AM/FM, CB radios | |
| Plumbing current | GPS systems | |
| Electric Fields - TEST WITH ELECTRIC FIELD METER | | |
| Magnetic Fields - TEST WITH GAUSS METER | | |

As you see, there are three basic kinds of frequencies.

**A. Lower Frequencies:** (electric and magnetic)

**Electric fields** are emitted by:

- Household electrical wiring in ceilings, walls and floors; wiring that powers lights and appliances
- Everyday power cords, extension cords, and power bars when plugged into an outlet, even if the appliance is not turned on
- Electric blankets, waterbeds, TVs, computers and all other electronic devices
- All electrical appliances, lamps and lighting
- High voltage power lines

**Electric fields** are tested by:

- An electric field meter

**Magnetic fields** are emitted by:

- High voltage power lines
- Electrical wiring errors and current on the electrical grounding system, water and gas pipes
- Electric meter and fuse box, dimmer switches, all power transformers/AC adapters
- Fluorescent and low voltage halogen lighting, alarm clocks
- Heating elements in stoves and ovens when heating
- All appliances (refrigerator, washing machine, furnace, hair dryers, exhaust fans etc…)
- All CRT (cathode ray tube) VDT (video display terminal) televisions and computer monitors (in some cases, LCD displays are a better choice but some still emit hazardous levels of EMR.)
- Automobile engines

**Magnetic fields** are tested by:

- A magnetic field, or Gauss, meter.

**B. Higher Frequencies:** (the middle window, including wireless)
**Microwaves/Radio-frequency fields** are emitted by:

- Baby monitors, wireless security systems, wireless game pads, and microwave ovens
- Cellular tower base stations, cellular phones, hand-held mobile devices, all cordless phones, wireless technology

- Wireless computer networks and Internet access routers
- All other wireless communication devices
- Some other sources include: fluorescent lights, PUC (under counter lights), some remote control toys, laptops in wireless mode, and some hydro, gas and water meters

**Higher Frequencies** are tested by:

- An RF meter.

## C. The Highest Frequencies:

The third kind of energy shown on the chart is a powerful force, which can create significant cell damage if there's enough power, proximity and duration. This is why it is now recommended to limit X-ray exposure to medically-urgent situations. Other sources include: radioactive mineral deposits, radon gas, nuclear facilities and fallout, depleted uranium such as some troops deploy in combat, and household smoke detectors that contain americium dioxide.

We are all exposed to cosmic radiation to some degree; it's most significant at high altitudes, or in airplanes. At 36,000 feet the levels can be hundreds of times higher than on the ground.

**The Highest Frequencies** are tested by:

- Instruments that measure X and gamma rays, instruments such as a Geiger counter or a scintillation counter.

Whether or not these or any other exposures are harmful depends on some significant variables. With each exposure you want to consider these factors.

**Six Key Factors:**

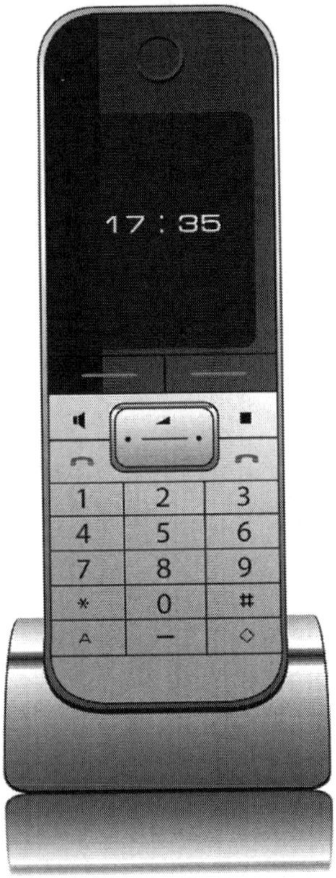


**Evidence of harm** – as we have discussed, even electro-magnetic levels far below existing 'safe' standards, not high enough to heat human tissue, cause adverse biological effects.

The evidence? See the first section of this book, or some of the Resources' websites. The Resources are at the end of the book.

**Intensity** – the power of the specific source: the type and power of your cordless phone – analog or digital – 900 MHz to DECT 6.0; and the range of the cell towers, broadcast antennas, power lines, wireless networks etc.

**Proximity** – how close you are to the source. Is the cell phone against your ear; the wireless laptop on your lap; the cordless phone base nearby; the cell tower, transformer, electric sub-station, or power lines near your house/school/workplace? Your neighbors' wireless network is exposing your family, but is less harmful than having one in your own home – due to proximity.

**Duration/frequency** – if you have a high-powered electric heater (intensity) on for 10 minutes to take the chill off the room, no big deal. If you sleep beside it, or have it on for hours every day (proximity, duration and frequency) that's more of a concern.

**Vulnerability** – fetuses, infants, children and teens, all with thinner skulls, still-growing brains and more aqueous brain tissue, are at greatest risk. Older people, cancer survivors, and individuals with compromised immune systems, learning disorders and other medical and neurological conditions, are also more vulnerable.

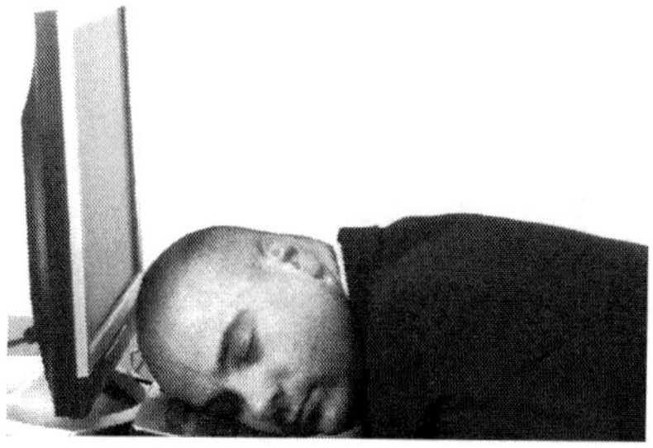

**Combination of factors** – the more of these factors that are present, the greater the danger, as you would presume. A baby sleeping near a wireless monitor, an electric outlet, and a cordless phone, in a home with a wireless security system and wireless Internet is surrounded by multiple, accumulating exposures.

Before I knew about all this, I gave my 85 year-old mother a heating pad to improve her circulation. She began sleeping with it held against her tummy. Shortly afterwards she began to experience uterine bleeding and was taken to hospital to be checked out.

Fortunately, this was about the time I found out about EMR, and that it could cause internal bleeding. My mother's doctor dismissed quickly this information, but we removed the heating pad anyway, and the bleeding stopped within 24 hours. (As with our daughter's metal canopy bed frame, I couldn't bring myself to give the heating pad to anyone else.) All factors were present: the EMR intensity of the heating pad, the proximity of having it next to her body, the duration and frequency of using it all night every night, and her vulnerability from age and health conditions.

Another example: a fragile premature infant in an incubator, hooked up to all kinds of life-saving electrodes and monitoring equipment. Adding to the infant's exposure is the hospital's electro-magnetic load – fluorescent lighting, wireless systems etc. The hospital may even have a large cell antenna on its roof.

Before we go to Strategy 3 – Safer Solutions, here's our library mum:

> Made a few changes since reading Strategy 2 last night. Thought about how I also use my new multi-task cell phone to listen to music, and for a bedside alarm. Turned it off for the night, as well as both computers which were humming away. Put 'get battery alarm clock' on my to do list. Am contemplating getting rid of this all-in-one phone and scaling back to the simpler cell phone.
>
> And I am feeling like we need to get outside more. Unplug.

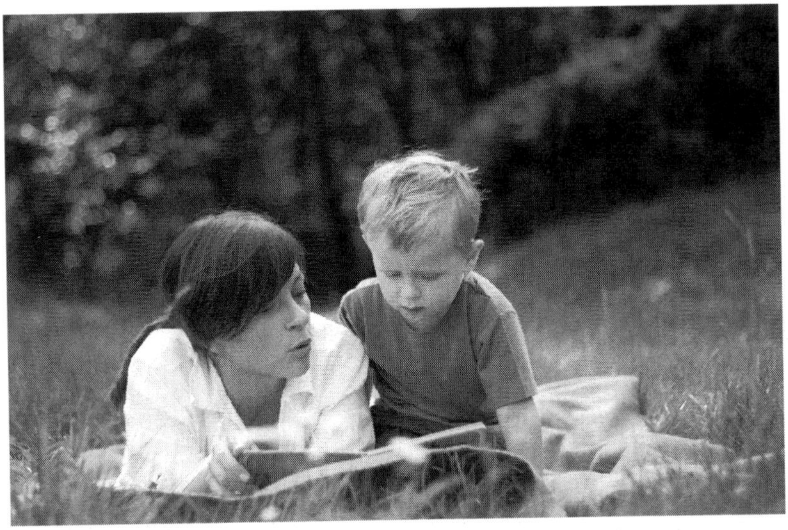

*2 Minute Quick Read Summary*

## Strategy 3 Safer Solutions

TO REDUCE THE RISKS of electro-pollution is our goal. In Strategy 3 you learn about the emitting devices/exposures and what to do about them. They are grouped into wireless and wired.

**Includes the safer use of:**

- cell phones
- tablets, mobile devices
- headsets, earpieces
- cordless phones
- Internet access
- laptops
- computer screens
- baby monitors
- video gaming
- microwave ovens
- fluorescent lights
- diagnostic X-rays
- plasma TVs
- electric/hybrid cars

You might know a lot about cell phones but the health benefits of replacing your cordless phones with corded landlines may surprise you. May I suggest you try it and see if your sleep improves.

Look here for our definitive guide to wired earpieces and headsets. Wireless ones are *not* the safest, our technical team tells us.

Learn about Smart Meters and wireless radiation in schools, and how to make sure our children are healthy. Read about WiFi in transportation and why we don't want pilots exposed to any more radiation, even if it's convenient for us to be online while flying.

You don't need to tackle all devices/exposures at once. Every reduction lowers long-term risk, and there are short-term benefits.

**See Strategy 3 for more details.**

## Strategy 3. Safer Solutions

**Here's all the information you need to know about the EMR-emitting devices in your home, office, school ...**

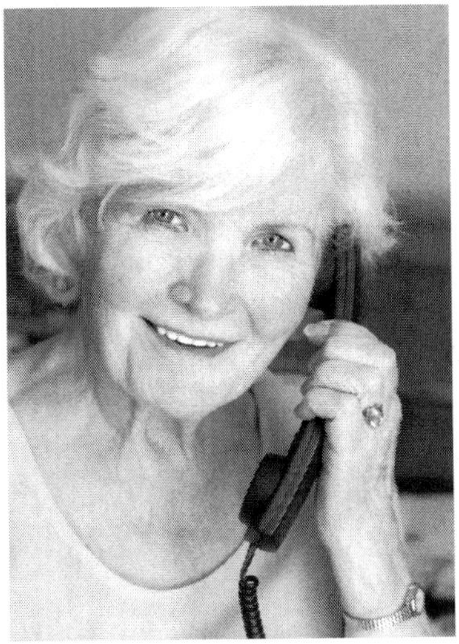

In this section we look at the specific devices – cell phones, earpieces, headsets, cordless phones, baby monitors, Internet access etc. – and hear from some world leading technical experts including: Alasdair Philips, Rob Metzinger, Larry Gust, Stan Hartman and Katharina Gustavs. This is what we, the consumers, need to know.

This is probably more than you *want* to know about many of your favorite things. I'm hoping that you won't go from techno-crazed to techno-phobic – there is a healthy balance in the middle way. The technical truth about these devices has been an eight-year discovery for me; I have had time to go through my stages of denial, anger, action and adjustment.

I don't want you to feel so swamped with these details that you abandon this rescue project altogether. If you find yourself feeling exasperated – "Oh no, not my hair dryer" – please take a break and come back to this another day.

Over time, if you can just tackle a few of the 'biggies' – such as the cordless phone – you have done a lot to safeguard your family.

## How can you decide whether devices are safe or not?

Let's use the analogy of sun tanning. You know that while we need some exposure to the sun (evidence of benefit), too much can be hazardous (evidence of harm). It follows that caution is advised when being outside in the mid-day sun (intensity), or using sun lamps or tanning beds (intensity and proximity).

According to our experts, if you are using a powerful device (intensity), on a regular basis (duration), wearing it on your body, sleeping near it, or holding it in your lap – or against your head (proximity), you are at risk. You can see why there's so much concern about cordless and mobile phones.

## Mobile Alert: Even Higher-Powered Tech Toys on the Electronic Horizon

An eye of awareness can wake us up when we see advertisements touting the latest high-tech toys: a compact wireless "netbook," a formidable DECT 6.0 cordless phone station to control all the functions in your home, a pink pendant cell phone that nestles in your cleavage, a wireless exercise pad for "WiFi fitness," and mobile online banking services – all from your cell phone.

Here's one to jolt your alert button: we are promised a 4G multi-function mobile that will "be like your very own butler in the palm of your hand. It'll do everything but tuck you in at night."

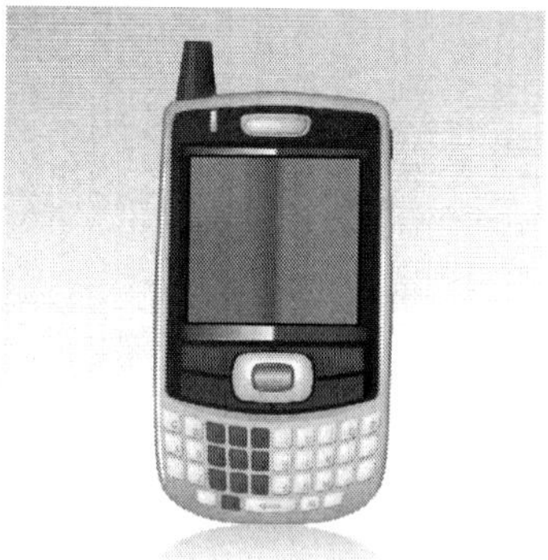

Get your radiation-testing meter ready.

## The Key Question: Does it work without wires?

Many people are concerned about living near power lines, or electric sub-stations. This risk is validated by extensive research. However, we are just learning of the risk of the radiation from cell towers.

Somehow these massive structures do seem menacing (of course, that's why they are often concealed in metal church crosses, or disguised as palm trees). Yet, the digital cordless phone sitting on your kitchen counter looks so benign. The new digital baby monitor seems to be essential for safety-minded parents. And in this digital age it seems an educational advantage to start our children young in becoming at home with computers – usually with wireless connection to the Internet.

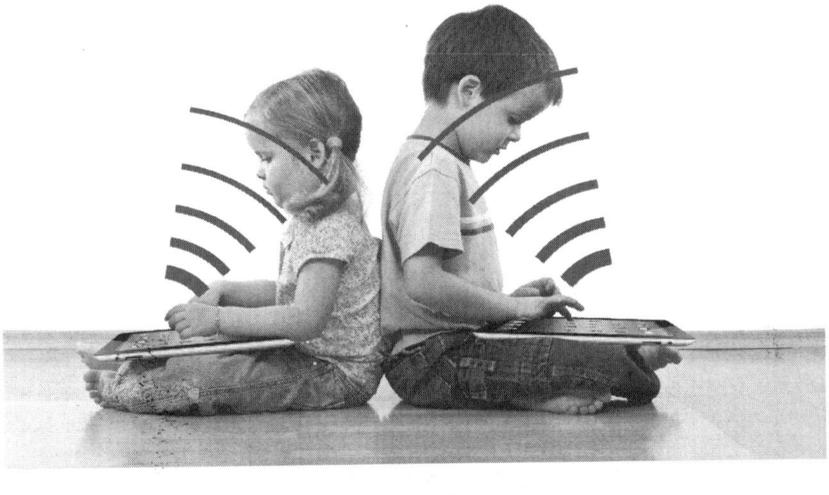

For something to communicate without wires, it uses some form of radiation to send and/or receive data through the air. Most of these waves travel easily through cement walls. This means they are also going through the skull, and the rest of the body.

## The Key to the Safer Solutions

Stan Hartman, an environmental health consultant, offers us key advice:

> The most important thing for people to keep in mind when trying to reduce electro-smog is, first of all, to replace all wireless technology (except infrared remote controls for TVs and other things) with wired alternatives.
>
> Get rid of all bluetooth devices, and replace other wireless gear like cordless speakers, headphones, keyboards, mice, etc.

If the data transmission is going through a hard-wired cable, a plugged-in phone line, or a fiber optics system, then it does not present that kind of exposure. These differences form the basis of the safer solutions.

When you have this awareness these decisions seem to arise instinctively. And wiser choices become obvious. You can decide, for example, how to set up your online banking.

If you're using a device that has a thin LCD screen (vs. the larger cathode ray terminal) and hard-wired Internet access (instead of wireless), you can enjoy that convenience with much less risk than using your cell phone or other mobile devices.

## The Sources and Recommendations

In this section we'll look at exposures from various sources, explain the experts' concerns about them, and suggest safer solutions.

It is important to know the difference between making something safer, and making it safe. For example, when you add a filter to a plain cigarette does it make it safe? If it is a low tar cigarette does it make it safe? If you only breathe in second hand smoke, does it make it safe?

As you read through this section, you will get an idea of the exposures you want to reduce. At the end of this strategy there is a preliminary Action Plan to help you prioritize; you'll find a more detailed version at the end of Strategy 4.

We are going to start with the devices from the higher frequencies – the middle of the EMR Spectrum.

### Microwave Ovens

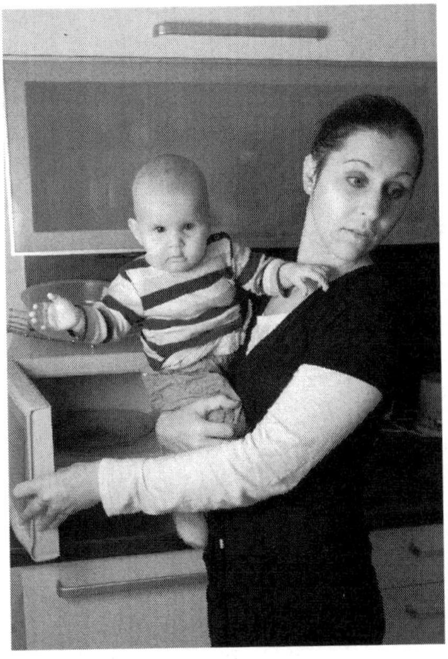

**The Concern:** Larry Gust, an electrical engineer, tells us why that handy appliance is not as harmless as it looks.

(LG) "All microwave ovens leak RF radiation (radio-frequency, microwaves) when they are in use. This radiation covers a surprisingly wide area – as much as 3 to 30 feet, and in older models up to 60 feet. Most people think that microwave ovens do not have any negative health consequences.

After all, if they did the government would not allow this product on the market. Think again.

The Soviet Union conducted extensive microwave research after finding German microwave ovens and research data at the end of WWII. Unhampered by capitalistic trade associations, Russian research has been more extensive than that in the US. This article summarizes early Russian and other more recent research.

Microwave ovens use electromagnetic energy that vibrates 2.4 billion times per second. This energy acts on the molecules in food, particularly water molecules, causing them to vibrate rapidly. This rapid movement generates friction and thus heat. Vibration is so violent that molecules are often torn apart or distorted, thereby changing the chemical makeup of the food. Additionally, this appliance leaks microwaves into the environment around it.

Studies of the thousands of Russian workers exposed to radar microwaves in the 1950's showed health effects so severe that the Russian microwave oven leakage limit was set at 1,000 times less than the US government leakage limit.

In 1976, microwave ovens were banned in the Soviet Union after researchers discovered that these devices caused a breakdown in the human (and animal) energy field. They also found degeneration of cell membranes and electrical nerve impulses in the brain, disruption of hormone production, and disturbance in various brain waves, leading to memory and concentration loss, slowing of intellectual process and interrupted sleep. Microwave ovens were allowed after 1987 when, under Perestroika, business interests pressured Gorbachev into changing the regulations that did not fit in with free-trade practices in the West."

Microwaving baby milk is not recommended. In the December 9, 1989 issue of the British medical journal, *The Lancet*, Dr. Lita Lee reported that heating formula in a microwave oven converted some of the amino acids in it into synthetic forms that are not biologically active. One was converted to a toxic form.

Dr. Lee is concerned:

> It's bad enough that many babies are not nursed, but now they are given fake milk (baby formula) made even more toxic via microwaving.

## Microwave Ovens – Safer Solutions:

Rob Metzinger (RM): "Replace microwave ovens with safer appliances and methods."

- If you absolutely must have a microwave oven get a smaller, lowered powered one and stand at least 15 feet away – even farther, to be on the safe side – when it is in use.

- Avoid heating baby formula in a microwave, and keep infants and children far away when it is on.

- Better alternatives: keep a small pot or pan with a lid for quick heating/reheating of food and liquids. Avoid non-stick coated pans. (As soon as they are the least bit scratched, you can ingest the toxic little flakes.) At work, heating your lunchtime leftovers in a toaster oven, or on a hot plate with the small pan and lid, takes a couple of minutes longer, but is a safer solution, the experts advise us.

- If you need something defrosted, take it out of the freezer a night or two beforehand and defrost in the fridge.

## Cordless Phones

**The Concern: You may have known about the hazards of microwave ovens, and been wary of cell phones, but did you know about the health hazards of cordless phones?** These conveniences emit high levels of radiation, particularly the newer ones, even when not in use.

Did you know that multiple cordless phone sets that come with a base station, and a charger for each handset, emit two kinds of radiation? The charger sends out harmful magnetic fields within 1 to 3 ft. (The emission of magnetic fields applies to all phones, cordless or not, that come with a cube-style adapter.)

The main base station of a cordless phone, however, is the more dangerous, as the antenna radiates microwaves continually for hundreds of feet/meters. Microwave radiation is also coming from the handset antenna. This is why all the experts urge us not to allow young children near cordless phones. Replacing them should be a key factor in your Action Plan.

From a January 2006 report by the German Federal Agency For Radiation Protection, *The Radiation Source at Home – cordless phones radiate unnecessarily:*

> A cordless phone (of DECT standard – 5.8 GHz or DECT 6.0) is often the strongest source of high frequency electromagnetic radiation in a private home. To renounce your cordless phone as a precautionary measure will contribute to minimizing your family's radiation exposure.

## DIGITAL CORDLESS PHONES – ALWAYS RADIATING

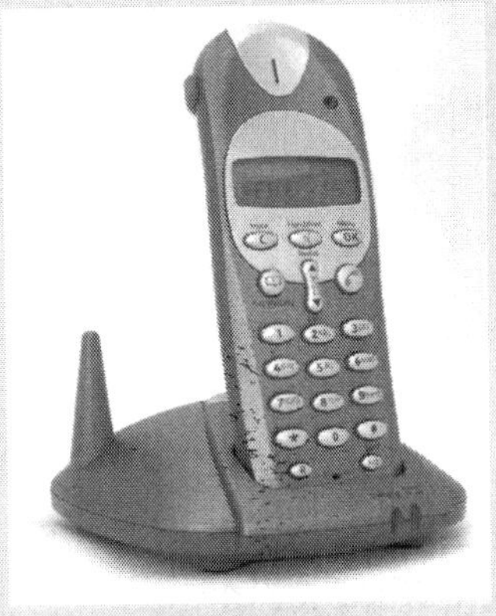

Beginning in 2008, phones of the DECT 6.0 generation started flooding the US market. DECT is the abbreviation for Digital Enhanced Cordless Telecommunication technology. In the last decade, only Europeans used this technology and were confronted with its headaches.

The 2.4 GHz band has been used by the majority of cordless phones in the last five years. However, this band has become crowded with devices such as microwave ovens, wireless area networks (WLAN), Bluetooth, cordless phones and remote control devices. This has led to interference and performance issues so the manufacturers moved to the 5.8 GHz frequency band and then to DECT 6.0 technology.

The problem with the DECT phones is that the base station is permanently sending (radiating) 24 hours a day, no matter if the system is in use or not. Indoor environmental consultants have rallied against their use for decades. There were so many outcries that it had an impact. Major European manufacturers now offer environmentally safer versions, with sleep mode or reduced output in standby mode.

**Case Study**

Clients are concerned about the installation of a new cellular base station to be erected on the roof of a recreation center across the street from their house and asked to have their home assessed prior to the installation.

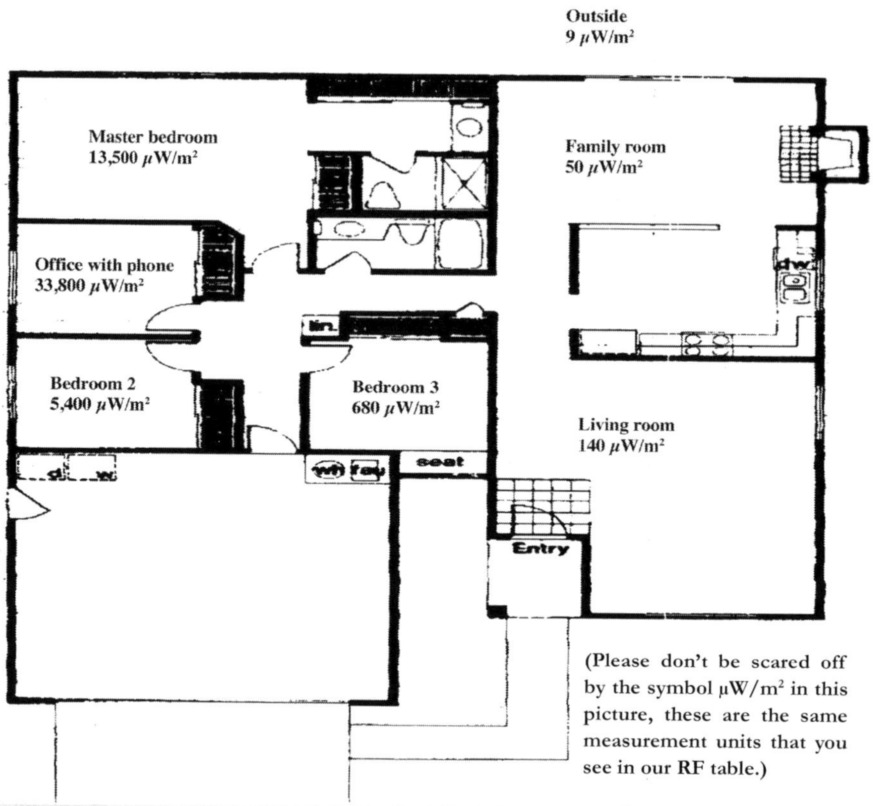


(Please don't be scared off by the symbol μW/m² in this picture, these are the same measurement units that you see in our RF table.)

## RF Exposure from One 2.4 GHz Cordless Phone in a House (these levels are *only* from the cordless phone)

When Peter Sierck sent me this paper on cordless phones, with the RF levels you see in this graphic, I couldn't quite believe that these readings were coming from *one* cordless phone.

He assured me that, "yes, these RF levels are from one 2.4 GHz cordless phone in the house, no wireless, cordless or other RF sources."

Can you just imagine the levels with a few 5.8 or DECT 6.0 phones in a similar house equipped with wireless Internet?

Another widely respected technical expert, Alasdair Philips, the director of Powerwatch in the UK, cautions:

> It's likely everyone in a house with a (DECT) digital cordless phone will be constantly exposed to levels of microwave radiation far higher than safe levels.

Dr. Hans Scheiner, the physician in Munich, also warned us about digital phones (virtually all new/recent cordless phones):

> Digital signals are more aggressive than analog. Both are harmful. However, digital signals are more aggressive, and more harmful, because they pulse and have peaks. This is a problem as the body's cells react negatively to the sharp peaks.

I know; all these health hazard alerts about cordless phones were a shock to me too. I invite you to consider this as good news and bypass the stage of remorse at having placed these phones throughout the house, and choose instead to hear this message.

Ready for another story? A good news one? I have a dear friend who moved into a small duplex near the waterfront, several years ago. She was thrilled to have found this 'fixer-upper' with a wide porch where she could sit and watch the waves; until she discovered that those were not the only waves hitting her haven by the sea. Since moving in, for no known reason, she was not sleeping well and her Chronic Fatigue symptoms were worsening daily.

Right across from her, not too far from shore, was a small island sprouting several broadcast antennas. This was around the time of the dawning of my wireless awareness so I shared with her what I was learning. She is a doctor with a keen and curious mind so she delved head first into the data. And soon took action.

My friend hired an EMR assessment consultant to do some testing. He identified what we had both suspected – radio-frequency radiation from the antennas across the water, and the wireless network in her home. She replaced her wireless with an Ethernet cable, and that seemed to help, but not enough. The consultant had also discovered another source that surprised us, but not him.

The person living in the other half of their duplex had a digital cordless phone that was blitzing the whole building, and way past the surrounding garden. (This may seem more credible to you after just seeing Peter Sierck's diagram of the house plan.)

Fortunately, the elderly woman who lived there was open to hearing about this, although she couldn't quite believe it, "My dear, I have had a cordless phone for years. I keep it beside my chair, and my bed, as I am slow getting up."

After she replaced it with a landline – with a sufficiently long cord – she and my friend both reported sleeping much better, and a reduction in several previously unexplained symptoms.

What similar benefits might there be for you and your family? Read on ...

## Cordless Phone Models:

There is a huge difference in radiation exposure from lowest to highest power. **Note: One gigahertz (GHz) is equal to 1,000 megahertz (MHz).**

The 900 MHz analog cordless phone (if you can find one) emits much less radiation than the newest DECT 6.0 model. Evidently, you can walk three blocks with this new mega-powered unit.

This list goes from the least to the most harmful according to our technical experts:

**900 MHz analog** – cordless phone is hard to find but a good option. The picture on the right shows this older model.

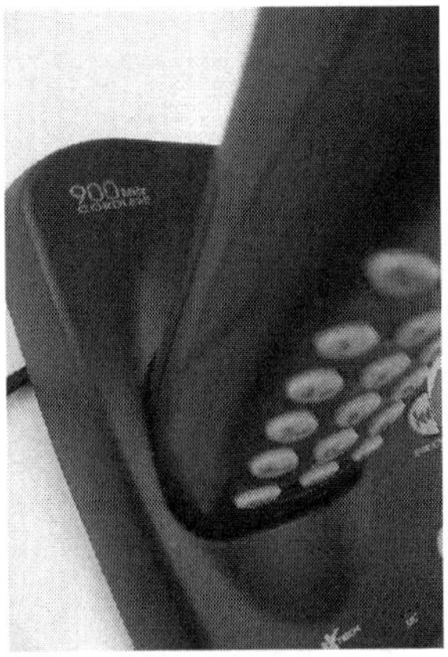

*900 MHz analog: Emits RF only during use*

Unlike digital cordless phones, the base of this one does not radiate all the time, only when you are on a call. I look for these at second hand stores. A wise health strategy.

**900 MHz digital** – avoid the DSS (digital spread spectrum). Better than the more powerful models below.

**2.4 GHz analog** – higher levels than the 900 MHz, but the analog signal is less of a concern than the following digital ones

**DECT: 2.4 GHz, 5.8 GHz, and 6.0 DECT (1.9 GHz)** – all use the same pulsing digital technology and the base station emits RF all the time. Radiation levels vary depending on model and manufacturer.

**The 6.0** models (the worst) emit extremely high levels – similar to the exposure from cell phones.

The environmental consultant, Katharina Gustavs, advises us that, "some of the DECT cordless phones operate at a higher frequency, which is not detected by all RF meters. In this case, the meter may show nothing, or give a false low level."

**Children and Cordless Phones:**

Many researchers warn us that children are more vulnerable to the effects of radiation. The child's small size will encourage whole-body exposure, and rapidly dividing cells that are part of the child's growth processes are highly vulnerable to radiation damage.

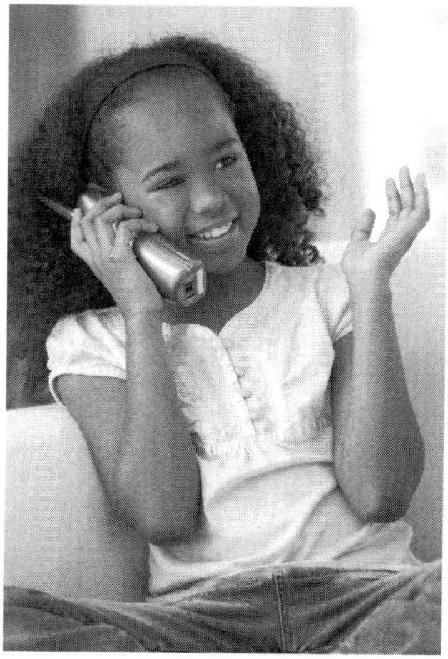

**Do not let a child use a cordless phone**; never put the base near children's sleeping or playing area, and don't use one near them.

Accepting the experts' advice that cordless phones are harmful is most challenging, do you agree? We lived with them for ages. But not with this digital signal and powerful intensity.

Remember, constantly amped-up electronics are not being tested for biological effects. And, there are slews of hyper-smart techies firing on all cylinders to flood the market with wireless gadgets. Unsupervised. Try testing the EMR levels in an electronics store.

**Cordless Phones – Safer Solutions:**

(RM) "Replace all DECT/digital cordless phones with landline telephones."

Every one of our technical experts, as well as the other contributors, advise replacing cordless phones. This might seem daunting? Tiresome? But as you learn more it will seem like an essential step and worth the hassle of stepping over a phone cord now and then.

**Safer-Tech – The Essentials**
**Corded Landline Phone – A Must-Have for a Healthy Home**

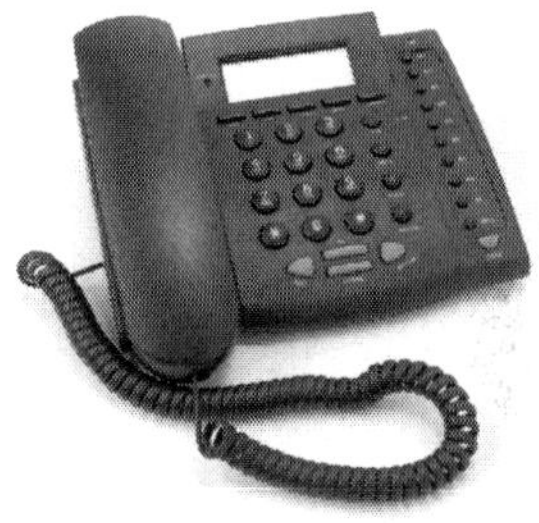

- No microwave radiation
- Replacing cordless phones (and/or mobile phones) with corded landlines may be the best step you can take to reduce your family's health risks
- Battery-operated ones are even better than those with an electrical cord and they keep working in power outages

Every expert I spoke with agrees on this. And if you test cordless phones for microwave emissions (yes, the same kind of radiation) you will understand, and dust off your old corded landline phone, or go out and buy one. You can get them with call display, call waiting etc.

If you want call display, you need a power source; best option is the battery-operated model, as I just advised; you don't need to plug it into the wall. You can also get good ones with speakerphone function, and long handset cords so you can still multi-task.

An extended coiled cord on the handset enables you to wander even farther while talking on the corded phone. No, it's not as handy as a cordless phone, but there's no comparison in terms of radiation risk.

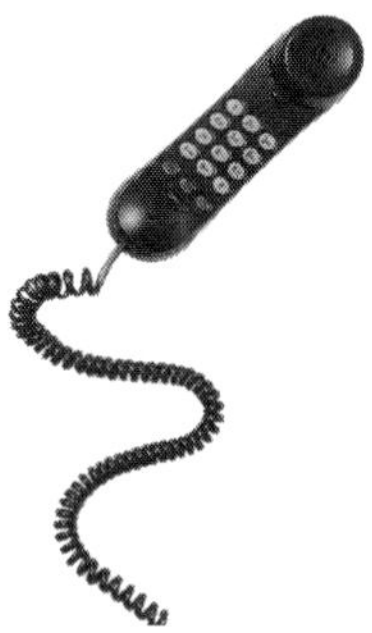

If having a cordless phone is non-negotiable for you at this time, consider choosing a 900 MHz analog model – if you can still find one.

The advantage is that it doesn't radiate 24/7. It does radiate when you are on a call, so it's recommended to keep those discussions brief, "I'll call you back on the corded landline."

I went to see if you can still buy the lower-tech 900 MHz and the salesperson looked at me as though I had asked for two soup cans and a string. Standing beside a stack of bright blue and black boxes of the hottest DECT 6.0 with a base station and three handsets, she declared, "Oh, I don't think they make those anymore; no one wants them. People want the latest, the most high-powered." If they only knew.

## Replacing My High-tech Cordless Phone

Here's a story about a woman who heard our wireless wake-up call: "I attended an eye-opening talk by Dr Crofton and her colleagues Dr Martin Blank and Dr Stephen Sinatra. I was shocked at the evidence of harm to our health from everyday Smart appliances and wireless conveniences. Had no idea. My son who is in the computer business got me this new fancy cordless phone and a super-strength wireless router. I had not made the connection but this was when my sleeping and immune system problems got much worse. After their talk I went home and unplugged these gadgets and slept better than I had for ages. Three months later my sleep is still good and my health continues to improve. I don't miss those 'conveniences' and now have safer ones."

## Cell Phones, Mobile Devices

### The Benefit:

In emergencies mobile phones can be life-savers, literally, and are unlikely to be harmful if use is very brief, limited to urgent calls, and the phone is kept powered off at all other times.

### The Concern:

### Near Field and Far Field – another bit of crucial information

Cell phones/mobile devices emit a plume-like beam of radiation from their antennas, which may be sticking out or embedded in the device. The near field radiates from the antenna for about 1-foot distance; the most intense plume is in all directions within 7 inches of the antenna.

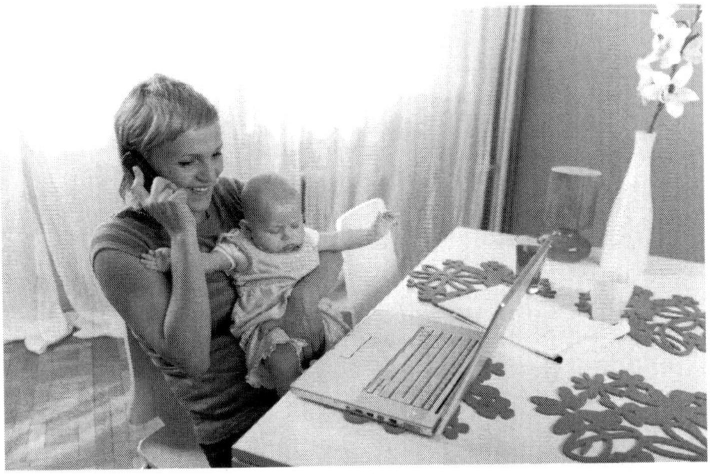

This powerful blast of near field radiation goes into your ear canal and directly to your brain. It harms your eyes, and nearby people and pets.

Un-knowingly and un-necessarily at risk. We can change this.

The far field, also radiation that causes concern, goes through everything in its path.

The reason you hear that a headset is recommended is that it removes the near field exposure from the area closest to your head and brain. While in a relative sense, it's safer to keep the antenna's near field as far from your brain as possible, as Rob Metzinger explains, the conventional wired and wireless headsets can work against us by increasing the exposure to other sensitive tissues. (There's more about headsets and earpieces later.)

Whether or not you're using a headset, when your mobile is clipped to your belt, or carried in your pocket or shoulder bag, you are radiating breasts (remember the pink pendant cell phone?) testicles and other sensitive body parts including organs like liver, kidney and ovaries. There are also concerns about the effect on the blood-producing bone marrow in your hip.

The intensity of radiation lessens with distance, but even the far field is not considered safe, as the information-carrying radio waves are still pulsing through your body for quite a distance.

The more powerful the device, the more intense the near and far field exposures, as you would imagine. Before you grab the latest multi-function mobile, consider testing it with a RF meter. Make sure the phone is transmitting when you test it.

(KG) "The concern with cell phones is not only the very high levels of RF radiation but they also generate very high pulsing magnetic fields, even in standby."

## Pregnant Women, Children – Cell Phones and WiFi

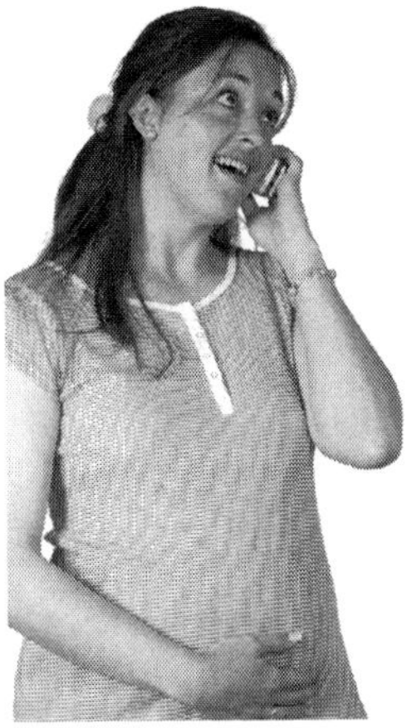

### The Concern:

Ronald Herberman, MD was the first director of the University of Pittsburgh Cancer Institute:

> The developing fetus or child are the most likely to be sensitive to any possible effects of exposure to electromagnetic fields. Do not allow children of any age to use a cell phone, except for emergencies.

*(See also pages 39, 41, and 275, and the Index references for Dr. Klinghardt.)*

Dr. Carrie Hyman reported:

> Children's developing brains, immune and endocrine systems between conception and their mid-twenties, particularly the brain and nervous system, are more vulnerable than ours to many toxins, including EMFs.

**BabySafe Project:** In June 2014, a Joint Statement on Pregnancy and Wireless Radiation was issued by Grassroots Environmental Education and Environmental Health Trust (EHT). It was signed by 44 physicians and scientists from thirteen nations and by 13 educators who have studied wireless radiation health effects. These experts urge pregnant women to limit their exposure to protect themselves and their unborn children. Any of your loved ones pregnant?

EHT Founder, Dr. Davis stated, "As a public health expert, I am deeply concerned about the experiment we are conducting on our pregnant women and young children today". Adverse effects of wireless radiation include interference with normal fetal brain development, which can lead to impaired communication skills, learning deficits, and behavioral problems. Alert your loved ones, without alarming them.

June 2014, MedPage Today: Obstetrician, Jacques Moritz, MD, director of gynecology, Mount Sinai Saint Luke's in New York City, reported advising his pregnant patients "to avoid keeping their cell phones around the fetus; that's just common sense. Also, I do advise them to go for the patdown with the Transportation Security Administration (TSA) at the airport." Does your OB-GYN know this? Tell him/her.

Assistant Professor Jennifer Hoskovec, MS, of the University of Texas, "The concern regarding risk associated with wireless radiation is becoming more frequent. A few recent studies have suggested a possible association between wireless radiation exposure during pregnancy and neurodevelopmental and behavioral differences. Although these studies have aimed at quantifying this specific risk, there is still much to learn about it." This is why Dr. Davis warns that global WiFi exposure is "an experiment on pregnant women and young children".

Alasdair Philips (AP): "Microwaves from mobile devices penetrate the head, and the younger you are, the further into the brain they go. Keep children away from anyone using a mobile and don't have one on standby anywhere near a child – on the stroller, etc. **Children should not hold any wireless device on their laps**, particularly when it is online accessing the Internet, sending or receiving, text messaging etc."

Outraged yet? You can't smoke or eat peanuts near schools but most schools are WiFi'd. Safer options are available. Why are most children using mobiles and most homes filled with microwaves? Why haven't teachers and parents been warned about this radiation?

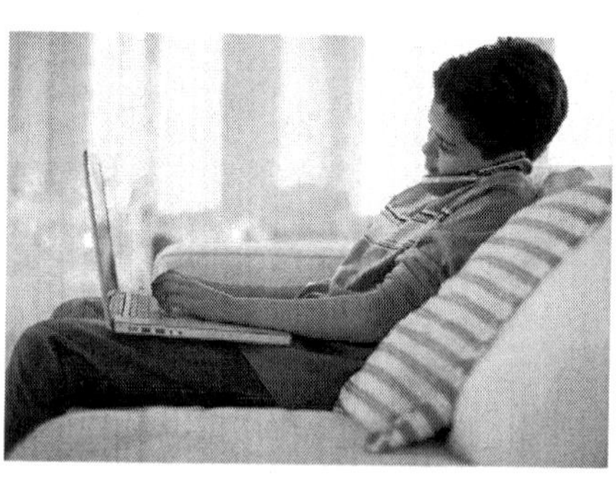

Use safer wired connections and don't use mobile phones for your home service: may save money but at what cost to your health? Best choice: a corded landline.

## Safe in Standby?

Have you noticed that when people in an audience are asked to turn off their cell phones, most put them on mute/vibrate? This prevents annoying rings, but not the harmful exposure.

When your phone is on standby, it communicates every three to five minutes, at full power, with the nearest base station to ensure it has the best signal. If you are in a poor reception area, the phone may transmit as often as every 30 seconds as it tries to get a better signal. If you are on the move, it will transmit even more frequently.

### The various modes of your mobile phone

This list sets out the various settings of a cell phone/mobile device, in order of exposure from lowest to highest.

### Not emitting radiation:

- battery out – YES, there is still a tiny bit of energy coming from a mobile that is powered off. Perhaps not a concern unless you are electro-sensitive. The only way to reduce the radiation to zero is to remove the phone's battery.

### Emitting radiation:

- powered off – be in this safe mode as much as you can
- charging
- on standby – you can receive calls
- sending receiving text – less harmful if only powered on for a moment to send or receive messages
- sending and receiving voice, online Internet, downloading movies

## Cell Phones – Safer-tech Solutions

Obviously, the safest is not to use a cell phone, and try to avoid others using them. Not very possible these days. When landline phone communication is not possible, the following suggestions will reduce your exposure. Consider these key factors: age (younger skulls are thinner), location (RF power when in cars/buildings/elevators/planes, and for distance from the connecting network), the number of bars on the mobile's screen (how much the battery is charged), frequency of use, how you use it (against your head, or speaker?), its features (does it have a good speaker?), and the radiation emission level (SAR).

## Specific Absorption Rate (SAR)

SAR describes the rate at which living tissue absorbs radiation, often used as a risk level indicator for the radiation-emitting device.

**As you can imagine, the more 'bells and whistles', the more power, the potential for more harm, we are told.** Choose the most basic phone, with a speaker, that you can find. As well as taking other precautions, it may be better to choose a device with the lowest SAR. These SAR ratings, however, may not be reliable. Powerwatch is a leader in this field; the organization's opinion is that SAR ratings are only minimally useful as they are based only on thermal effects. As you may remember, from Know the Evidence, the radiation from cell phones produces harmful biological effects far below thermal levels and existing government standards. For these reasons, relying on a low SAR cell phone could give you a false sense of safety.

(LG) "The way the SAR standard is being subverted to allow more power output has been explained to me that the dimensions of the tissue measured for this test have been altered to have 1/10th the surface area. Therefore the power per unit area is reduced allowing 10 times the power for the same SAR value."

However, it's still advisable to use a lower SAR cell phone (dealing with relative risk). As the word gets out about the evidence, we can expect to see manufacturers' revised ad campaigns: "this low SAR mobile phone ..." Our tips begin with choosing a mobile with a low SAR *combined with* other recommendations found here.

If you want to know the SAR of your mobile, CNET.com has comprised a list of the 2014 lowest and highest emitters based on their radiation absorption levels.

Sorry, your iPhone (1.38) and Blackberry (1.42) are near the top. Motorola's Droid Maxx leads the pack with 1.54, getting perilously close to the US limit of 1.6. The lowest on their list start at 0.18. With the advent of dazzingly-apped smartphones we entered into a new realm of increased use and increased radiation levels. Better to go back to a low SAR flip phone. Still not safe, but a lot less hazardous, and still want to keep away it from your head; use the speaker instead

## Frequency of use

(RM) "**Use cell phones as little as possible. Biological effects occur after 30 seconds**. Only use your cell phone to establish contact, or for conversations lasting a few minutes, as the biological effects are directly related to the duration of exposure.

Your phone communicates at full power when it is connecting to a number, so hold it away from your body when you have finished dialing, until the person answers. This limits the power of the electromagnetic field emitted near your ear and the duration of your exposure. For longer conversations, use a land line with a corded phone, not a cordless phone.

When you are not using your cell phone, turn it completely off (powered off, not on standby) to avoid exposure that is the result of your cell phone transmitting its location through constant signaling.

If you must have your cell phone on, carry it in a purse, backpack or briefcase. Never carry a cell phone that is turned on in any pocket, as the radiation from the phone will couple with your body's natural electro-magnetic field and trigger whole-body adverse biological cascades. There are also effective shielding carrying cases for mobiles.

If you must carry your phone on you, make sure to position the keypad facing your body so the back (where antennas are visible or embedded) is toward the outside, so that more of the transmitted electromagnetic fields move away from you rather than through you.

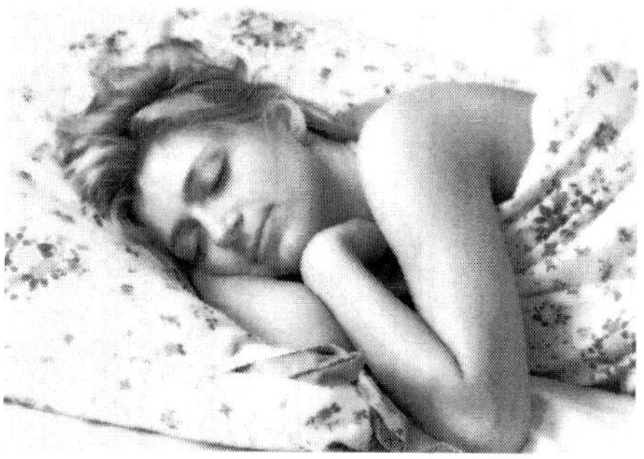

Avoid having a cell phone near your body at night, under the pillow, or on a bedside table.

If you need an alarm consider a much safer alternative such as a battery powered alarm clock."

What's a health-savvy gift? Give your loved one a battery alarm clock.

## Type of use

Here are some of the recommendations you need to know: **Never use a cell phone when the antenna is within 6 inches of your body**. As much as possible, prefer to use speakerphone mode so that the antenna is in a position further away from vulnerable tissues and organs. **Never wear your cell phone in a pocket, or carry it near your heart.**

As a cardiologist, Dr. Sinatra is aware of this concern and reinforces this recommendation, "I would avoid having any wireless device near the heart; this includes a wireless microphone."

Switch sides regularly while communicating on your cell phone to spread out your exposure. It is advisable to use text messaging instead of talking when possible. Hold the phone away from you until the text is sent. Then power it off.

Is your mobile 'amping up'? The bars indicate the strength of the network signal in your area; the maximum number of bars is preferable.

It's best to keep your cell phone fully charged, and best not to use it with low battery, and/or in an area of poor reception. And don't talk on the phone when the battery is being charged – that amplifies both the low frequencies (from the electrical connection) and the Information Carrying Radio Waves (the wireless communication).

Charge the phone in an area away from people and pets.

## Location of use

Evidently, if you're standing somewhere and turn your cell phone on, and the base station is behind you, the signal goes through you. Yes, through you.

(CA) "When you use your cell phone in an environment where WiFi or Wi-MAX signals are present, the body is subjected to 2 major assaults… these signals tend to couple forming new waveforms, which cause more harm."

We are also advised to refrain from using a cell phone, or other wireless device, in a car, truck, train, boat, airplane or other confined metal perimeter space. When you're inside a metal box your mobile is continually trying to reconnect to the nearest relay antenna, and the signal is trapped inside and bounces around, concentrating the exposure and amplifying the radiation.

And it is not recommended to use your cell phone when moving at high speed, in any mode of transportation, as this automatically increases the mobile's power to a maximum as it makes repeated attempts to connect to a new antenna.

If you must have a phone on in the car, an external roof-mounted antenna will make it less harmful, though dividing your attention between a phone conversation and the road is never a good idea.

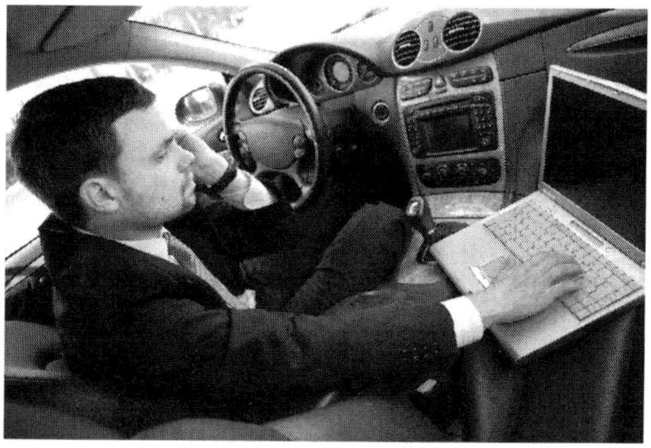

(CA) "Hands free cell phones are reportedly no safer than hand-held ones, as some studies show them being 50% more likely to cause accidents. Moreover, science shows that cell phone radiation impairs reaction time and brain function, so it is clear that the main culprit is not the 'distraction' factor – as claimed by the wireless industry – but the phone radiation which causes impairment and more accidents."

Also, please think about this: other drivers using phones may be suffering from similar impairment, so drive defensively.

Japanese physicists have also found that radiation hot spots often emerge in reflective areas, such as elevators. These researchers say passive radiation exposure is similar to second-hand smoke.

When using a mobile in a building, it is recommended to stand by a door or window and to hold it between you and the outside so less radiation goes through you as the signal blasts to connect with the nearest antenna.

## # 1 Guideline – Limit use of your cell phone.

Have a "no frills" cell phone with speaker function – use it outside of cars and other confined spaces. A wired headset is recommended if you cannot use the speakerphone.

- **Keep it turned off as much as you can.**
- Use standby mode only when expecting an urgent call.
- Turn it off when it's charging – so that it isn't connected to receive.
- Use a limited service plan. If you have young people using a mobile device, make sure you check the bill often. Your idea of their having a cell phone to keep them safe, and in touch with you, may not match their communication objectives. The bill will tell the true story. Remember the risk of 500 minutes per month.

## Pagers

Stan Hartman (SH) "If you have to be accessible by phone it's safer to carry a pager. Then when you are paged you can turn on your cell phone to make a quick call, if there is no landline nearby."

Remember this is "safer," reduced risk. Not "safe." Some doctors report people who have pagers have symptoms near where they carry them.

**10 Safer Guidelines for Mobile Phones – Best Practices**

1. Use a landline whenever possible – "May I call you back from my landline?"

2. Use a low-tech, lowest SAR rated phone with a speaker function – avoid the hands-free in-the-ear phones.

3. Use on speakerphone or with an accessory corded handset.

4. Limit calls, and keep powered off whenever possible.

5. Carry away from your body – at least with the keypad or front of the cell phone facing toward the body, and the back or antenna side facing away from the body.

6. Use outside of a car, train, elevator, airplane or other confined metal space.

7. Use a computer (desktop or mobile) with wired Internet access and with its wireless function disabled to surf the Internet, watch movies, download music etc.

8. Keep it fully charged (it has to 'amp' up power if the battery is weak and/or if signal reception is poor.)

9. Use a battery-operated alarm clock to wake you up. Never sleep with your cell phone powered on in your sleep zone. Charge away from humans/pets and turned off (not on 'standby').

10. Internet Phones (Skype) carry a risk if you're on wireless Internet access. It's great to talk and see the grandchildren; switch to wired-only connection to make it safe.

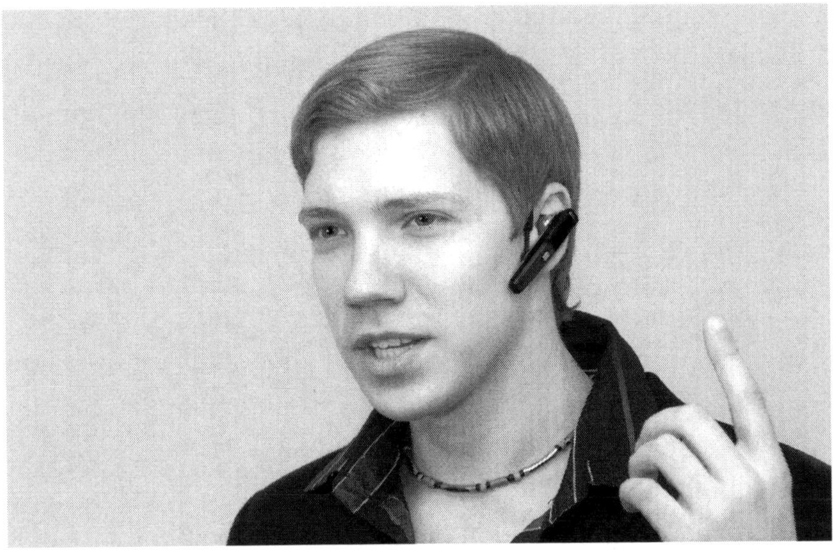

**Wireless Earpiece Phones**

**The Concern:**

One website marketing these all-in-one microphone and speaker wireless ear buds trumpets the advantages: **"Boosting sound and channeling it directly into the ear, reducing interference and noise."** This is *not* all they're channeling.

And, yes, these do keep your hands free for driving, which seems a good idea. However, these devices may be the most harmful of all to your vulnerable eyes and brain.

(RM) **"It is important *not* to have the speaker IN the ear, as with the microphone kind of phone. Magnetic fields go right through the surface so they are active in the brain at close distance."**

Think about the pulsing digital radiation blasting to its host, or base station, and then on to a cell tower every few minutes, even on standby. And where is it also going from its snug position wedged in your ear?

Technology writer Stewart Fist reported from Australia that lab testing of wireless earpiece phones shows **the radiation they give off exceeds current government standards**, and we know about those.

## Hands-free While Driving

Oprah Winfrey is on a worthy campaign to make cars a "No Phone Zone" after hearing about a young girl killed by a distracted driver. "A call or text isn't worth taking a life," said Winfrey. "My biggest hope is that it becomes mandatory that no one uses their phone in the car or texts while driving—just as seat belts are mandatory, I'm hoping that this becomes not just law, but second nature for all of us."

Bringing such high-level media attention to this issue is much needed and not always easy to do as the wireless industry is massively powerful.

And Dr. McKinney sent me this – an increasing trend in transportation:

> POLICY: The use of interactive wireless communication devices by employees of The Pennsylvania State University while on University business is prohibited while operating any vehicle.

As we know from the research, wireless radiation can cause cognitive impairment, so this isn't just an issue of multi-tasking. Hands-free is a positive step, but not with a wireless earpiece. The "No Phone Zone," and pulling over to make your brief call, using the speakerphone, are better, our technical experts advise, and could save a life. Maybe yours.

## Wireless Earpiece Phones – Safer Solutions:

As noted above, it is highly recommended to use the speakerphone function on a low-tech cell phone – see other headset recommendations on the next few pages.

## Cell Phone Headsets, Wireless Earpieces

## The Concern:

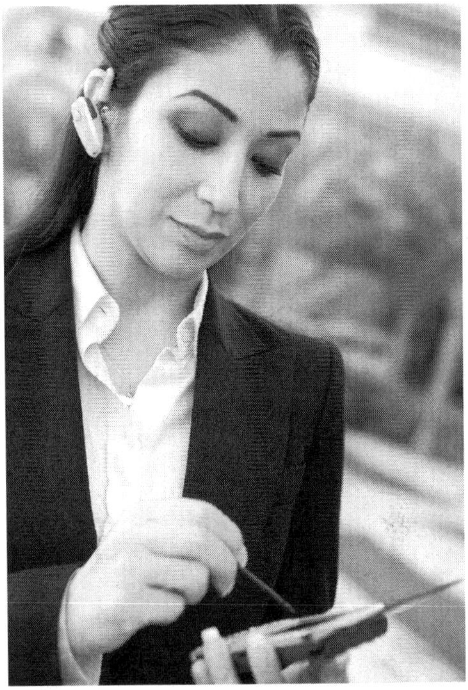

People often ask whether using a headset is safer than holding a mobile phone at your ear. This seems to make sense. And most experts do recommend using some kind of wired headset, if you cannot use the speakerphone.

However, **all advise against wireless headsets**. You will see the difference here again between the various levels of reducing exposure, and something being considered relatively safe.

## Wireless Headsets, Wireless Earpieces

Many experts advise us that most headsets are not safe and that wireless listening devices worn in the ear dramatically increase whole-body radiation exposure and trigger systemic adverse effects.

(RM) "I would not recommend using a wireless headset. Even if they have relatively low power, as compared to the mobile phone, your head's exposure to the additional digital RF-signal will still be above the values recommended in 2008 by IBE (Institute for Bau-Biologie®). It also adds another signal which can increase risk."

## Wired Headsets, Wired Earpieces

These are much better than wireless ones, and helpful if your mobile has no speaker function. However, wired earpieces are not the safest solution as they are only reducing the **near field** of the microwave radiation emitted by your mobile. Yes, the stronger near field is the radiation plume's highest intensity closest to your vulnerable eyes and brain, but the far field is also considered harmful. Larry Gust explains:

(LG) "The wired headset does get the phone away from the head. So the big hammer is removed because you are out of the near field which is 4 times stronger than the far field. However, I have heard commentary that the radio signal (wireless microwave radiation) follows the wire from the cell phone to the head set."

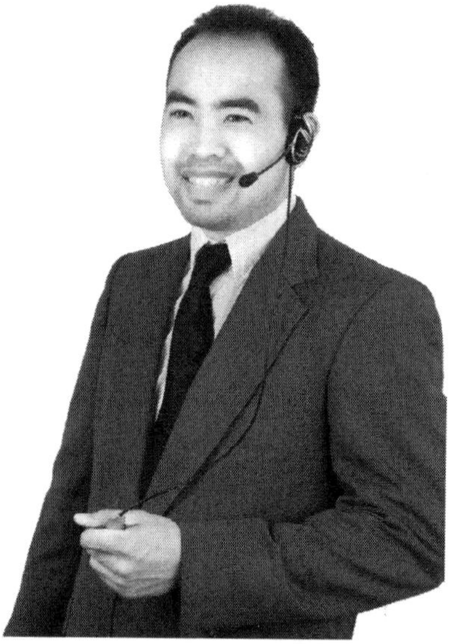

(RM) "I have concerns about using conventional wired headsets. The high frequencies emitted by the mobile phone will tend to follow the direction of the wire and 'lead their way' up to the ear/head.

This is a concentrated emission and can be just as strong as holding the mobile phone directly to the ear. Also, the generation of sound in the earphone speaker produces low frequency AC magnetic fields in the range of 5 Hz to 20,000 Hz – not a good thing, as these AC fields will easily penetrate the skull since the source is the earphone, directly inside the ear. This is why using an air tube headset is advantageous." (See next page)

## Headsets, Earpieces – Safer Solutions:

(RM) "Here is a summary of options – worst to best:

**Worst** – Cell phone held against your head, up to your ear, or using a wireless headset, then slightly better – the wired headset

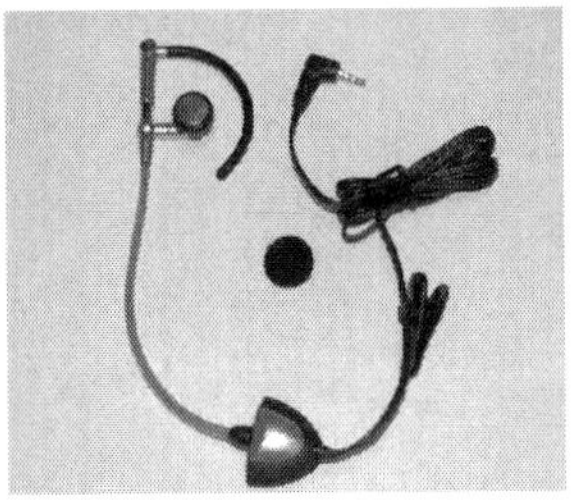

**Better** – The air tube headset is non-conductive thus separating you from the wires and speaker. This makes it better than a wired headset, and certainly much better than a wireless one. For best results, ensure the phone is at a distance and you are not in contact with the wire or the phone. Note: compatible adapters for your particular model of phone may be challenging to find.

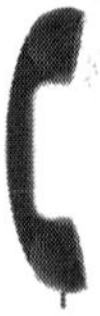

NativeUnion.com makes this 'Retro' POP handset for mobiles; it looks just like a corded phone handset and plugs into your mobile phone, or computer, to reduce radiation exposure. The bluetooth model is not advised.

**Best** – Using a phone with a good quality speaker (away from the body without contacting it) is a safer option but most speakers are poor quality sound and don't allow privacy. This is where the air tube headset comes into play. Note: these steps reduce radiation but mobiles are still not safe.

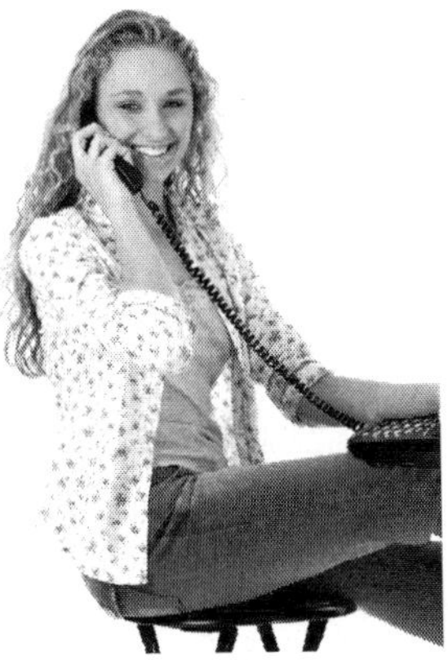

**Safe** – Standard landline phone – corded not cordless. (If you are electro-sensitive, use the speaker function on this corded phone.) Switch from cell/cordless phones to corded landlines to maintain your health. Best kind has batteries; isn't plugged into a wall socket."

## What did we learn about headsets/earpieces?

(SH) "An ordinary wired headset will reduce radiation by many magnitudes. The air-tube headset is a kind of speaker that's a lot closer to your body than the speaker if you used that function. Using the mobile phone's speakerphone is recommended."

Even with the POP handset you're being exposed to EMR. The desk set model is used with Skype; your mobile sits on a desk away from your body – a good idea if you have given up the landline. Please get a *battery-operated*, *corded* landline – a wise health investment. Most mobiles have poor speakers and there's no perfect headset/earpiece. It is prudent to use precautions: limit calls; use a low SAR phone with a speaker; power off the signal when you can; never have it on at night (use a battery alarm clock); use a corded landline as your regular phone.

## 'Protective' Stick-on chips, diodes, discs – not enough proof

There is no solid science to show that claims of 'neutralizing' the radiation are true, or that serious adverse effects like DNA damage are prevented, even if thermal images were done. Perhaps you talk/text away thinking you are now protected. Maybe not. More on that later.

There's a mobile phone holder with a radiation blocking pocket as well as a pocket that allows connectivity. If scientifically designed to be a physical barrier, holders that are RF shields are advised. LG handed out a mobile phone 'radiation shield' at the 2014 Mobile World Congress, to mixed reviews from the attendees. Imagine the stratosphere levels of microwave buzz in that place? Not sure how much radiation these LG shields reduce but it's good to see the "Life's Good" company is thinking this way. As consumers demand safer tech solutions, we will see more 'radiation-reducing' products. The key principle that all of our experts agree upon is: when any mobile device is communicating data through the air, wirelessly, use caution. The signal is harming you.

## It's Not Just Children at Risk

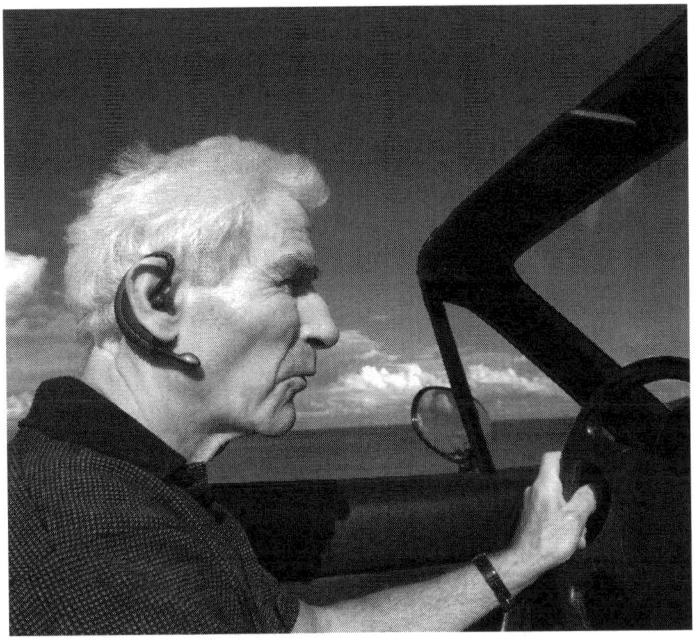

When we are exposed to the radiation from mobile phones, and other wireless technology, we must consider the intermediate massive impairment of our micro-circulation, and therewith the oxygen supply of our inner organs and brain, caused by the tendency of our red blood cells to stick together under the influence of radio waves (DR. PETERSOHN 1998, RITTER UND WOLSKI 2005). In addition to this Prof. Kind (Environmental Hygienic Department of Vienna University) found a high increase of heart attacks, strokes, thromboses and embolism in people who live near (cell towers) transmitter masts.

Hans Scheiner, MD

## A Summary: the Safer-Tech Communications Kit

- Corded landline phone – use for all phone calls, whenever possible
- Low-tech cell phone with speakerphone function – for quick, urgent-only calls (see Safer Use Recommendations)
- Wired headset
- Pager – only on at times you must be reachable
- Cable/wired Internet access

## A Great Gift

Consider this kit for your family at home, and when your young people leave to set out on their own. Graduation gift?

As you know, many of this young generation are using mobile phones for all their calls and have never had a landline installed where they are living.

A young woman who works in our office is getting married, and we are giving her the first corded landline phone she has ever had since moving away from home.

Of course, it is much more convenient, and less money, not to bother installing a landline and just rely on mobile phone service.

But at what cost to our health? And, there is the consideration that a battery-operated, or not-plugged in, corded phone will keep working during power outages, and when your cell phone is not charged.

Mobile phones have their benefits, as well: great if your car breaks down. Many of our experts told me they keep a fully-charged cell phone – powered off – in the glove compartment of their car.

## Video/Wireless Games

### The Concern:

Many of these games use wireless technology, both on any size handheld or bigger computers and gaming systems. Much as you may hate the thought of trying to wrest the controller away from the young gamer, there are some concerns you need to know about.

A paper published in 2004 in the medical journal *Human Reproduction* reports some devices when held close to the genitals raise the temperature in the testicles as much as 3 degrees Celsius. Temperature changes can occur within 15 minutes. Repeated exposure can reduce fertility.

The researchers say that after a few years of daily exposure, the damage may be irreversible, and others report this exposure may be a factor in the increasing rate of testicular cancer in young men.

### Computer Game Consoles

(AP) "The transformer which plugs into a power socket emits very high levels of magnetic fields, and should be unplugged when not in use. The hand controls can give off high electric fields."

Other than the considerable health concerns, there's another problem with gaming etc. It keeps our children – of all ages – inside.

Not only is this an unhealthy sedentary lifestyle, they are missing out on being outside. After the rapid-fire explosiveness of the 3-D games, strolling along the beach can seem tediously dull.

Nature, in all its wondrous simplicity, can hardly compete.

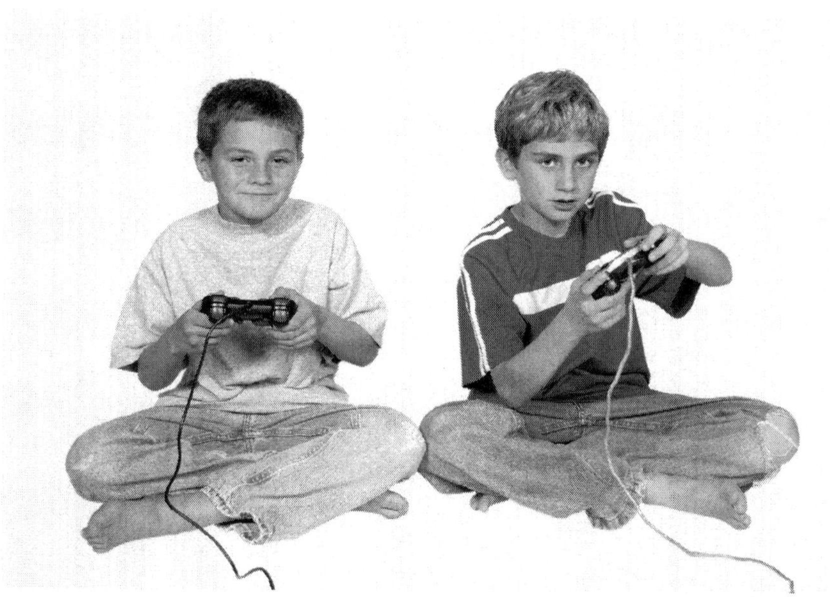

**Safer Gaming Solutions:**

(RM) "Hard-wired is much safer than wireless. Disable the wireless component and replace it with a cable. Encourage your children to use their game systems and laptops on a table or desk, not directly on their laps. And limit use."

(KG) "There are gaming consoles, which will still emit substantial amounts of RF radiation even when the RF antenna from the back is removed and the control devices used are wired! The popular XBOX, for example, will keep radiating as long as it is plugged in."

(AP) "It is advisable to add a grounding wire, and limit use of all video games."

## Wireless Internet Access – Global Electro-pollution

Even the most humble coffee shop offers "free wireless Internet." Hard to believe but we will see signs: "No WiFi here!"

## The Concern:

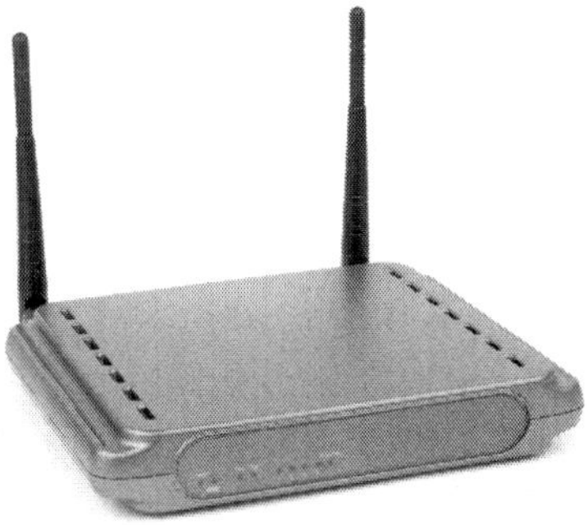

It used to just be cell phones. Now WiFi is everywhere and the background level is reaching a dangerously high level. Alasdair Philips, the electronic engineer who heads Powerwatch, cautions: "With wireless Internet access the space is filled with pulsing microwave radiation all of the time even when the computers are not in use. (Your techie may not agree.) **We believe that you should avoid using wireless Internet at all costs.**"

## Travel in Our WiFi World

Virtually all accommodation now offers WiFi – in your room, at the pool, meeting places and even the spa. If you operate a hotel or B&B, consider replacing this with safe hard-wired Internet access, at least in the guest rooms. You will lead the way as more people request this. And you, and your guests, will get a better night's sleep. Some day we will look back on this WiFi era and it will remind us of the days of asbestos and tobacco.

**Renting/owning an RV/motorhome** is a good option if it has a metal body that blocks outside WiFi (in most RV parks). Inside, make sure all electro-magnetic fields are low (test with Gauss meter), and there's no WiFi or microwave oven. In some refuges for electro-sensitive people, metal "Faraday cage" shelters are their only way of surviving in this electrified world.

## Safer Internet Access Solutions

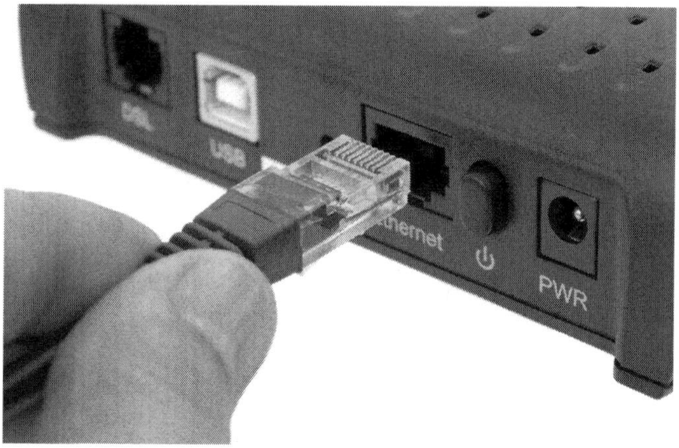


### Best Option:

This is a situation where you really need to weigh the risks and benefits, of convenience and your health.

(AP) "It is better to get a cable or ADSL modem/router and run network cables to the rooms where you wish computers to have Internet access. This is not expensive and will avoid irradiating your living and working environment with pulsing microwaves."

(RM) "Replace wireless Internet routers with hard-wired units. Some wireless router models allow the user to shut off the wireless component and convert it to a hard-wired unit. To ensure conversion, test the area around it with a RF detector.

When using a notebook/laptop computer use a hard-wired network connection. Settings to disable the wireless connection are found in Network Settings on a PC, or AirPort on a Mac." Some tablets can connect by hard-wire (a small portable adapter may be necessary).

As you may know, all computers nowadays are shipped with a default setting that ensures that all wireless networks and systems are turned on as soon as you start your computer. These functions need to be deliberately disabled: go to the Control Panel, click on 'wireless connections', and actually 'disable' the wLAN as well as the 'bluetooth' system.

On a personal note: during my EMR reduction frenzy, I replaced our wireless router with the hard-wired kind. Well, the phone company only had wireless ones, but the techie assured me that there would be no RF/microwave radiation if it wasn't being used wirelessly. Guess what? I had been sitting here at the computer for long hours wondering why I was getting headaches, (of course, there are always other reasons – eye strain etc).

I decided to test the hard-wired router with an RF (radio-frequency) meter. Even though I had disabled the computer's wireless settings, there were really high RF radiation levels coming from the router. Not good. Evidently, you have to go online to modify the router's settings. Now they tell me!

### Another Hard-wired Option:

### Networking your Ethernet and your home's power lines

If you cannot use the recommended cable hook-up – wired Internet access – you might consider this new set up where you access the Internet through electrical outlets in the wall. This is not inexpensive, but safer than having all the wireless radiation going through your house, and neighborhood. Make sure you get the non-wireless model.

(SH) "This is not as good as an ordinary wired modem using Ethernet cable, but way better than WiFi, because the signal is going through the wiring, not through the air. Even if there is some radiation leakage from the wiring, it will be much, much weaker than the exposure from WiFi."

(RM) "This solution may be a bit dicey because of the dirty electricity issue, which is a bit of an unknown at this point." Suggestion: also power off this type of router at bedtime.

**Another Internet Access Option:**

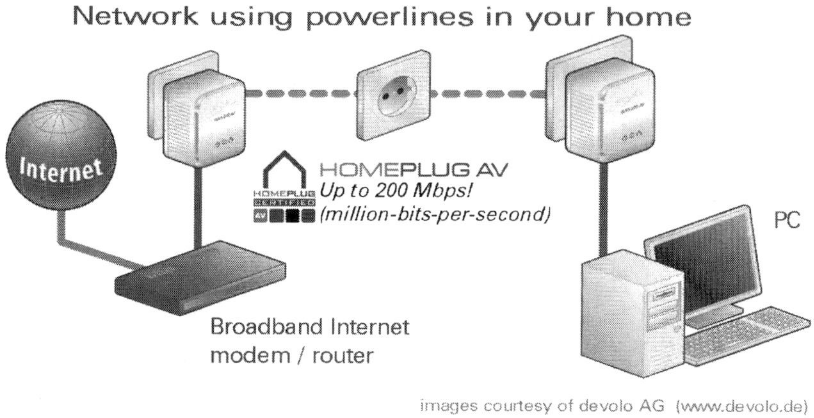


Have at least one computer hard-wired. If you have someone in your house who insists on a wireless computer, turn on the router for that time, then shut it off. **Make sure a WiFi router is turned off at bedtime**. A quality power bar may be helpful, maybe with a timer.

**A Caution About Power Bars**

Chris Cowan of Source Holdings Ltd., an electrician who worked as a safety inspector, rescued me when a power bar with a surge suppressor flamed up in smelly smoke. He advised a top quality power bar without a surge suppressor as this feature can be a fire hazard – who knew? – and to have an electrician add a surge suppressor at the main panel.

The following safer solutions list is from leading experts in this field:

**How can I protect myself from wireless radiation?**

The following tips help to avoid or reduce your personal radiation exposure to wireless networks:

- Always prefer wired data transmission systems to wireless networks (even though you may have to run some wire), especially in residences, schools, and preschools.
- If at all, wireless networks should be run at the lowest possible power output actually required to get the work done (which usually can be set in the software).
- Have access points only transmit for the short period of time required to transfer data, otherwise keep it always turned off, especially during the night. Simply turn the switch at the wireless device off or, better yet, unplug it.
- Preferably, keep transmitting antennas a large distance (>10m or 32.5 ft) away from areas of frequent human use.
- Transmitting antennas should NOT be installed in the rooms they service but rather in hallways, attics or less used rooms farther away.
- Also keep your neighbor in mind!
- Strategically place access point antennas in such a way as to minimize the radiation exposure in areas of frequent human use. Never connect sector antennas with high antenna gains (and their increased directivity) to access points and never point them towards areas of frequent human use.

- Laptop or PC: Keep your distance from the wireless card; if at any time larger amounts of data are transferred, leave the area. Always turn off the wireless card with a separate switch or disable it in the control panel (PC) or at the task bar (Mac) when not in use.

Perhaps rooms or walls could be specifically shielded if the wireless radiation comes from outside or a neighbor; though it is imperative to have a RF radiation survey conducted prior to any shielding project.

With an external source any solid masonry wall or concrete ceiling reduces RF levels by about 50-80 %, wood frame wall constructions, however, provide hardly any reduction.

One can also cover the wireless device with shielding cloth at night or to reduce the emission level.

W. Maes, F. Mehlis: Wireless Network. A Flyer by the Building Biology Association (VB), 2009. Used with permission. (www.verband-baubiologie.de)

## Wireless Systems in Schools

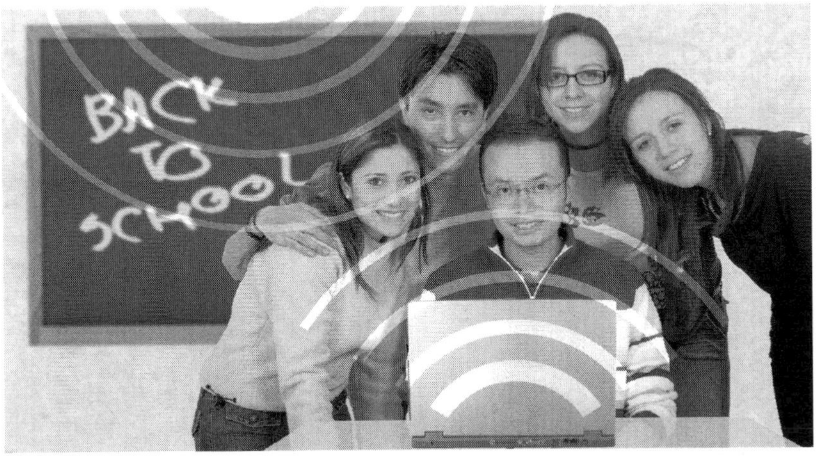


As the Principals of my children's schools will tell you, I am a "mother warrior" on this issue.

Another concerned parent, director of a large information technology company, used this analogy:

> If someone put a glass of drinking water in front of you and said we think it's OK to drink and it meets current government standards but there is a substance in it that some credible scientists say may be carcinogenic, would you give your child a glass of that water day after day?
>
> The scientists and organizations in Europe that are taking positions and actions against WiFi are, in my opinion, highly credible.
>
> There is no conspiracy here; our governments and institutions have simply not kept pace with the rapid roll out of new technology. Anyone who spends time educating themselves would err on the side of caution.

> Anyone who says 'I am not convinced there is a problem with wireless technology' and turns a blind eye is being imprudent. By the time they are convinced, the damage will have been done.

This issue is a dilemma for schools. On the one hand, they're told that information technology gives students an essential educational edge. There's also pressure to go wireless since it's cheaper to install than hard wired systems. On the other hand, what's true of cell phone radiation is equally true of wireless Internet: children are more vulnerable to the biological damage.

## The Concern:

Dr. Martin Blank is taking the lead in alerting communities:

> There is enough evidence of a plausible mechanism to link EMF exposure to increased risk of cancer, and therefore of a need to limit exposure, especially of children. (Radio-frequency) RF in any form – cell tower radiation, WiFi networks, cell phones etc. – is potentially bad, especially if one is exposed for extended periods (e.g., asleep in bed at home, seated at a desk in school).

Epilepsy is one of the associated EMR conditions, including adult onset. A young man told me about his first seizure – on a transatlantic flight that had WiFi. Maybe no connection. Sadly, I heard recently that he died of a seizure. His last few years had been a struggle as being highly electro-sensitive, he had difficulty finding places where he could work, and live. It seems likely we will see an increase in electro-sensitive youth, as most of them attend WiFi schools and are immersed in it.

Many eminent scientists, including Dr. Gerd Oberfeld and Professor Johansson join Drs. Blank and Havas in calling for WiFi – free schools.

Dr. Magda Havas, Associate Professor, Trent University, sent an open letter to Canadian parents, teachers and school boards:

> I am a scientist who does research on the health effects of electromagnetic radiation and I am becoming increasingly concerned that schools are installing WiFi networks and are making their school grounds available for cell phone antennas. Both the federal government and the WiFi provider say this technology is safe and the exposures remain below federal standards. This information is outdated and incorrect based on the growing number of scientific publications that are reporting adverse health and biological effects well below our Safety Code 6 standards (see www.bioiniative.org) and the growing number of scientific and medical organizations that are asking for stricter standards to be enforced. For these reasons, it is irresponsible to introduce WiFi microwave radiation into a school environment.

Dr. Havas has developed a questionnaire to monitor a child's health in a WiFi school – to track symptoms that may, or may not, be related. Ideally, safer-tech Internet access would be used and not WiFi. Contrary to what some WiFi-promoting parents and educators think, we are *not* against technology. We know our kids need to be tech-savvy in this 21st century. They can be connected to the Internet more safely.

Frank Clegg has an extensive background in technology – he headed Microsoft Canada for fourteen years – and now leads Canadians For Safe Technology. Mr. Clegg is calling for caution, "There are already children who can't go to school because of headaches, nausea and heart problems from the wireless systems. This is a real hazard and we shouldn't wait for the government to catch up to the technology. We should exercise caution, especially with children." (More at: c4st.org)

Dr. Sarah Starkey, a UK neuroscientist, set up a website out of concern about the rapid spread of wireless technologies in schools. She has studied the mechanisms underlying learning and memory, circadian rhythms (like our sleep/wake cycles), epilepsy and depression.

According to research on www.wifiinschools.org.uk many of the health risks may only become apparent after years of exposure. Some students and staff could be susceptible to more immediate effects, such as symptoms of electro-hypersensitivity. There are studies that suggest that people with epilepsy have an increased chance of seizures when they're exposed to cell phone signals.

Our international advisory board, Doctors for Safer Schools, is asking legitimate questions about wireless radiation in schools, and requesting accurate answers. We acknowledge we are all part of this biological experiment, as Dr. Salford has warned; however, we must consider our children. How much more evidence do we need before taking protective action?

### Wireless Networks, Immune Systems and Viruses

Do you remember that Dr. Scheiner and other medical experts have reported wireless radiation suppresses the immune system? With the current spread of the H1N1 virus, and its threat to schools, wouldn't you think that school Principals would be more than keen to go back to hard-wired Internet connections and reduce all other exposure levels?

These precautionary steps also make sense in other public spaces, including confined ones like trains, buses and airplanes. Also, you'll read later on what one of our scientists, an immunologist, has to say about wireless radiation and the immune system.

## Safer-Tech Solutions for School Trustees, Library Boards

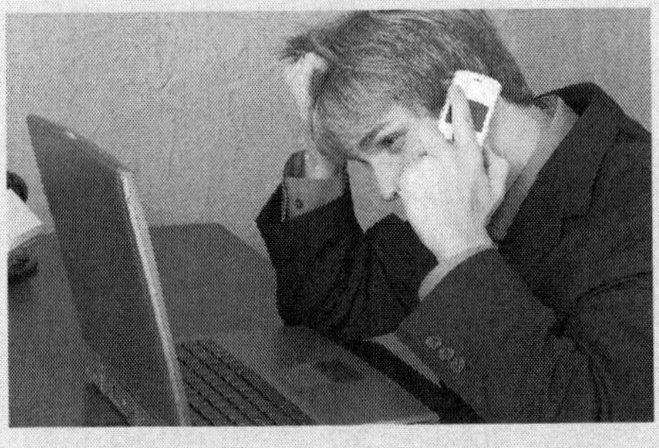

In this time of WiFi debate, do you want to continue this time-consuming battle with opposing experts and evidence that could go on for years? Or, are you ready for the precautionary principle? Until you install a safer system for Internet connectivity – wired and/or fiber optics – why not choose a still-effective system in areas where you rely on WiFi? – *not* around pregnant women or young children who are too vulnerable.

**Consider this stop-gap option**: WiFi-free zones; use hard-wired computers as much as possible; avoid Bluetooth® and the wireless keyboard/mouse; avoid interactive whiteboards; limit duration of WiFi exposure with router on/off switches; place routers far away from all humans; educate staff and students about the safer use of mobile devices; keep them away from the body; make sure laptops/iPads/tablets are not on the lap; never hold a cell phone against the head; whenever you can, select the safer, 'no-signal', airplane mode.

For WiFi, choose a signal strength as low as possible – below a *maximum* of 1,000 microwatts per square meter (and this level only in close proximity to an access point.) Ensure levels below 10-100 everywhere else. This allows connectivity and avoids the 'overkill' radiation exposure now in place (between 10,000 – 100,000).

**Risk-benefit ratio?** Extreme levels can enhance signal strength but are not essential. Is it worth the significant health risk, especially when there are many electro-sensitive people – and there's evidence it is needlessly placing *all* students and staff in harm's way? And, there's another benefit to a lower signal strength – energy-savings.

*Disclaimer: We have concerns about all WiFi levels. There are harmful effects far below 1,000 microwatts per sq meter, but this maximum is preferable to the worst option – what we have now – unregulated levels and un-monitored exposures.*

## Decrease in Memory, Attention and Ability to Learn?

Electro-magnetic radiation can alter the electrical activity in the brain – with unknown effects on the still-developing brains of children and teens.

As we have seen, scientific studies also show a decrease in cognitive abilities such as memory, attention and decision-making.

Does it makes sense to radiate an educational environment when this exposure has been shown to damage our children, including their ability to sit still, and to learn?

(AP) "School libraries and IT facilities usually have wireless local area networked (wLAN) computers. These can give a high background level of microwaves to which teachers and pupils will be exposed for most of the day.

We are against every pupil having a wireless enabled computer to do his or her school work.

This is because 20 or more computers, with wireless access, fill the classroom with several volts per metre of pulsing microwave radiation electrosmog. Electrically sensitive children will react very badly to this exposure, which is associated with memory and concentration problems and increased aggressive behaviour."

(AP) "**Laptops wired by Ethernet using standard cables are fine.** The pupils can use their laptops on their own for most work and plug in a network cable when they need to access files on the school server computer or on the Internet. Infrared data connections are also believed to be safe."

(AP) "Interactive whiteboards, used to display computer and video images in the classroom also use microwave technology. The whiteboard display (using back or front projection) should be connected by wire to the teacher's controller PC and will not then be a problem.

However, some are now being sold with built-in wireless networks to connect to the teacher's PC and to wireless connected interactive pen displays that can be moved around the classroom and operated by pupils.

These wireless options will increase the ambient level of electrosmog in the classroom."

**Wireless Internet in Schools – Safer Solutions** (see page 167):

The obvious solution is to remove the wireless network and go back to the hard-wired system. Dr. Starkey advises parents to take a stand on wireless in their children's classrooms:

> Schools will only use wireless computer networks if the parents want this for their children. Obviously it is not desirable for a few children to be isolated, or to miss out in their education.
>
> But if parents en masse decide together that their children will only use wired technologies then schools will need to revise their communications technology provision.

How about the safest option – fiber optics?

Visit our website SaferTechSolutions.org for more information on this important issue: the wellbeing of our children *and* of teachers and staff in WiFi schools.

## Reducing your child's EMR exposure

- Minimise the time your children play computer games.
- Monitor the type of games they play.
- Keep children at least a metre (3.25 feet) away from working electrical appliances in the kitchen.
- Make sure your child sits at least a metre (3.25 feet) away from the front of a TV screen while watching.
- Position the television set so children cannot spend time to the side or back of it.
- Make sure transformers are kept away from chairs, beds and anywhere a child sits and plays regularly.
- Consider your use of battery-operated equipment. Use rechargeable batteries where possible and dispose of them as toxic waste.
- Position your child's bed away from cupboards containing electric equipment, meters, heaters and the like.
- Make sure all music/entertainment players are plugged in with a grounded cord.
- Make sure your child sits well away from the transmitting unit of a cordless phone system.
- Make sure desk and bedside table lamps are grounded.
- Check your garden for EMR sources and build play areas where field levels are low.
- Make sure your child sits in seats that are not exposed to high EMR in public transport.
- Check your child's nursery and school for sources of EMR.
- Monitor your child's health, behaviour and achievement levels and check school EMR exposure if these deteriorate.

Check whether your child's school has a wireless system or interactive whiteboards. Measure the EMR in the classroom to see if it is at an acceptable level.

(Source: Powerwatch)

## Fluorescent Lights

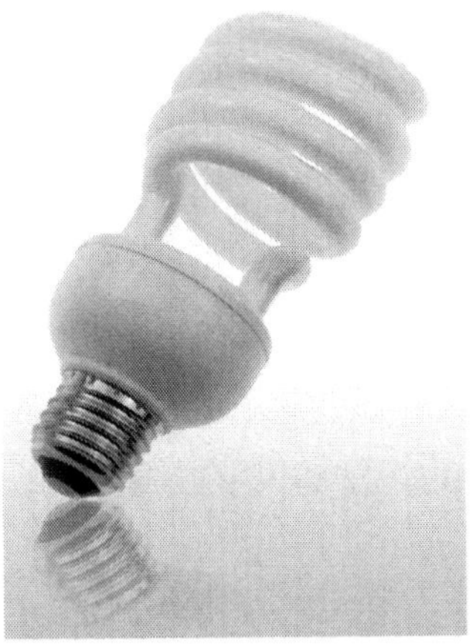

Most people working in offices with overhead fluorescents, whether they are buzzing or not, report eyestrain, fatigue and headaches. The recent promotion of compact fluorescent lights for their energy efficiency causes the scientific community concern. There are two problems with the compact fluorescent lights – one EMR assessment technician calls the CFL "chronic fatigue lights" for their negative impact on our energy. The second problem is they feed what is called dirty electricity back into the electrical system.

Dr. Magda Havas (MH): "Don't use CFL bulbs. These energy efficient compact fluorescent lights generate radio-frequency radiation, ultraviolet radiation, and dirty electricity. Dirty electricity has been shown to adversely affect human health. A recent study of cancer clusters in a school in California associated the increased risk of cancer among teachers to dirty electricity. **CFLs contain mercury – a known neurotoxin** – which can be dangerous once it is released into the environment through breakage or in landfills. With thousands of bulbs sold around the country and inadequate disposal facilities we are setting ourselves up for a mercury time bomb. Compact fluorescent lights are making some people ill, including those who suffer from migraines, epilepsy, skin problems and electrical sensitivity."

Many environmental groups, and governments, are advocating a ban on incandescent lights and mandating the use of CFLs. When you read the science it seems evident we need to find safer ways to cut our energy costs and consumption.

(AP) "Many schools (and workplaces) use fluorescent lighting. The flicker can trigger electrical hypersensitivity and increase antisocial behaviour. If your child develops headaches and/or eye strain, check the school classroom lighting."

**Fluorescent Lights – Safer Solutions:**

(AP) "Ensure lights are full-spectrum – not fluorescent – as it has been found that people are much healthier and thus able to learn better (and work better) in lighting that approximates daylight as closely as possible."

(KG) "If using fluorescent lights – standard or full-spectrum – be sure to have them electrically shielded with a proper grounding connection."

(RM) "Incandescent light bulbs are a better alternative. LED (light emitting diode) technology looks promising as well."

(MH) "Instead of promoting compact fluorescent light bulbs, governments around the world should be insisting that manufacturers produce light bulbs that are electro-magnetically clean and contain no toxic chemicals. LEDs are a safer option." Unlike compact fluorescent bulbs, LEDs contain no mercury and they work well in cold weather. They may provide a more pleasing light than fluorescents and appear to be the greenest and potentially healthiest option.

(KG) "Watch out for poor quality electronic drivers in LEDs that increase electro-magnetic field emissions and may cause flickers. Models with a proper grounding connection are preferable."

The high cost of LED light production has meant that their use has been limited to commercial and outdoor lighting, but that is changing. Soon they will be more available, and more economical, for use in our homes, offices and schools.

## Halogen Lights

### The Concern:

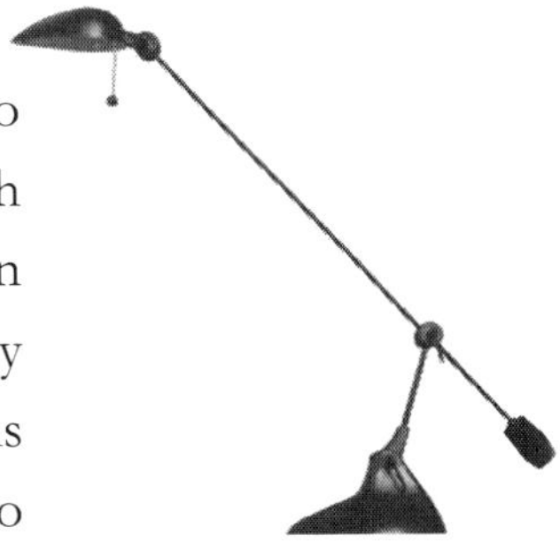

(AP) "Low voltage halogen lights are also not recommended as they give off high electric fields, and many have their own built-in transformer. This is usually poorly constructed and gives off very high levels of power-frequency magnetic fields close to them."

### Halogen Lights – Safer Solutions:

(KG) "If using low-voltage halogen lights, the transformers should be located away from high-occupancy areas and the wiring shielded. Since most transformers in low-voltage desk lamps emit magnetic fields even when turned off, avoid these. Line-voltage (120V) halogen lamps are better, especially for bedside and desk lamps. See the lighting recommendations in my paper on low-emission office environments: www.buildingbiology.ca/healthyoffice.php"

## Night lights

### The Concern:

(AP) "There is plenty of strong scientific evidence that shows that even quite low levels of light stop the production of melatonin, a hormonal chemical synthesised in the pineal gland. It, and its associated chemicals, 'mop up' dangerous free-radical damage. There is good evidence that low levels of melatonin increase the likelihood of cancers and other serious health problems developing. It is often your anxiety about seeing your child that starts the 'light at night' habit."

## Night Lights – Safer Solutions:

The only type of night light that you should use are the very low power (usually plug mounted) orange or red ones that just glow gently as these colors hardly affect the production of melatonin. White and blue-white lights are likely to stop the pineal gland's production of melatonin for the whole night.

(KG) "I am very concerned about light exposure at night, no matter what its color. Darkness is best."

## Dimmer Lights

## The Concern:

(RM) "Dimmer switches produce elevated magnetic fields and power line transients, which are high frequency noise on the power lines."

## Dimmer Lights – Safer Solution:

(RM) "Remove dimmer switches."

(MB) "Get rid of instant-on devices."

(SH) "Do not have dimmer lights or touch-on (clap-on) lamps near where you sit or sleep."

Even if you choose to be wary of cell phones, cordless phones and wireless Internet, you are still being exposed to EMR in all kinds of ways that have never occurred to you, and some are ways that you may not be able to control (except by suggesting others control them).

Consider the following. Just because diagnostic tests are ordered by your doctor or dentist does not mean you don't get a second opinion, or a second thought to weigh the risks and benefits.

## Medical Technologies

One of Dr. Becker's concerns was that our conventional medical system relies on powerful testing and treatment technologies that may administer high doses of EMR. Dr. William Rea, also a surgeon and a highly respected pioneer in this field, reports that he became electro-sensitive from being immersed many hours a day in the radiation around him.

At what point do the risks begin to outweigh the benefits?

## Pre-natal Ultrasound

This snapshot of your unborn child can offer a magical moment for expectant parents, and also crucial medical information. I just want you to know that some experts have advised caution. How it works: ultrasound is a sound wave transmitted in water or biological tissue. A low energy ultrasound is used in medicine as a diagnostic imaging technique, especially in obstetrics.

**The Benefits**: finding out whether a fetus is growing normally.

## The Concern:

Some expectant parents are subjecting their babies to multiple ultrasounds for reasons that aren't medically necessary. The Federal Drug Administration (FDA) in the US, and the Society of Obstetricians and Gynecologists of Canada are among the medical experts who caution:

> Although there have been no fetal abnormalities linked directly to diagnostic ultrasound, it involves targeted energy exposure to the fetus, and there remains a theoretical risk for subtle effects on fetal development.

This is suggested by some biological effects of ultrasound observed at, or near, diagnostic intensities in both human studies and animal models.

Source: Non-medical Use of Ultrasound – SOGC Policy Statement April 2007

There is also concern that some technicians may deliver a stronger exposure than required, or may try to reposition the fetus for a better viewing angle.

(KG) "The sound level of an ultrasound scanner is 100 dB; in the human audible range, this would be comparable to subjecting your fetus to the sound level of a jackhammer at 1 m distance."

### Ultrasound – Safer Solution:

The experts' recommendation: have ultrasound only when medically necessary.

## Dental/Medical X-rays

Electro-magnetic waves at this very high frequency – called ionizing radiation – may damage or kill cells through the production of free radicals.

### What are free radicals?

You'll need a small dose of science here if you want to know what this means. The high-energy waves from X-rays interact with DNA in your body tissue and dislodge electrons, splitting the atom into negatively charged electrons and a positively charged ion.

This ion, or free radical, behaves wildly seeking to replace its missing electron. (I once heard this described as 'recently single, seeking a mate'.) The unleashed reaction of free radicals in the body can lead to the disruption of intra-cellular metabolism and interference with DNA repair.

As you may know, many forms of cancer are thought to be the result of free radicals reacting with DNA, resulting in unwanted cell mutations. (Antioxidant nutritional supplements are considered by many physicians to reduce the production of these free radicals.)

## Dental X-rays

Again this procedure has its benefits – and risks. I was often told by a dentist that there was no concern about these levels of radiation, "Just like a day in the sunshine." Not true.

Our new family dentist does not have the digital X-ray machine, but I found one office that does, so if any of us need a dental X-ray we go there to have this lower-exposure kind.

How dental X-rays work: a beam of radiation is focused to go through your teeth and onto a small piece of photographic film. Dense structures such as teeth and bones absorb more X-rays than the soft tissues. Cavities and infections will show up as lighter areas because more radiation has passed through them before striking the film.

**The Benefit**: finding decay and diagnosing periodontal disease in impossible-to-see areas, such as under fillings or between teeth.

### The Concern:

While the amount of radiation in any one X-ray is reportedly 'small', exposure is cumulative – it builds up with each one. In the head and neck, areas exposed to dental radiation, X-rays increase the risk of damage to, or cancer of, the lens of the eye, thyroid, salivary glands, bone marrow and skin. Scientists in the UK have found that about 0.6% of the cumulative cancer risk in people under age 75 – about 700 cases per year – could be attributed to diagnostic X-rays. In Japan, which has the highest frequency of diagnostic X-ray exposure in the world, the risk was more than 3%.

Source: *The Lancet*, Vol. 363, Issue 9406

## Dental X-rays – Safer Solutions:

Question your dentist – is the X-ray essential? Why? I switched dentists when one insisted our children needed whole mouth X-rays "on file." Find a practitioner who uses newer digital X-rays, which evidently beam out 90% less radiation.

## Medical X-rays – Safer Solutions:

It's a similar situation with medical X-rays, used, among other reasons, to check for broken bones, or in the case of chest X-rays, to diagnose pneumonia. I don't want to scare you away from essential medical tests, but to encourage you to discuss with your practitioner whether there's another way to get the information needed for diagnosis. Again, is this X-ray essential? Do people with recurring sinus infections really need to have their heads X-rayed? What is the effect on their eyes? Brains?

Medical thermography emits nothing – there is no radiation. It only takes an image and these thermal readings can be a useful tool in detecting and monitoring a number of diseases and physical injuries. This FDA approved test can show physiological change and metabolic processes and is used with back injuries, for example. Thermography can also offer early detection of breast abnormalities and monitor changes. This is an option with, or instead of, mammography. More research on the safety and effectiveness of mammograms is needed.

## CT and MRI scans

I also hesitate to sound an alarm about these tests, as it seems unlikely anyone would have them unless it was medically crucial – when the benefits would outweigh the risks. Or so I used to think!

Private clinics are now marketing full-body CT and MRI scans to the general public, even those who have no other signs of disease.

Health authorities agree there is no scientific evidence that using these scans on people without symptoms is useful in catching diseases early. If the tests produce suspicious findings, this could lead to having more unnecessary procedures, exploratory surgery, medications, etc.

If the scan shows nothing, you might then ignore signs of an actual illness that can't be detected by scans. And that's before you even consider the potential side effects of the procedures themselves.

### The Concern:

In December 2008, American researchers, developing tools to help doctors weigh the risks and benefits of CT (computed tomography) scans, reported that as many as 7 percent of patients from a large U.S. hospital system received enough radiation exposure from scans over the course of their lifetime to slightly increase their risk of cancer.

The researchers raised the concern that repeated scans of people who had cancer could increase the patients' chances of developing another tumor.

And in February 2009 a paper in the *Journal of the American Medical Association* reported that one CT angiogram, widely used by cardiologists to find potentially fatal blockages in heart arteries, could deliver a radiation dose equivalent to 600 chest X-rays.

Researchers caution that whole body CT screening exposes you to radiation levels that up to 1000 times as high as those from an X-ray, increasing your risk of developing radiation-induced cancer.

MRI (magnetic resonance imaging) is a different technology, as you may know. Its powerful magnetic field excites the molecules of the body's tissues, causing the nuclei in these molecules to emit a radio-frequency. The MRI scanner transmits these radio signals to a computer, which translates them into a 3-D image of the area being examined.

Unlike CT scans, or other kinds of X-rays, this process does not involve the highest power – ionizing – radiation. Some companies are marketing MRIs as having 'no radiation'; this is not completely true. And, some people claim they became electro-sensitive only after having had an MRI.

Unnecessary scans could increase the risk of bringing on the very diseases you're worried about and trying to detect early. So the recommendation is to have these tests only when medically necessary. Even if your doctor is ordering them, you have the right to question. And to a second opinion.

Mark Baerlocher, MD, a fellow in interventional radiology offers his concern about, "the lack of awareness, and the general misinformation regarding the radiation risks associated with Medical Imaging and related exams, and procedures, among both health care professionals and patients."

This concern led him to develop the Radiation Passport, a computer program to help patients, physicians, and dentists track lifetime exposures and better understand the risks. One can look up the estimated effective radiation dose associated with a given Medical Imaging exam or procedure, and the associated estimated risk of developing cancer due to that radiation.

## Medical Scans – Safer Solutions:

Cardiologists say CT angiograms are indispensable in some cases. I was relieved to read that techniques are being developed to reduce the radiation exposure in valuable tests. Some physicians who practice complementary medicine recommend a protocol to reduce exposure impact of X-rays and scans. See *Prescription for Nutritional Healing,* Avery, New York, by James Balch, MD and Phyllis A. Balch, CNC.

## Other Exposures:

## Radio-frequency ID tags/wristbands

Wireless chips are spreading like viruses, everywhere: in store tags on clothing, in security access cards, passports, tollbooths, library books and bus passes. Recently, I saw little devices handed out at a pharmacy prescription counter so staff could beep customers when their prescriptions were ready. I walked past the beeper station quite quickly. Some of these devices only emit signals when run through a scanner. The ones causing more concern are those that send out signals constantly. Obstetrician Jacques Moritz, MD tells pregnant women, "Avoid the RF that is used in stores to prevent shoplifting, i.e., don't linger near the door of the Gap". One day we will have warning signs.

## How they work:

The chips "communicate" with each other by generating radio frequencies. In hospitals they're used to track medical supplies, equipment, and even people. A hospital in Israel used RFID wristbands on babies in the neonatal ICU as one way to make sure each preemie was fed from a container of his or her own mother's milk.

## The Benefit:

Better inventory control, faster service. In hospitals, RFID bracelets is one way to help keep track of people with dementia, for instance.

**The Concern:** According to a study published in the June 2008 *Journal of the American Medical Association*, tests show these devices may interfere with pacemakers, ventilators, IV pumps and anesthesia machines. And even though evidence exists that tumors can develop at the site of implantation, some pets are still tagged this way. Why?

### ID Tags – Safer Solutions:

Hospitals should check all new technology, including wireless chips, to make sure they don't interfere with medical equipment, and should know the potential adverse biological effects – including cardiac effects. Be aware of this if you have an implanted defibrillator or pacemaker.

## Airport Security Scanners – Your Dignity or Your DNA?

### How they work:

Metal detectors can't locate plastic explosives so now there are more invasive methods: millimeter-wave scanners that use non-ionizing radiation and the more intense backscatter X-ray technology that uses ionizing levels. These scans produce digital images of our body, and any weapons or explosives. There are privacy and health concerns.

### The Benefit:

Avoid the supposedly dreaded "enhanced" patdown, speed up security screening, and theoretically keep us safer. Everyone wants safe skies. However, this technology itself may not have been properly screened!

### The Concern:

We are told that "the scanners are safe," the emissions levels are "within safety standards" and lower than what we receive from "cosmic radiation during a flight, or being in the earth's magnetic fields." However, natural-source radiation is more diffuse, usually goes right through us, and we've adapted to it. Artificial radiation from scanners is more focused – like a laser beam. We already know about the safety standards. And Professor Olle Johansson questions,

"If airport scanners are safe, then there must be peer review-based scientific publications clearly showing it. If not, then you must ask why not?" Dr. Sinatra queries, "Are there any adverse effects in patients with vulnerable hearts, or in patients with pacemakers and defibrillators?"

The biochemist Dr. David Agard and others from the University of California urge caution. And Alasdair Philips tells us, "The key point is the bombarding of the skin with a mass of high-energy electrons. That may, or may not be a significant problem, but there has been almost no work done to test it on animals (or humans) at these relatively low energy levels. This technology should not be used until it has been shown over several years not to cause cancer-related problems."

Skin cancer is a concern as the dose is concentrated in the skin and underlying tissue. Eyes, testicles and breast tissue are also vulnerable. Dr. Henry Lai found DNA damage from non-ionizing radiation and Dr. Singh (and other researchers) from ionizing levels. There's serious concern about effects on pregnant women and damage to reproductive DNA. Obstetrician Jacques Moritz, MD advises, "go for the patdown at the airport." Vital for pregnant women and best choice for all of us.

And there's increased risk for flight crews' high occupational exposure and for frequent flyers – both groups repeatedly pass through security. And there's wireless radiation at airports and in-flight WiFi on planes.

**Security Scanners – Safer Solutions:**

You may have to put up with the indignity of the intrusive patdown to avoid being scanned. If you are electro-sensitive or pregnant, have a pacemaker or heart condition, or have had skin cancer, inform security staff that you need this alternative; also a prudent choice with children.

(KG) "It's not just scanners; flying increases radiation exposure. During pregnancy or with babies, it is best not to travel by airplane, certainly not on an intercontinental flight. The ionizing radiation exposure from the cosmic radiation is rather high, especially at higher altitudes."

## Smart Meter ™

A Smart Meter is a remote way the electric, gas or water company reads a meter. There are several ways these meters work. Some use radio waves that can cause some people to feel ill. Contrary to what your utility company may tell you, technical experts report these emit very high levels of RF – certainly strong enough to cause health problems. Find out what method is used for yours. If it is a radio wave method, ask that the SmartMeter be replaced with a regular mechanical meter. You may have to pay a bit more, but your exposure is less, and given the evidence of adverse health effects, and some people's medical electro-sensitivity, we should have a choice – a right to health issue to fight for.

## Wired Devices

Let's look at the devices from the lower frequencies – the first part of the Spectrum. (As you may remember, we examined the third category – X-rays, etc. – in our last section with the Risk Survey information.)

## Computers

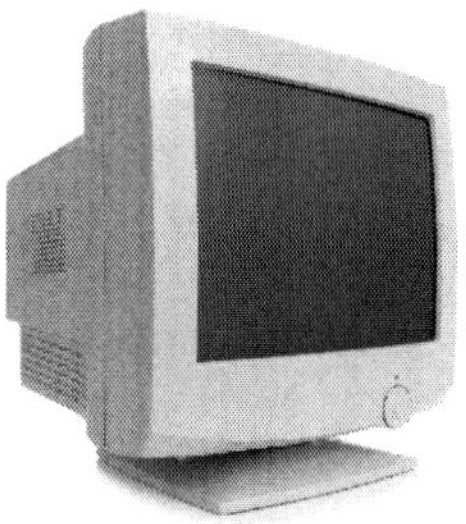

Computer screens are an EMR issue. The older standard monitors, with cathode ray tubes (CRT), emit high levels all around them. These are the curved back chunky kinds that were often found in school computer labs. Outfitting them now with wireless computers and tablets is even more harmful.

All CRT monitors give off higher fields at the back and sides. Always sit more than 1 metre (39 inches) from the rear. I have been told by EMR technicians that if you have a bank of computers, it is better to put them back to back to minimize this exposure.

Magnetic fields travel through walls, so be alert about use in the next room (for instance, don't let it be your child's sleeping room).

Smaller monitors are not necessarily better than large ones, because the field's strength depends more on the internal design than on the screen size.

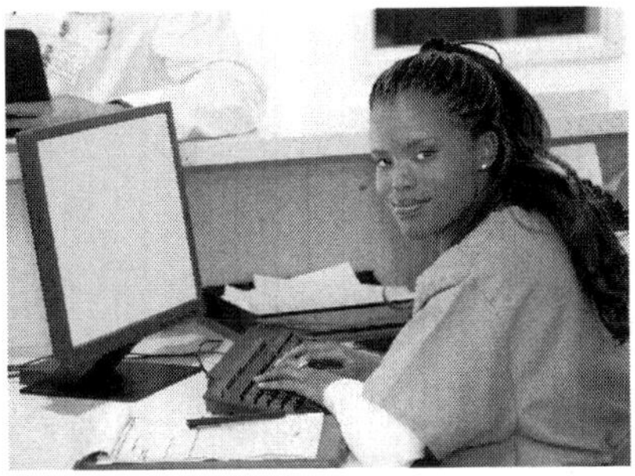

The flat LCD screen is a better choice. I chose the low-tech LCD model that had small speakers and no other frills. It also has a good-sized screen so that I could place it far back from where I sit - more than an arm's length away.

(SH) "Infrared computer gear is okay, including some keyboard and mouse connections."

Choose a wired (not wireless) keyboard, mouse, printer, speakers etc. An optical mouse, because of its design, has a higher electro-magnetic field than a laser mouse. I use a laser, corded mouse. I tested a Bluetooth® mouse and it emitted a significant amount of wireless radiation.

## Laptop computers and iPads

### The Concern:

(AP) "These handy computers can emit significant levels of electric fields from the back illumination and scanning processes. When run from the plug-in adapters, they can give off very high electric fields next to the keyboard and display, of several hundred volts/metre."

A woman asked me if the numbness in her legs might be caused by sitting for long periods with her wireless laptop on her lap. She did

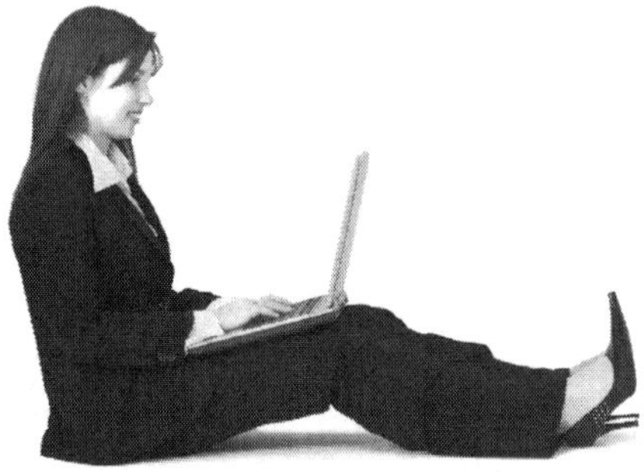

a trial of sitting in the same position for the same amount of time without the laptop, with no numbness in her legs.

Best to keep laptops, and iPads/tablets, **off** your lap and use an external keyboard.

**Laptops – Safer Solutions:**

(AP) "Charge laptops away from where you sit, then run them off their internal recharged batteries, and keep them off your lap."

**iPads – The Concern (Un-knowingly, Un-necessarily At Risk)**

Here's a wake-up call: when the WiFi antennas are turned on (there's more than one) the tablet emits a burst of radiation (e.g., iPads approximately every 4 seconds – 900 blasts an hour) even if a child is just drawing. The radiation levels are close to a cell phone's but we don't hear similar warnings – most parents and teachers have no idea. Dr. Davis speaks strongly about the iPad health hazards, "They are even worse than cell phones." How I wish these experts could speak directly to parents giving dangerous devices to their children, including children with autism (the educational apps seem ideal) and to the schools investing in this technology. We want students to be tech-savvy and to survive – why that picture is on the front cover.

**iPADS – Safer Solutions:**

There's a safer way to connect an iPad to the Internet: in airplane mode with the Bluetooth turned off. You need a Lightning to USB adaptor; a USB to Internet adaptor and a USB to a powered-on hub. More complex than an Ethernet connection (as with the Mac Air) but better than the standard iPad setup which can only go online with WiFi.

The user, too often a young child, is exposed whenever the iPad, or other wirelessly-connected device, is in the sending/receiving mode. Best to keep it on airplane mode, and far away from young people. Better still to choose a device that can easily be Ethernet connected.

There are many good reasons to limit computer time; as you know gazing absentmindedly, or even mindfully, at a computer screen can be a factor in a myriad of eye symptoms and conditions. Again, there is a real concern with the amount of time children spend staring into computer/video screens.

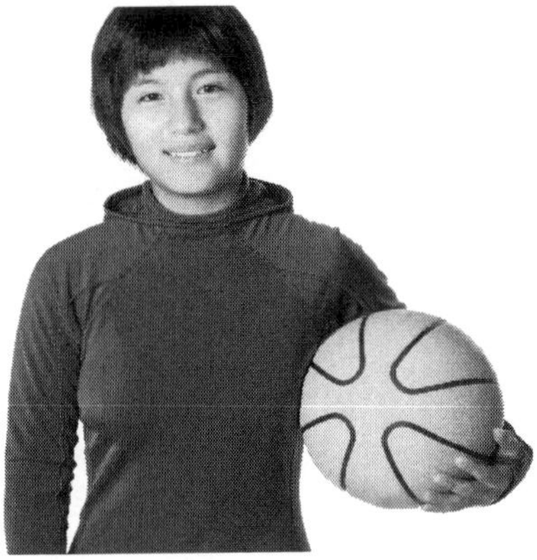

Encourage your children to get outside, whenever you can. Maybe even wander outside with them. Doesn't matter if it's not a bright sunny day.

As Richard Louv wisely remarks in *Last Child in the Woods,* "There's no bad weather, just wearing the wrong clothes."

With so much time sitting at a computer, many of us suffer from repetitive strain injuries, such as carpal tunnel syndrome, headaches and muscle pains in the low back, shoulders and neck. All in all, it's not the best activity for our wellbeing.

On my computer I keep a sticky note reminding me to:

Stretch. Breathe. Blink. Take a Break. Get outside.

In your office at home or at work, there are many electrical devices you may want to move farther away from you, downgrade to a lower tech version, or remove altogether.

### Other office equipment

How many times a day do you see people clustered around a huge, humming photocopier waiting for a long document?

### The concern:

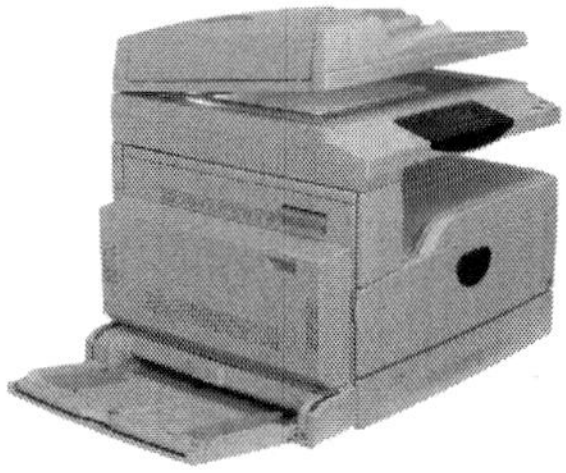

(AP) "Photocopiers give off quite high levels of EMFs from the motor. It would be advisable not to stand immediately next to the motor while it is working. Photocopiers also emit significant levels of ozone, and should always be in a well-ventilated room, or in a corridor. Volatile organic compounds (VOCs) are released, which increase with warmth, and double-sided copying. VOCs are given off even when the photocopier is not working, but is still switched on."

(AP) "Printers, scanners and fax machines can all give off significant levels of EMF near them, and some laser printers also release ozone."

### Office Equipment – Safer Solutions:

It's obviously best to place printers, fax machines, copiers etc. as far away as possible from where you sit, and don't stand next to them while they're in operation. This is the basic recommendation with all electrical equipment.

If you have a wireless printer, consider replacing it with a wired one. Ink-jet printers are more ecologically friendly than laser printers and do not give off ozone.

## Entertainment Devices

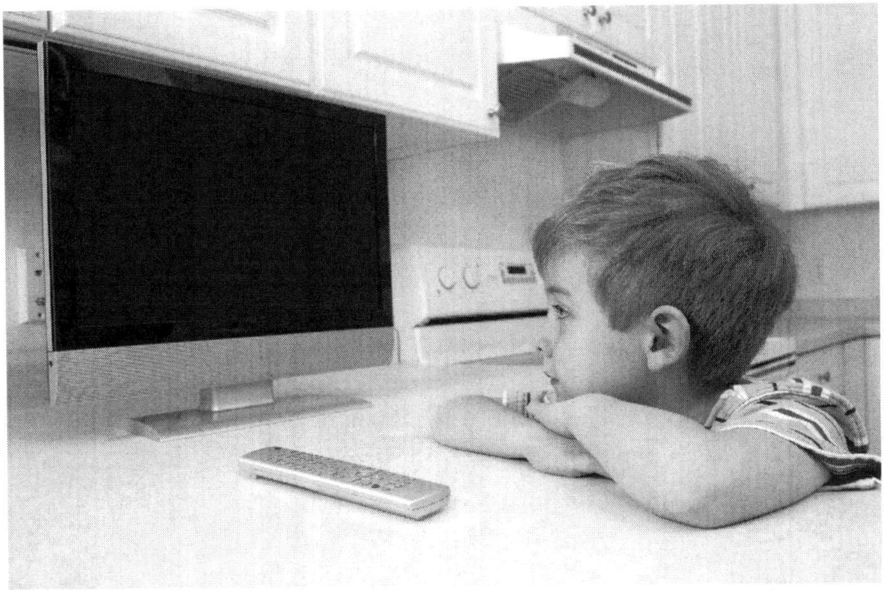

### The Concern and Safer Solutions:

**Consumer Beware**: Most new TVs have built-in wireless Bluetooth.

(AP) "**Televisions** give off high magnetic and electric fields up to 1.5 metres away (about 4 feet). Remember that magnetic fields travel through walls. EMR from **digital TVs** is not much different in level from older analog models, though some people with EHS say that they are more affected by them. Children should not sit close to any size television. Watch TV, including plasma screens, from a distance of at least 2 metres (7 feet).

**Plasma screens** give off high levels of electric fields. Use the main switch on the set to switch off the television. Some types of remote control leave the TV on standby and it continues to consume up to a quarter of the energy it uses when switched on."

(KG) "LCD TV screens usually have much lower EMF emissions than plasma TV screens."

Most TV and video remote controls work using very low-power infrared light, and pose no problems.

(RM) "Some high tech remote controls do use RF but are only transmitting when buttons are pushed."

**Analog TV reception signals** are relatively low power and are believed to have fewer adverse biological effects (but not none).

(KG) "It is true that digital TV radiation seems to be more biologically active than analog TV. But if you happen to live in the vicinity of an analog TV tower, levels are so high that this will also cause major adverse health impacts."

(RM) "TV reception signals are switching to digital and these will pose a health threat."

**Digital TV receivers** can give off high electric fields if the TV system, or satellite decoder, is not connected to the building's electrical grounding wire. Most TVs, video recorders and satellite systems are not grounded when you buy them, as they only have a two-wire power cord, rather than a grounded three-prong plug. Walls will give some protection from the electric fields; windows are less effective at screening them.

**DVD and video players and recorders** have transformers in their power supplies, which can generate strong magnetic fields.

**TV, video and Hi-Fi microwave transmitter boxes**, used to transmit pictures and sound from your main entertainment system to all other rooms in the house with a suitable receiver box, should be avoided. They are another source of microwave exposure in your home environment.

## Personal portable music players

(RM) "Personal music players can affect the electrically sensitive even if not WiFi. Recommendations are to keep electronics off of the body."

Note: The new 'improved' wireless-enabled music players are not recommended for the obvious reason that the listener is now exposed to wireless radiation. Listening to music from a laptop that is wirelessly connected is also not recommended.

## Electric Heating Pads, Electric Blankets, Electric Mattress Pads, etc.

Electric blankets and heating pads seem comforting and health-enhancing. Or at least, we think they are. Remember my surrounding my dear mother with this electric warmth to keep her sluggish circulation moving?

### The Concern:

(RM) "These heating devices have wires threaded through them, and electricity is used to create heat. I think it is easy to see the issues when they are plugged in and turned on. While operational, extreme levels of AC Electric and possibly AC Magnetic Fields can exist.

If they are turned off and still plugged in there still may be a high electric field because of the mere presence of electricity on its power cord. And the wires that run throughout the items can act as an antenna for radio waves and also re-radiate other electric fields from other sources."

Dr. Andrew Weil, (AW), a respected physician and health educator advises on his website: www.drweil.com:

(AW) "Household appliances such as heating pads, electric blankets and mattress covers, plug-in hair dryers, computers, and coffee-makers all generate EMFs that surround electrical equipment, power cords, and power lines.

Some research has suggested that exposure to low-level magnetic fields emitted by such appliances as hair dryers, electric blankets and electric razors can damage DNA in brain cells. The data come from a study in rats at the University of Washington (conducted by Henry Lai, PhD) which found DNA damage in animals exposed to a 60 hertz field for 24 hours; more damage was found after 48 hours."

## Electric Blankets, etc. – Safer Solutions:

On his website, Dr. Weil also suggests: "Because we can't say for sure that electro-magnetic fields pose no risks, I would advise you to use a non-electric heating pad, such as one that you warm up in hot water."

(RM) "Find non-electrical methods for heating your bed, like an organic wool/cotton comforter. And it is recommended to keep wires and metal away from the sleeping area. Also use a non-metallic mattress and foundation like natural latex with an organic cotton/wool topper."

## Healing Mattresses, Sleeping Pads, Mats

There are several kinds, all with testimonials and some with claims of turning harmful AC into healing DC electro-magnetic fields – not so sure as some technicians have found high AC. Yes, there are healing frequencies and some mats seem to provide benefits. Best to do your research and try it for yourself. Test with the proper meters. Power off all other electronics. Assure you can get a full refund if you feel worse.

## Your Sleep Zone – Another Reminder

As we have mentioned, all experts advise making our sleeping areas electronic-free zones, as much as we can. This is especially important if anyone is vulnerable due to age, illness, electro-sensitivity etc. or is experiencing any of the symptoms or conditions we have listed as being related to EMR exposure.

If anyone is having trouble sleeping, lowering the levels, as low as possible, is strongly recommended. Most electro-sensitive people have sleep disorders. Meters can measure to help determine the best place in the house to sleep and monitor the effectiveness of interventions.

While having a low-EMR sleep zone is very important for us all, it is *crucial* for babies and young children.

## Baby's Room – Must be a low-EMR environment

(AP) "Arrange your baby's sleeping area so that he or she is at least a metre (3.25 feet) from the nearest electric appliance and about that far away from the wall. Don't use a dimmer switch to provide a light in the baby's sleeping room, unless it is well away from the baby's head. Ensure the bulb it is lighting is red or orange, not white or bluish."

You know, of course, that it's prudent to avoid electronics in a baby's, or young child's room. These precautions include avoiding plugged-in clocks [prefer battery power], fluorescent lights [use incandescents] and cordless phones [use corded phones.] And it's best to avoid digital baby monitors – see the next few pages for details. It is especially important if you are pregnant, or want to be, or if you have a newborn or young children, to also make sure your Internet access is wired, not wireless, as a wireless router radiates for hundreds of feet (metres) in all directions. Cautions also include avoiding exposure to cell phone radiation and microwave ovens, as you know by now. Your whole family will benefit.

(RM) "Be aware of what is in the room below or beside the baby's sleeping area. I find many houses have fluorescent light fixtures mounted underneath the bedrooms, which may be on when the children are sleeping. Make sure no one, especially a child, is sleeping close to appliances in adjoining rooms. Smart Meters are also a concern."

(CA) "I recommend not having a fuse box, television, fridge or other electronics on the other side of the wall from a crib or child's bed."

**Baby Monitors**

## The Concern:

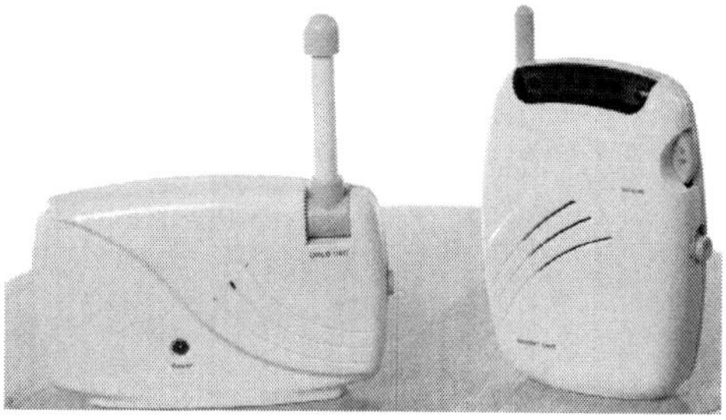

Now that you know a lot about the health hazards of wireless radiation and digital DECT cordless phones, imagine this kind of radiation-emitting device near a newborn. If you know parents who have a digital/wireless monitor in their child's room, please let them know. Let's alert the companies that make these, and the retail and online stores that sell them. When they hear that we won't buy digital/wireless monitors they will bring back the safer analog/wired ones.

Larry Gust comments: "The baby monitor signal used to be run through the house electrical wiring to where mom or dad were listening. Then 'progress' was made and the monitor went wireless using analog radio waves. This was okay as long as the monitor was not placed within six feet of baby. Then came more 'progress' using digital radio signals. A component of this signal is unhealthy for the cells in the baby's body, and yours. Now virtually all baby monitors are wireless and digital – emitting digital microwave radiation throughout the baby's room."

(KG) "Digital baby monitors measured one foot away (30cm) emit RF levels up to 20,000 (microwatts per sq. metre) – very high levels."

## A Factor in SIDS?

I read a report about an increase in sudden infant death syndrome – tragic deaths. Pre-natal EMR exposure has been shown to cause harm to organs of the developing fetus. Could this and/or exposure to the infant from digital baby monitors, mobile phones and WiFi in the home be a factor in SIDS? Is anyone looking into this, or monitoring the cumulative effects on a fetus, or infant, of unprecedented EMR levels? Until the research is done, we need to take protective action.

A grandmother who read this book, with increasing horror, evidently, told me that she insisted steps be taken to reduce EMR in her grandchildren's environment. The children's parents balked at the perceived loss of convenience but soon adapted, and she reports all are well and sleeping better. Never underestimate a determined granny.

## Baby Monitors – Safer Solutions:

(AP) "Avoid the 2.4 GHz (gigaHertz) and 5.8 GHz digital baby monitors. Use the old fashioned plug-in or analog type. As long as the analog monitor unit is six feet away from the baby, it does not appear to present a risk. Find older ones at garage sales, thrift stores, eBay, etc. Look for the antenna to be about 6 inches or more long. If the antenna is not visible, or is one inch or less, the unit is the 2.4 GHz or 5.8 GHz and should be avoided."

## Baby Sensor Pads/Crib Bedding

(AP) "Sensor pads are put under the mattress to monitor the baby's breathing. One well-known UK make was found to produce significant levels of pulsing microwaves around the baby's body."

(LG) "Some parents use sensor pads as extra protection against crib death. Wireless systems are a problem and the type of the baby's bedding is also an important concern. Dr. Jim Sprott, a New Zealand scientist, states that SIDS is caused by toxic gases. These gases can be generated from the mattress when a fungus, that commonly grows in bedding, interacts with fire retardant chemicals that are added to mattresses (Richardson 1994).

Depending on conditions, these heavier-than-air gases, generated by the fungus acting on the retardants, are concentrated in a thin layer on the baby's mattress, or dissipated into the surrounding atmosphere. If a baby breathes or absorbs a lethal dose of the gases, the central nervous system shuts down, stopping breathing and heart function. These gases can fatally poison a baby, without waking the sleeping baby and without any struggle. A normal autopsy would not reveal any sign that the baby was poisoned (Sprott 1996 & 2000)."

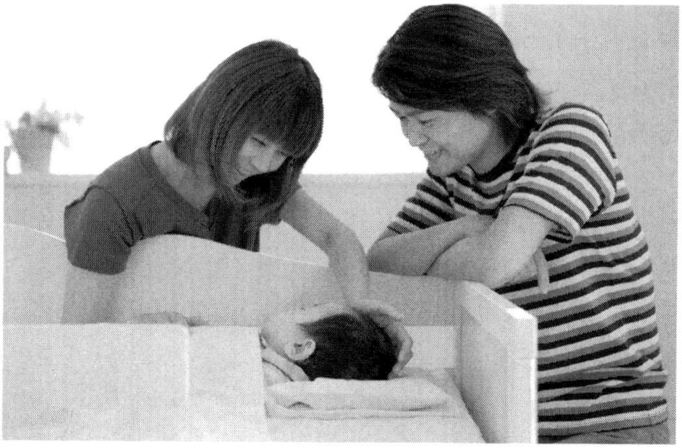

(LG) "Eliminate all sources of phosphorus, arsenic and antimony from mattresses. Putting the mattresses in a gas-impermeable cover made from high-grade polyethylene can prevent exposure to these gases plus insuring that bedding used on top of a covered mattress does not contain any phosphorus, arsenic or antimony."

Dr. Sprott specifies a pure cotton flannelette under blanket, with only cotton, or poly-cotton sheets and woolen, or cotton blankets over the baby. No other bedding should be used. Do not use synthetic sheets or blankets, duvet, sleeping bag, or sheepskin.

## Baby Sensor Pads/Crib Bedding – Safer Solutions:

The safer choice is a wired system. I tested a wireless sensor pad and the RF readings were very high, the RF readings were zero on the wired one. You need to check the magnetic fields with a Gauss meter.

## Crib toys

Battery-operated stuffies/toys look so cuddly but are they safe?

(LG) "The level of radiation of these little toys is small. Yet, newborns are in a critical phase of life. I wouldn't give one to an infant."

(AP) "I would have these toys outside, not inside, of the bed/cot. Be aware that increasing numbers of these toys have a microprocessor inside that will generate some EMF very close by."

## Baby Apps on the iPad/tablet? Or a safer screen-free baby?

All of our experts have strong views on babies being around these very high levels of microwave radiation – this is a highly dangerous way to amuse your precious child. Wise parents go screen-free and low EMR.

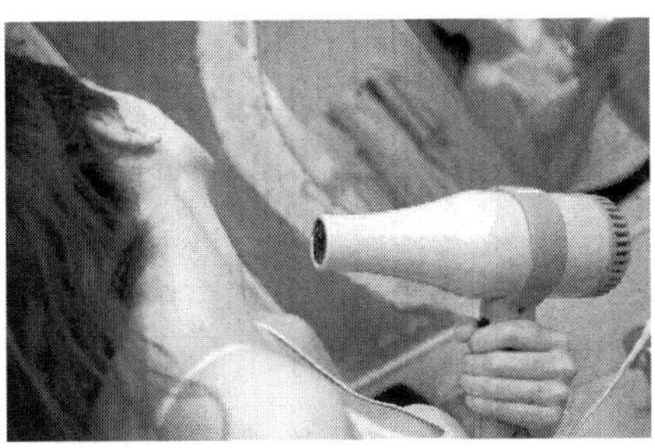

## Hair Dryers, Electric Razors The Concern:

If you are a stylist, or use a hair dryer frequently this is a concern. Remember the key factors of intensity, proximity and duration?

Dr. Henry Lai cautioned:

> Data suggest that the effects of EMF exposure are cumulative and may build up in humans over time as a result of repeated brief use of common plug-in appliances. I suggest limiting exposure to as little time as possible, particularly with devices used close to the body.

(AP) "The motor of a hair dryer gives off very high fields near the handle, dropping only a little at normal drying distances (6 to 18 inches). The fields are slightly higher on high heat, than low heat. Any metal hairpins will increase exposure. It's recommended not to use hair dryers etc. after 7 pm. High magnetic fields near the head in the evening could interfere with the production of melatonin – needed for sleep – by the pineal gland for the rest of that night.

The heating units for electric hair curlers give off significant levels. Sit away from the heating unit while it is still working. When you have removed the curlers, switch off the heating unit.

Hair curling tongs and flattening irons give off quite high fields. It is best to use them with care.

Sitting under a hooded hair dryer regularly is not recommended as they emit a high field. Metal pins will increase EMR exposure.

Electric razors also give off high fields. Again, this is more of a concern with professionals who are handling them all day."

Having read this far, no doubt you are now leaping ahead to your own safer solutions considering proximity, duration etc. There are also lower-EMF hair dryers advertised. What meter would you use to test the field around them? Yes, the Gauss meter that measures the non-communicating type of radiation.

## Hair Dryers, Electric Razors – Safer Solutions:

(AW) "The strength of EMF falls off exponentially as distance from the source increases. So hold the hair dryer farther away."

Non-electric razors are an option if you are concerned about this exposure.

## Electric Alarm Clocks/Clock Radios

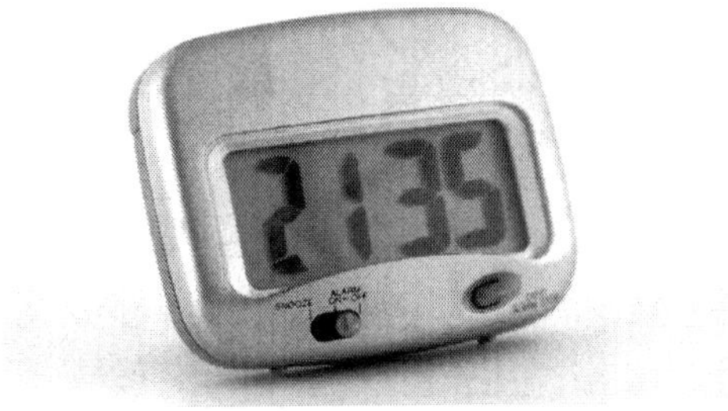

Imagine my consternation when I saw a fully-loaded bedside unit: a sleek silver wireless router, alarm clock and CD combo unit for sale, in a pharmacy, no less!

## The Concern:

If a plugged in clock, or any other electronic gadget, is lying within a few feet of your head all night, you're receiving that exposure when your body most needs a low-EMR environment. This is not a minor concern and may have significant impact on our health over time.

## Clocks – Safer Solutions:

(SH) "Plugged-in clocks, radios etc. should be kept at least 6 feet away from where you sleep."

The best option is a battery-operated alarm clock. The next best is a small electric alarm clock placed at least six feet from you; those of us older than 40 may have to get one with larger numbers!

## Other Electric Equipment

**Hot Tubs/Whirlpool Baths** – Yes, these tubs of hot swirling water are relaxing, but we should know the powerful motors produce electro-magnetic fields.

(AP) "Most have pumps and motors built in to the base resulting in high EMR exposure as you take a bath. It's recommended that the pumps and motors are at least half a metre (roughly 2 feet) away from the bath.

**Sunbeds** emit high electric and magnetic fields, as well as possibly dangerous levels of ultraviolet radiation. And many can give off five times as much UVA as would be expected from bright sunlight at the equator.

These will increase your risk of developing skin cancer, especially if you are fair-skinned.

**Sunlamps** – the EMR is not as high as sunbeds, but like sunbeds they give off ultraviolet light – a form of radiation that we know causes skin cancers.

**Exercise machines** – Motors (such as those used to power treadmills) give off high magnetic fields. You are usually not that close to the motor so they are generally not a problem. The exercise is probably more beneficial than the small level of potential risk.

**Vibrating muscle toners** emit both electric and magnetic fields. Probably all right if you are not electrically sensitive or pregnant."

(KG) "Depending an the device, muscle-toning machines can emit substantial amounts of EMF. A rebounder is definitely a safer option."

(AP) "**TENS** (transcutaneous electrical nerve stimulation) machines are used for chronic pain control and muscle stimulation. They work by passing short pulses of electrical energy though parts of the body. Not recommended if you are electrically sensitive."

## Power Tools

The problem here is much the same as with devices like hair dryers and electric razors. If you're a professional, using high-power versions all day, it's more of concern than if you're just doing the occasional odd job around the house. It may be possible to find some models with shielded power cords.

Obviously, if you're pregnant, electro-sensitive, recovering from cancer or otherwise immune-compromised, you may want to consider your use of these.

## Electrical – Wiring and Fuse Boxes

## The Concern:

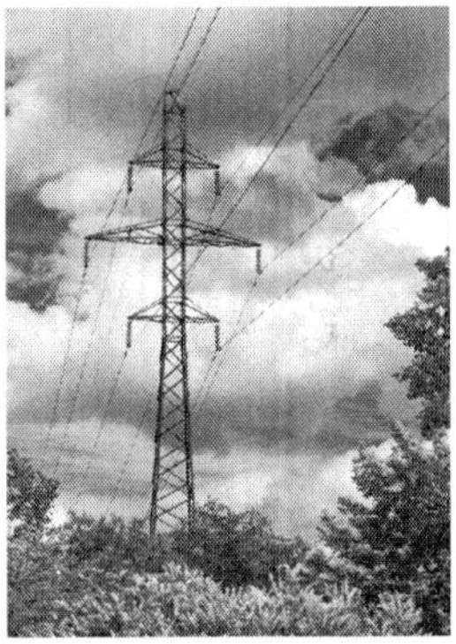

This was a surprise to me. Even when plugged-in things are not turned on, they emit an electrical field. This includes the miles of wiring in buildings.

You can test these lower frequency exposures, from the first window of our Spectrum, with a reliable electric field meter. It is worth it to have a professional testing of your home, office and school for these fields as the radiation can 'pool' in spots and the professionals know where, and how, to test for these fields. And their instruments are highly sensitive and reliable.

An EMR-qualified electrician can advise you and do the work on your house wiring – for instance installing demand switches to turn off circuits when they're not being used. Then you can retest on your own to assess the effectiveness of your interventions. This is certainly something to keep in mind when you're building a new house or about to do a major renovation.

(KG) "Demand switches should only be installed if proper testing was done first to identify the contributing circuits. To my knowledge, there is no consumer electric-field probe that would give you reliable readings. Body voltage testing can give you false readings, depending on the electrical conductivity of surrounding building materials e.g. in close range to grounding pads, stucco on wire mesh, metal roofs, etc."

### Electrical Wiring – Safer Solutions

Building or renovating?

(CA) "Ideally, it is preferable and far less expensive and problematic to have an EMR professional create a low EMR wiring design and implementation – before the construction stage – using shielded cable throughout the building. This eliminates all electric fields from wiring sources."

### Fuse Boxes – Safer Solutions:

(RM) "Locate household power meters and fuse boxes away from main living areas. They may be a source of high magnetic fields."

### Power Bars – Avoid cheap ones

Good option if you must keep your WiFi router and want an easy way to power it off at night. A quality power bar with a timer is convenient. Best to choose one *without* a surge suppressor (can be a fire hazard). If you want a surge suppressor have an electrician install one on the main panel. He/she can also make a light switch to power on/off the router.

### Power Cords

(RM) "Do not have power cords near your feet, or under your bed. Where power cords are necessary, use shielded ones as they reduce the EMF levels drastically."

### Power Lines

If you live close to power lines, you should test inside, and outside, your house and property to know how much radiation you're being exposed to. Best to hire a professional, or get a Gauss meter and do it yourself.

Experts warn that these high-voltage power lines should not be close to schools, hospitals, or where people live.

Environmental health consultant Stan Hartman tells us:

> People should also know that neighborhood power lines are a concern, as they can have stronger fields than huge towering transmission lines. Be sure to check the lines at different times of day and on different days.

Here is an example of what we are up against. In British Columbia, the official response to Moms Against Power Lines, from a chief medical health officer, was "I've been following this thing for my 35 years in public health and there is no real danger."

### Power Lines – Safer Solutions:

Ideally, you choose a neighborhood after you've checked out the radiation levels emitted from cell phone base stations, or radio or ham broadcast antennas, radar, or some power lines. Stan Hartman suggests the only solution is to paint all the walls and doors with shielding paint, and cover the windows with metal screening or metallic sunshield or shielding fabric. There's more about these products later in this section. All shielding must be properly used or it can worsen the situation.

(KG) "If properly installed, metal screenings/shielding fabric could protect from the electric field exposure (and potentially from wireless transmitters if specified for it). One of the major components of power line emissions is magnetic fields, which the shielding paints and metal screenings would not address. The safest solution for power lines is to keep sufficient distance."

## Vehicles

### Electric/Hybrid Cars

Unfortunately, the energy-saving strategy of hybrid cars may have significant risks for human health. A hybrid vehicle combines a regular internal combustion engine and an electric motor powered by batteries. When you start the car, and at low speeds, the car runs just with the electric motor and battery. At high speeds the gasoline engine kicks in. The electric motor and batteries help the conventional engine work more efficiently, so far less fuel is used compared to even very efficient gas-powered vehicles. A good goal.

### Electric/Hybrid Cars – The Concern:

However, these vehicles have big battery packs just behind the rear seat, with cables running underneath the passengers toward the front of the car. Some drivers have used Gauss meters to check inside their hybrid vehicles for the EMR levels from the flow of electrical current to the motor. They reported very high levels – hundreds of times higher than our scientists consider safe.

There are also anecdotal reports of drivers of hybrids complaining of new health problems including rising blood pressure, excessive fatigue while driving, and other symptoms of electro-hypersensitivity. I hear hybrid trucks and buses are being developed – very big batteries. Good to consider global warming, but what about health of the occupants?

(LG) "The magnetic fields are approx. 10 times higher in hybrids than in conventional vehicles, depending on the measurement location."

The back seat reading can be extremely high. Is this really where you want to put your child's car seat?

### Hybrid Cars – Safer Solutions:

Shielding for the batteries is crucial. Unlike in mobile communications, there are no information-carrying microwaves here, so the batteries can be completely covered with a special metal that blocks the EMR, without disrupting the efficiency of the battery.

(KG) "In order to block the magnetic fields from the batteries, the current-carrying wires would also have to be shielded."

The Nissan Leaf seems to have shielded cables as the magnetic field readings are lower than other electric cars. Test with a Gauss meter before buying. Ensure the Bluetooth is disabled and can't turn on; use an RF meter to test for that exposure, as you may know by now.

### EMR in your gasoline-powered car?

Even in the non-hybrid vehicles, there are hundreds of electrical devices producing strong fields. Our car has electrically-heated seats. I used to think this was a great winter feature.

### The Concern:

(KG) "Most cars emit substantial amounts of magnetic fields. Depending on the tires and the location of electronics and wiring, exposure levels can vary greatly in conventional cars, and can be just as bad as in hybrid cars."

(AP) "Cars have electrical and electronic equipment (power wiring, fan motors, computerised controls and dashboards) that can disturb electrically sensitive people. The front seat can be a risky area.

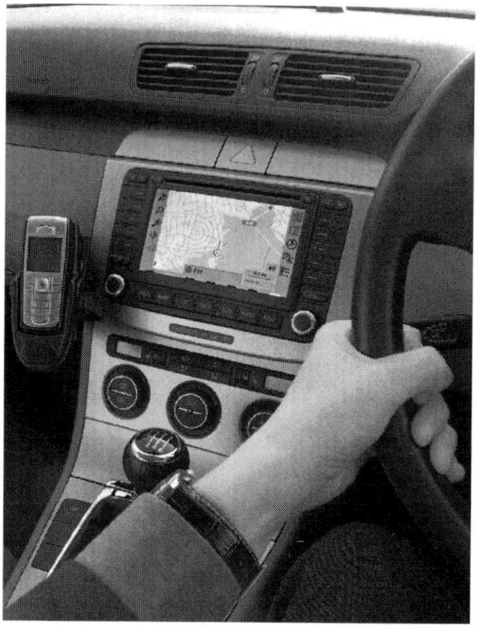

Some upscale cars have electronic control units under (or even as a part of) the driver's seat. These will give off high magnetic fields. Also worth checking is whether the angle and position of car seats are electrically controlled. These have higher EMF/EMR than mechanically operated seats."

(LG) "Other features in conventional cars can cause discomfort e.g. an air conditioning system control that sits in the ceiling right above the driver's head and puts out a high magnetic field. This has given some a blinding headache. When the cause was discovered and the equipment disconnected, the headache never returned."

(CA) "In gas-fuelled vehicles, spark plugs firing repeatedly a few feet from occupants causes RF exposure. Many EMR-sensitive people react to this. Diesel cars without spark plugs do not have this problem."

Newer vehicles present more exposure than older cars, because of on-board computers, and other high-tech additions. And we are exposed to more and more microwaves as we travel. I found a powerful WiFi router right behind the head of a hotel bed – a mere 5 inches from the sleeper's, or more likely the non-sleeper's, brain. Wake-up IT designers!

## Wireless on the road and by rail?

Most trains, cars, boats and planes are "wireless hot spots" whether you want this or not. Bluetooth/WiFi systems are activated with the ignition. Having a conductor, driver or pilot texting is an obvious distraction, but WiFi-enabled transportation presents other hazards, particularly worrying in a high-speed train or car, or aircraft. A confined metal space increases harmful effects; as you will see in the next section, and this kind of radiation impairs cognitive abilities including reaction time, as Professor Mosgoeller and other researchers have shown.

## More microwave madness: WiFi in and between vehicles?

Check out the latest "What are they thinking?" It's not hazardous enough to have vehicles packed with high-tech distracting devices and cognitive-impairing microwaves, now the US Dept of Transportation is evidently quite serious about this innovative technology – "a built-in transponder would continually transmit the vehicle's position, heading, speed and other information **10 times per second in all directions using radio signals similar to WiFi**, and then receive the same information back from other vehicles. A vehicle's computer would alert the driver to an impending collision. Some systems could automatically brake to avoid an accident." Seems risky and not just from the WiFi.

"It will change driving as we know it over time," said Scott Belcher, president and CEO of the Intelligent Transportation Society of America. "Over time, we'll see a reduction in crashes. Automobile makers will rethink how they design and construct cars because they will no longer be constructing cars to survive a crash, but building them to avoid a crash."

Intelligent transportation? How many drivers slumping over the wheel will it take before they see the transportation hazard they've created?

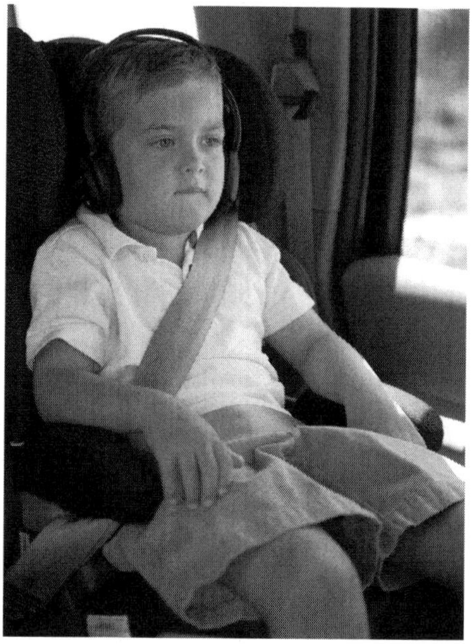

A mom asks good questions:

"I just read about a study showing WiFi is safe. Our high-tech car has Bluetooth for hands-free calls and online access – a safety feature. The kids think this is very cool. And we got them wireless headphones. Thought we were doing the right thing – so handy, so safe. How are consumers to know? Where are the regulators? Who trusts the industry to monitor itself? What can we do?"

### Non-hybrid Cars – Safer Solutions:

If you're considering buying a new vehicle, or renting one, look for fewer electronic bells and whistles, – and no Bluetooth. Use an RF meter to detect WiFi and a Gauss meter to detect the electro-magnetic fields (see Resources). It is still possible to rent a Bluetooth-free car – make sure they know you insist on this. Remember, otherwise the car becomes a WiFi hotspot when you turn on the ignition. And for our environment, opt for the most fuel-efficient conventional vehicles, limit driving, limit speeding, carpool etc.

### Global Positioning Systems (GPS)

Here's some good news. The on-board GPS is *not* so much of a concern, unless it gets 'amped-up' for sending and receiving functions.

(LG) "The GPS is a receiving-only device emitting a small amount of radiation – more like a radio."

## Airplane Travel, WiFi – Safe in the Sky?

Alasdair Philips, an electrical engineer, has done onboard testing of the electro-magnetic fields in aircraft cabins and cautions:

> Most airlines now provide in-flight mobile phone and WiFi service. They are installing a picocell base station – effectively, a small mobile phone mast – onboard the aircraft. Passengers web-browsing and video streaming greatly increase the RF levels in the cabin.

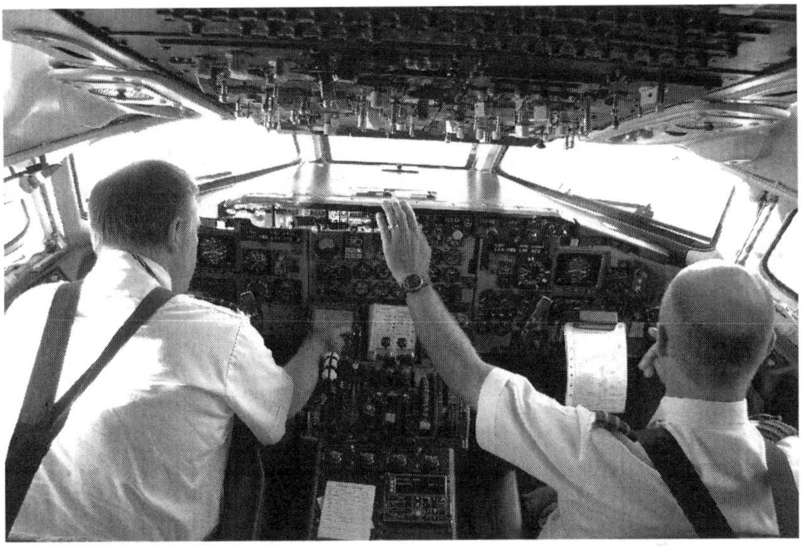

Many other experts are alarmed by this techno trend. A group of European physicians, the German Environmental Physician Initiative, headed by Dr. Scheiner, sent a letter to several airline companies about how in-flight WiFi can affect the passengers, and the crew – including the crew's cognitive functions. Now that's a scary thought. Stay tuned.

Yes, the proponents of this new technology have tested it for interference with aircraft navigation systems. Yet we hear of incidents where it has caused interference. And there are *no reports* that anyone has tested the impact on the pilot, other air crew, or the passengers.

## Radiation from Mobile Phones and Reaction Time

Here is part of Dr. Scheiner's 2008 letter:

"There are not yet any scientific studies of the biological effects on the crew and passengers, but there is enough evidence to cause concern. While the airplane is moving at an altitude between 8,000 and 12,000 metres, a reduced air pressure occurs inside of the plane, which equals the air pressure of 2,000 – 3,000 metres outside. Therefore the breakage of the blood-brain barrier is more likely because of the lack of oxygen and the well known altitude sickness. The severe consequences of the brain and nerve damages and safety of passengers are very concerning especially those of the pilots, because they are already highly exposed from radar. The symptoms caused by high frequencies include: headaches, drowsiness, vertigo, nausea are often connected with loss of hearing and vision; lack of concentration and memorization. (Johnson-Liakouris, 1998, Mild 1998, Santini 2001, 2002, 2003, Navarro, Oberfeld 2003). A British lab found that reaction time is much longer when someone is exposed to WiFi and mobile phones. This is particularly a concern with the pilot's reaction time, when these high frequencies open the blood-brain barrier. Researchers at the University of Toronto found that drivers of vehicles were nearly five times more likely to have an accident when people were using mobile phones in the car."

In 2012 Dr. Scheiner warned again, "Equipping aircraft with WiFi is a dangerous experiment. Even quite low levels of radio-frequency (RF) radiation – from WiFi and mobile devices – can open the blood-brain barrier and cause a lot of harm, including miniature edemas destroying brain cells which cannot be renewed. This damage presents an increased risk of neurodegenerative conditions including Parkinson's disease. At the actual RF levels which are expected to occur on board commercial airplanes equipped with WiFi, 100% of the animals tested had serious brain damage. Electro-hypersensitivity is another issue: People with this condition may faint, feel dizzy, or have impaired vision. It's likely these are signs of opening of the blood-brain barrier. People may also experience nausea, muscle weakness, skin reactions and lack of concentration. Review Dr. Mosgoeller's reaction time research that found disturbing changes in human brainwaves during RF exposure (from mobiles and WiFi) causing the subjects to make bad decisions more quickly." The last thing you want happening to your pilot.

Alasdair Philips explains some technical details:

> Most planes have in-flight video screens built into the back of each seat. The personal lights above the seats can be sources of significant electric fields. Turn yours off. With added wireless Internet and mobile devices, the RF radiation will bounce up and down the cabin 'metal tube'. There are also signals from various plane transponders mounted under the fuselage which make their way up into the cabin at surprisingly high levels. Many planes also have an emergency Iridium phone system that is internally active all the time they are in the air.

Have a heart condition or pacemaker? Or epilepsy? (In 2014 the Israel Ministry of Health warned doctors about iPads and epilepsy, an alert from Dr. Scheiner, as well.) High-tech aircraft and mobile devices can be even more hazardous to your health. If you have a medical incident on board a Wi-Fi-enabled aircraft you may have grounds for litigation?

## In-flight Incidents (Fainting Pilots?) Should Raise an Alert

A pilot had a mental breakdown and was carried off the plane yelling, "You can just email me." A few years later, a highly-experienced pilot has a mental breakdown screaming about terrorist threats and has to be restrained mid-flight, on a WiFi-enabled aircraft. And in 2013, there were two reports of pilots fainting in-flight – also on WiFi aircraft.

These incidents could have nothing to do with EMR. I asked pilot, air safety investigator and aviation expert Dr. Todd Curtis to review a document I prepared and sent to aviation officials. (Available at www.safertechsolutions.org) Here is an excerpt from his expert opinion:

"The issue of in-flight WiFi has recently been brought to my attention by Dr. Kerry Crofton, and her colleagues. Although the risk of RF radiation from WiFi routers and other equipment hasn't been looked at as a health and safety risk by the aviation community, the fact that some quarters in the medical and scientific communities have shown that this may be a risk is a concern to me. In reviewing the material sent to me by Dr. Crofton, it seems there is enough evidence to warrant further investigation. I am not aware of any tests on in-flight WiFi, or if there a requirement, with respect to potential health effects on flight crews. It appears this new technology has been tested on the electrical systems, navigation systems but not on the flight crews. It would make sense for the appropriate authorities – the FAA and elsewhere – to take a serious look at this issue.

Reportedly, there have been separate incidents of two pilots fainting in-flight – apparently on aircraft with WiFi installations. This could be a huge red flag. That sort of a medical event in the air, with pilots being medically incapacitated, isn't necessarily reported. If there were a common cause, the major concern would be if both pilots in the cockpit became incapacitated. In this event all the flight crew, cabin crew and passengers would soon be 'in a world of hurt.' The concern is not just the pilots; the cabin crew's biggest job is safety – if they are incapacitated that is also a potential problem. Should there be any factor that impairs the flight and cabin crews at once you could have a catastrophic situation.

As entertainment and communication technology advances in this digital age, passengers are looking for in-flight WiFi, and this is income generating for all airlines. I don't fault the airlines. It is the aviation regulatory bodies responsibility to ensure that any new technology that is introduced into an aircraft does not have a negative effect on the health and safety of the passengers, and especially on the health and performance of the flight crew (pilots) and cabin crew. As many of the experts in Dr. Crofton's document have stated – there is no evidence that this new WiFi technology has been tested on the crew, or is being monitored. I have to ask if anyone is tracking WiFi flights to monitor any potential adverse effects on pilot performance, fatigue etc? Was the radio-frequency radiation exposure from the onboard WiFi one of the contributing factors in the pilots' fainting? Is this factor even being considered?" – Dr. Todd Curtis

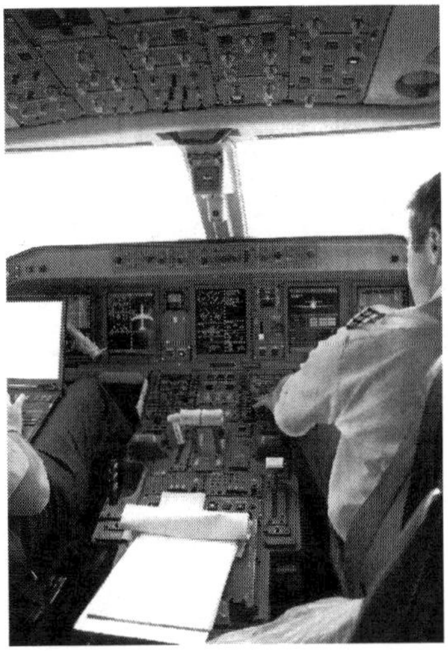

**WASHINGTON, October 2009** (Reuters) – "Pilots of a jetliner that overshot its destination by 150 miles last week told U.S. investigators they became distracted during an extended discussion of crew scheduling that included their use of personal laptops." Evidently, their airline offers in-flight WiFi.

Here's a comment from a commercial pilot on navigational interference: "I had an HSI spin around for about 10 minutes in cruise on the A320, until a business class passenger was asked to stop his cell phone call. The needles immediately stopped when he turned off his cell phone." So, maybe this aspect wasn't well tested?

Yes, most people are clamoring to use their personal electronics onboard. Airline marketing departments take note: Don't you think that most people value being safe in the sky more than convenience?

Airline litigation departments: consider the ramifications if there's an incident and it's proven that no one pre-tested the acute, or long-term, effects of this radiation on the cognitive and cardiac functions of pilots and that airlines ignored medical warnings?

I used to work in the aviation industry leading programs for pilots and air traffic controllers and was a member of the Canadian Aviation Tribunal. I predict a reversal on in-flight electronics. Maybe security concerns, not health and safety issues, will be the wake-up call.

**Aviation Security In The Digital Age** is a new challenge: online connectivity in the skies could facilitate communication between terrorists planning, or co-ordinating, an attack. In 2014, there's global concern with new explosives: bombs undetected by security scanners hidden in laptops and other electronics. In the US, the TSA banned battery-dead cell phones from flights. In-flight WiFi could be next?

**And there are privacy issues**. Also in 2014, there was a report that a Canadian spy agency collected personal data from airport passengers' smartphones and laptops over a two-week period and tracked those devices for a week or longer afterward. What else don't we know?

Then there's the annoyance factor: loud, endless chatter, or worse, on nearby mobile devices, and if you are electro-sensitive it is already difficult for you to travel. As more of us become electro-sensitive, we will need special areas set aside in airports that are "WiFi-Free".

**Safer Solutions?** Lobby the airlines, and regulatory agencies, to test the effects of EMR exposure on flight crews, and passengers, not just on the technical equipment. The marketplace responds to us, the consumers. Talk to pilots and other flight crew. I have worked with many pilot groups and have great respect for their professionalism. No one cares more about flight safety than they do.

## Hotel/Motel Accommodations

Even roadside motels tout enhanced WiFi. When more of us request *wireless-free* accommodations, this will change. Explain you are sensitive to, and/or concerned about, WiFi radiation – an opportunity to awaken them. Ask about the location of cell tower antennas and WiFi routers/access points. Secure a room with a weaker signal. I travel with small squares of shielding fabric to cover the router if it can't be turned off. A corner room on the ground floor, furthest away from routers, elevators and the electrical room – is best. Unplug cordless phones; I bring a small corded one. Then let go and relax and maybe use some natural melatonin and calcium/magnesium to sleep better.

## Tech-free Retreats – Off-the-Grid and Back On Track

No WiFi, digital devices or electronic gadgets here. Just fun and games and being outside. Wilderness experts, spirited camp leaders and guest instructors provide a 'back-to-the-earth' retreat for all ages. A digital detox is to break free of screen fixations and to reconnect with each other face to face. Remember that? The Mindful EYE contemplative photography is a creative way to slow down and tune in, and Simplicity mindfulness meditation, yoga, Tai Chi and Qi Gong quieten the most jazzed-up mind. Sketch, journal, wander in the woods, watch birds – this does wonders to de-stress and to enhance your state of mind, social interactions and relationships. Then for re-entry to the digital world look at safer-tech solutions to maintain this balance ongoing – connected and still on track. (See pages 314-321 for more inspiration.)

Visit SaferTechSolutions.org for details, and how you can host one; or how to make your existing retreat or program tech-free, or safer-tech.

Also see the Campaign for a Commercial-Free Childhood's screen-free week and to bring the whole family together again – tech-free.

## Other Ways to Reduce Our EMR Exposure?

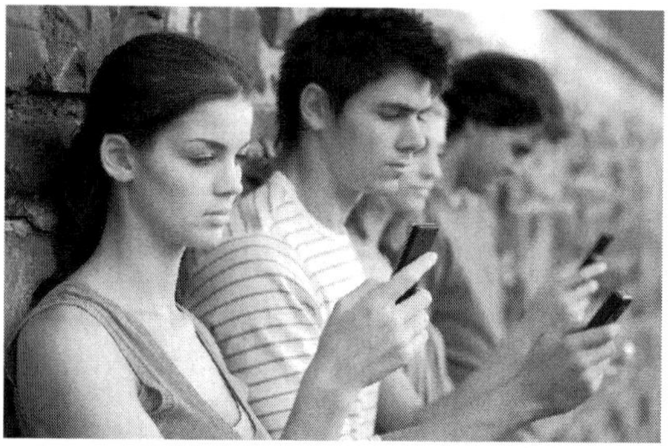

With so many of our younger generation using mobile phones, wouldn't it be comforting to think that there was a quick and easy solution to protect them from the radiation? At this point, there does not seem to be a scientifically sound way to prevent all harmful biological effects with 'protective' devices.

## Chips, Pendants etc.

People often ask me about the numerous devices on the market, such as radiation-deflecting/harmonizing chips that you stick on your cell phone or laptop, or about jewelry – pendants or bracelets – that you wear. These kinds of interventions are described as enhancing your own energy field in some way, and/or harmonizing/neutralizing the artificial electro-magnetic fields.

Some of these products seem to be helpful, for some people, at least for a while; many do not. I tried some of these myself, at one time. This technology, while promising, does not seem to provide the answer, just yet. Before investing, and trusting in this protection, you need to see some solid science on their effectiveness – not just testimonials. And insist on seeing the scientific evidence of how long the reported protection lasts.

And some clinicians advise that for some electro-sensitive people, these kind of protective interventions are contra-indicated because they may make symptoms worse.

The safety consultants I've talked with are concerned that 'magic bullets' like chips, pendants, diodes etc. may lull people into a false sense of safety – using their cell phones, cordless phones, iPads etc. and wireless routers without caution, believing they are now safe.

Having said that, some people report benefits from Swiss Harmony products that reportedly reduce EMR-related symptoms. To repeat myself – anything like this should be used with reducing EMR exposure, as there is no evidence the products prevent all adverse effects.

Technical experts also stress the need for proper testing and shielding. Sensory Perspective in the UK offers people information and tools to protect themselves, including the very handy Electrosmog Detector.

One of their technical directors explains:

> Sensory Perspective focuses on what it knows will work: certifiably calibrated measuring instruments for detection, EMF barrier products for protection. We simply suggest that one uses suitable barrier products (shielded curtain materials, wallpapers, paints) for the home or office. www.detect-protect.com

## Physical Radiation Barriers

These kinds of products work by deflecting/blocking the radiation in some way. Stan Hartman comments on one example, pocket protectors: "I haven't tested any of them, but assuming that they shield the high frequencies from the phone, that still leaves the low-frequency magnetic fields from the battery-saver technology, which they can't shield.

It's best to just keep the phone at a distance in a purse or backpack or something – or toss it, of course. Certainly don't put it in a pocket over your heart."

## Shielding Materials

If you've done everything you can to reduce your exposure, you may still want or need more protection from sources you can't control. In that case, you might have to do an EMR-repelling reno. This might include special window screens or films, wallpapers and EMR absorbing paints.

Stan Hartman gives us some expert advice on shielding:

> Keeping out microwaves is a little like trying to keep out blowing sand, though – you can do it, but you have to be sure there aren't any sources inside or any crevices for the radiation to get in through. That means no CFLs or other fluorescent lights, for instance, or CRTs – the old TV sets and computer monitors – or microwave ovens. If you have inescapable internal radiation sources, you could be better off not shielding at all and just trying to avoid radiation while you're sleeping at least, with a bed shield.

When it comes to shielding fabrics, wallpapers, paints, etc. caution is required. Shielding curtains, and bed canopies, are made from a fabric made of RF reflective fibers. This fabric is very effective at blocking RF – but you MUST use it properly, or you can get badly zapped! Some of these products have to be grounded. Do not use any of these without professional consultation, even if it's just a phone conversation with the supplier.

For example, the bed canopy fabric has to be properly draped away from the edges of the bed so it does not touch you, or any pet sleeping nearby. You cannot have any EMF/EMR sources inside the space draped by the fabric – no regular lamps, plugged in clocks, alarms etc.

So how do you read? A non-metal lamp, with an incandescent light bulb (not halogen or fluorescent) and shielded power cord is recommended.

And you need demand switches to reduce the electric and magnetic fields in the room before you use the fabric. A demand switch is a smart electronic device that automatically cuts off electricity when there is no demand for it. It also supplies electricity when there is a demand. Saves on your power bill, as well. This is one area where, unless you're a licensed electrician, you'll need professional help.

It's important to note that shielding devices, and therapeutic interventions, that may be very helpful for people without symptoms, can be devastating for electro-sensitive people, if not used properly.

At the end of the book, in Resources, I have listed sites in several countries, operated by qualified experts. You could begin your research there if you're considering adding these to your home.

## Where to Start?

As you contemplate changes you might want to make in your family's technology habits, this thoughtful message from our "library mum" may be useful:

> As you know, my life is very hectic but I am now taking a break more often to get outside with the kids. It's great for them, and for me. I'm not even texting at the beach.
>
> And, thanks for Strategy 3, it was lucid, well set out and not frightening, after all. After reading it last night, I became convinced that it is necessary for us to have the discipline to do something about our cell phone use.

> So, I see *A Wellness Guide for The Digital Age* can be read on various levels. It can lead to basic changes – but it can also lead to quite profound changes. It has already instigated these more philosophical reflections on our life choices in our family.

Yes, this book is packed with cautions and recommendations. This can be quite a lot to take in and may be more than you want to know?

I hope you have found this section useful and feel good about what you can do to protect your family. It's great if you can involve them and explain that when you were young there weren't all these digital distractions, that we played outside more often. Yes we had tvs but our screen time was nothing like today.

As we have said, it is not only the health concerns but also the importance of our connection with nature and with each other.

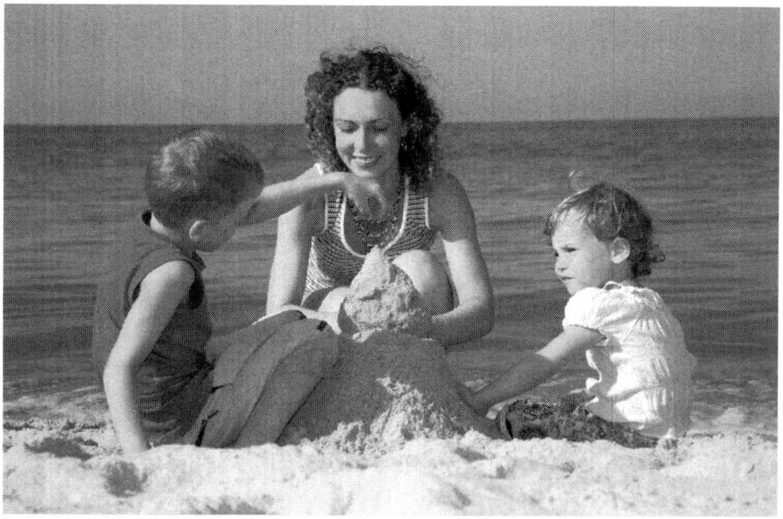

I'd like to summarize some of these best practices for you.

## 7 Key Reminders

### Key point: choose wired over wireless, and corded over cordless

1. Switch your cordless phones to corded ones. Please don't give up your landline phone (and they are also health-savvy gifts);
2. Seek wired solutions for all things wireless, including your Internet access, keep laptops and all wireless devices off your lap, and please do not use digital baby monitors;
3. Keep your cell phone simple (basic, low SAR), and away from heads, hearts, pregnant women and the young or frail. Limit use;
4. Use your mobile's speakerphone (rather than wireless or wired headsets), and remember the most hazardous option of all is holding a mobile device against your head;
5. Avoid using a cell phone as an alarm, and do not sleep near it;
6. Tell your airline and hotel that you want a wireless-free environment;
7. Talk to your local legislators, calmly and clearly. Provide some information (not overwhelming them) and ask for a response.

NOTE: If your child's iPod (or other digital device) can send and receive messages – in other words go online – the child is being harmed by microwave radiation when the device is transmitting. Leave it on airplane mode, as much as possible.

Keeping young people safe is our responsibility, so best to make sure music devices do not have Bluetooth or other transmitting mode, and you know by now giving them a cell phone is not keeping them safe.

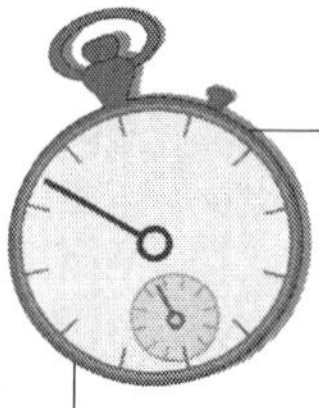

*2 Minute Quick Read Summary*

## Strategy 4 Your Action Plan

Now that you understand – from Strategy 1 – why so many experts are concerned, and know how to recognize the related symptoms and conditions – from Strategy 2 – and have learned what sources you need to address – in Strategy 3 – you are well-outfitted to draft your priorities here, then go to Strategy 4 for your Action Plan.

Strategy 4 includes a room by room EMR audit; medical information about preventing and treating many symptoms and conditions that can be related; details on biological dentistry, and more. There is also a section on the Safer-Tech Family.

First, you might want to try this.

**Our Safer-Tech Challenge Intentions**
Top Priorities - what I want to tackle first:

Secondary priorities – what I want to deal with after that:

I should consult a professional to assess the following:

Other environmental exposures I want to address:

**See Strategy 4 for more details.**

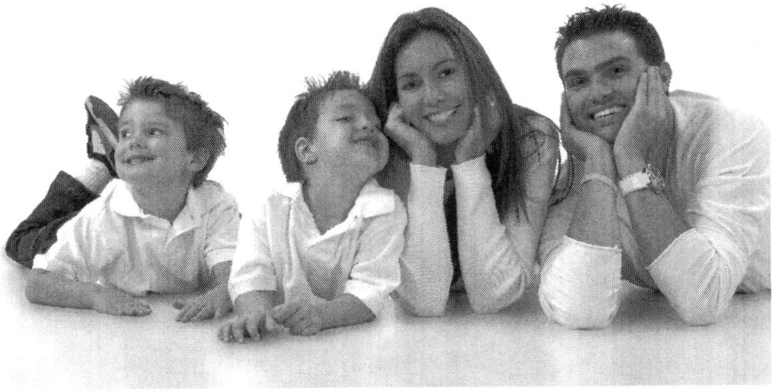

## Strategy 4. Your Action Plan

Is anyone in your family already experiencing a lot of possibly related symptoms – difficulty sleeping, dizziness? Or one of the conditions that may be connected – headaches, insomnia, learning disorders, autism/Asperger's etc.?

If so, you will want to approach this step more vigorously as these people are more vulnerable.

If no one is experiencing symptoms, it does not mean the radiation is not having biological effects. It does give you the opportunity to reduce your family's exposure and risk of these symptoms and conditions.

You will also want to keep in mind the factors like proximity, intensity, duration/frequency as you decide on your priorities for action.

## Room by Room – EMR Audit and Recommendations

Fairly soon I decided not to bog down in guilt, resentment or denial. I became determined to protect my family and sought help, as I have explained, from the best sources I could find. Now all of that is set out here for you. Keep in mind this is not a quick fix; it is a process that takes some time.

My family began with a professional assessment. I strongly urge you to do the same, particularly if you are considering shielding fabrics, or other interventions that can cause problems if not used or installed correctly.

In the case of retro-fitting your home, or anything to do with electrical wiring, or shielding technology, it's wise to consult with and hire qualified professionals. Some of these are listed in the Resources section.

### Testing of Your Home, Office and School

**The Do-It Yourself Assessment** – consumer devices to measure EMR are very helpful, not only in your own environment – but also vital when traveling (see Resources). You must know the basics, however, about the instruments, and what you are testing, or you can make your situation worse, not better. Like my friend with the microwave oven.

**The Professional Assessment** – this is key, in my view. Here is what Rob Metzinger (RM) advises: "Before the proper solutions can be implemented the primary sources of the problem – internal and external – must be identified."

Testing of Electric Fields, Magnetic Fields and RF (radio-frequency) should be done with the most sensitive testing equipment available.

The professionals' recommendations should look something like this:

1. Devices/sources to remove, perhaps in an order of priority for your situation: the urgent first-to-go, and then remove as you can, etc.

2. Devices/sources to replace, and with what ….

3. Alterations in position, use of the devices/sources etc.

4. Protective Interventions – shielding fabric etc.

Once solutions have been put in place the site must be re-tested to verify the efficacy of the products. Periodically the site should be retested to ensure the interventions are still performing and that new sources of contamination have not arisen.

## Some Tips on Having a Professional Assessment

Before you have the pros come in it is helpful to label your electrical control panel. Make sure the person turning the breakers on and off is wearing non-conductive gloves, and is <u>not</u> electro-sensitive.

Mark each light switch and wall socket (in pencil) with the circuit number, and the same number, obviously, on the control panel (in pen). The technicians will check this but it saves you money if you can get a head start on this step.

Then they will go room by room – and outside of the building – to test for the electric, magnetic and radio-frequency exposures.

As we move through your house, I'll offer what I learned during our audit and in the eight years since. Our experts' recommendations for safer/less harmful alternatives are in square brackets, like this [ ].

**EMR Testing Equipment:** Exposure levels are on pages 60 and 61 and see page 112 for various kinds of electro-magnetic fields.

If you are using testing equipment before, or instead of, a professional assessment, please be very careful. Three things to keep in mind:

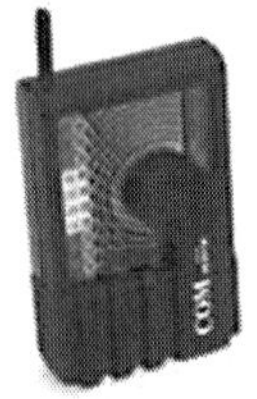

1. Do you know how to use the meter?

2. Is it reliable? Consumer models may not detect the higher frequency devices – your digital cordless phone, for example – and so you would have a false 'safe' reading.

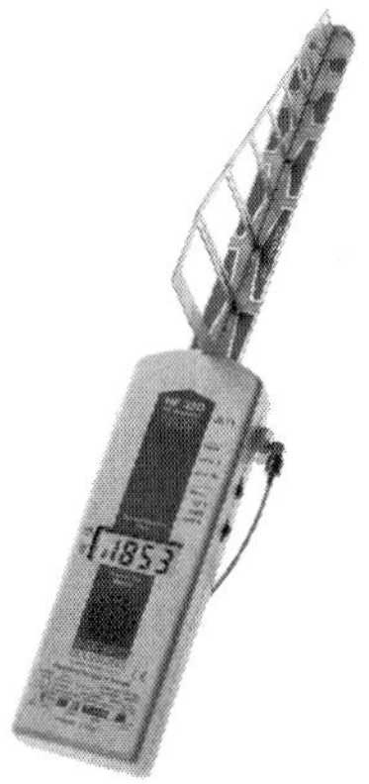

3. Are you using the correct meter? An RF (radio-frequency) meter tests: microwave oven; cordless phone (handset/base); cell phone; Bluetooth; WiFi; any wirelessly connected computer, game, baby monitor, sensor; cell tower; Smart Meter (some transmit intermittently). To roughly find hot and cool spots, I recommend the affordable effective Electrosmog Detector – useful when travelling to find the least hazardous place to sit and to sleep – available at www.detect-protect.com.

For electrical outlets, appliances, heating pads and other wired devices you need a Gauss meter. You need an electric meter to test built-in wiring and extension cords/power bars. You see why a professional assessment is best.

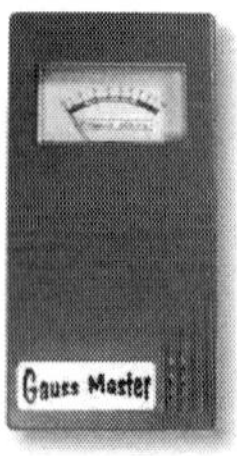

A professional assessment is crucial if someone in your family is having symptoms that may be related. Pregnant women, children and seniors are most vulnerable, as we have discussed. Refer to the Resources section for qualified EMR testing and remediation consultants, and for do-it-yourself testing equipment.

Most electricians don't know these specifics and may assure you "no need to test, there's no problem, it's all to code and within government standards". This is a sign to continue looking for a trained professional.

When looking for a new home (buying or renting) have EMR testing done. It's surprising how faulty electrical installation can harm health. And watch out for high-tech, 'smart' innovations, such as a wireless home security system, electrically-heated floors, or Smart Meters.

**Front Porch**

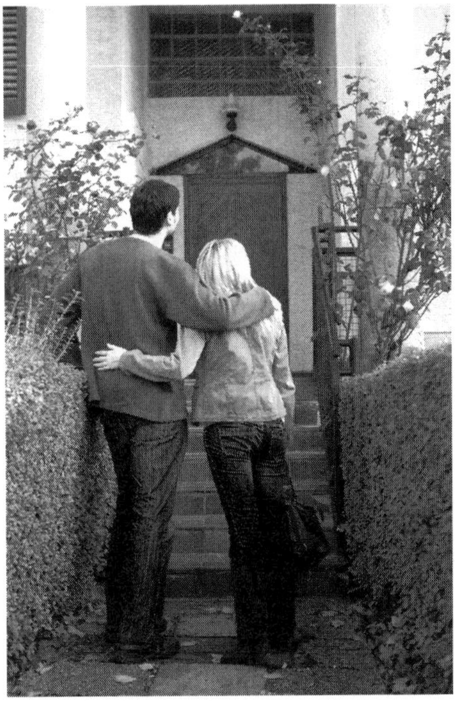

Let's start this house tour right at the front doorstep. First, is there a wireless home security system, or a wireless front doorbell [hard-wired options]? Is the outdoor light fluorescent [low wattage incandescent]? An automatic garage door opener communicates wirelessly but is not considered a significant risk. [Just be mindful of this and don't point the clicker directly at anyone standing between it and the door. Same recommendation for the TV channel changer.]

## Bedrooms

The sleep zone is crucial to your wellbeing. As you may remember, EMR is known to disrupt sleep in many ways. Is your bedroom a radiation hot spot, or a calm low-tech oasis?

Besides looking at your own sleeping area, check out the places where children and/or pets sleep.

You are looking for: everything wireless, everything electric – all things plugged in – including clocks, radios, portable phones, TVs, electric beds, heaters, heating pads, electric cords, battery chargers, wall sockets, fluorescent (including compact fluorescent) or low voltage halogen lights, dimmer switches, lamps with transformers or the clap-on, or touch-on feature, everything metal – lamps, bed frames, headboard, footboard, side rails and box spring mattresses. No, you don't need to toss all of these, just note them and identify the ones that are creating high EMR.

[To reduce your EMR exposure, remove or unplug electronic devices located in the sleeping areas such as: televisions, DVD/VCRs, electric clock radios/alarm clocks, stereo systems, heating pads, electric blankets, and waterbeds. Battery-operated alarm clocks are a good alternative, or at least put the electric one a minimum of six feet away from your head.]

[If you absolutely have to have a television or a computer – with hard-wired Internet – in your bedroom, put them as far away as possible from the bed, and put them on a power bar that you turn off at night – or on a timer power bar. Best to choose a quality power bar without a surge suppressor which can be a fire hazard.]

[Replace an electric blanket or heating pad with a hot water bottle or gel pack, or use the electrical kind just to heat up your bed, then turn off and unplug the cord before you get in.]

Metal is not recommended in sleeping areas as it reflects, and re-radiates, radiation from all surrounding sources, worsening exposures. Like most of us, you probably need to budget for many changes here. Science tells us that children are at least ten times more vulnerable to any toxic exposure than adults, so they need more protection.

[Making our children's bedrooms a priority, our technical experts urge us to: replace box springs with ones that contain no metal; replace coil and spring mattresses with foam mattresses made from low emission natural latex, or cotton mattresses such as futons (and to use natural cotton fabrics wherever possible to reduce static electricity); and to replace metal bed frames, metal cribs, metal bedside tables and lamps, metal bunk beds – with safer non-metallic types.]

[As we could afford it, I replaced these items, and our metal-framed bed with a solid wood one that even has wooden slats to hold the natural fiber futon mattresses.]

[My husband and I built a wooden reading lamp with a specially insulated electrical cord. We removed the halogen lamps with the transformers that had set the detector screaming.

And we replaced all fluorescent lights with regular incandescent ones.] Everyone in our family is mindful of energy consumption and we have many other ways to conserve energy and costs.

Ideally, and especially if you are suffering from any symptoms, shut off power in the rooms where you sleep and all the adjacent rooms, above and below this area, at night. This can be done by turning off the corresponding breakers, or by using a demand switch.

You may find inspiration in creating a low-tech, low EMR sanctuary where you sleep. Instead of a TV area, why not think about a space for calming practices like meditation, yoga or tai chi?

These have many benefits including balancing our life force energies that are so disrupted by electro-pollution – more on this later.

### Children's Room

You want to go through your children's room with a sharp eye of awareness. Check for everything that is plugged in, the lights, electronic equipment etc. [Move the beds/cribs away from the wall – from any wall sockets and even the wiring in the wall. Avoid the use of sensor pads under baby.]

I'm presuming you are onboard by now in removing everything that hints of wireless – Internet access, cordless phones, wireless baby monitors [replace with low-powered plug-in ones, if you must have one].

[Use wooden beds without metal box springs or metal coiled mattresses. Use incandescent lights and battery alarm clocks.] Remember what Alasdair Philips told us about night lights – it's best to sleep in as dark a room as possible and that [plug-in red or orange, soft glow ones are preferred over white or blue lights, if we must have one.]

You might discuss this safer-tech reno with your children before yanking out their electronic entertainments and explain why you want their bedrooms healthier and safer for them. As you know, these issues are not high on any child's priority list.

### Bathroom

You might test the electric toothbrush, electric razor and the hair dryer – using a Gauss meter. And check for microwave radiation around any mirrors or windows using a RF meter.

I realized the electric in-floor heating was not a great idea. Turning the dial down to "off" is not enough. [I had it disconnected.] Is the floor colder in the winter? Yes. But with a thick, cotton bath mat, it's fine. Also during that reno, I had found a quite large mirrored wall unit that we hung above the sink. It seemed like a great idea at the time. When the radiation detector "ghost busters" did our home assessment, the radiation bouncing off that mirror and metal cabinet was extreme.

(We may have to rethink some Feng Shui principles; while mirrors are considered good reflectors of energy, they do however also reflect what we could call the "negative energy" of EMR). [Now we have a small wooden framed mirror, and a small wooden shelf on the side wall.] After this EMR-busting retrofit, the radiation levels in the bathroom are now minimal.

As we've discussed, the health hazards in our homes are not all from EMR. Plastic shower curtains were found to off-gas toxic chemicals – and were still off-gassing a month after the package was opened! [I also replaced the plastic shower curtain with a fabric one.] And you may know about the chlorine and other chemicals in our tap water. [We have a filter on our shower head and another in the kitchen for our drinking and cooking water.]

You have the option of chemically- scented personal care products, cosmetics etc. [or the less toxic alternatives]. I discovered that virtually all standard brands of deodorant contain aluminum. Just 'trace amounts'. [All brands in natural health food stores are labeled "aluminum free."

Same recommendation goes for baby powder and baking powder – check for aluminum-free brands.] Dousing a newborn with sweet-smelling powder laced with aluminum? What are we thinking?

## A friend reports on her home testing

On the weekend I used the device that measures wireless radiation. The three "hot spots" were the portable phone, cell phone and the wireless router near the kitchen.

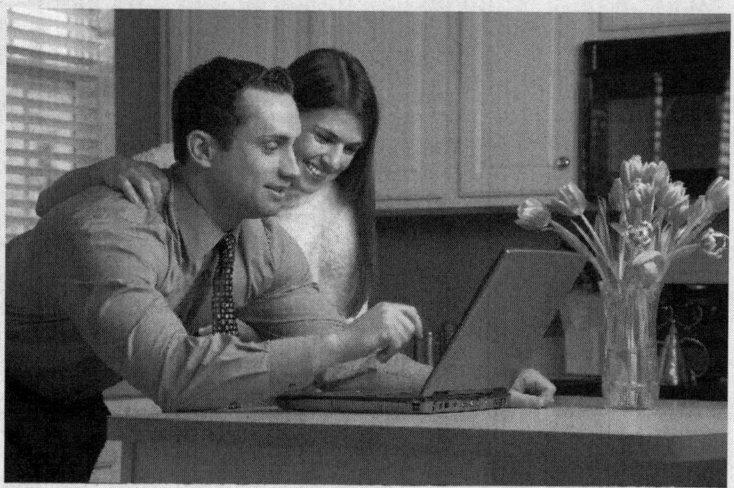

The biggest shock came when I measured the microwaves coming from our portable phone. I had been happily using it as an alternative to my cell phone – thinking that my exposure would be less. In fact, the readings from the portable phone were 10 percent higher. The take away message for me is to get a corded landline.

I was also surprised to find the elevated readings from my cell phone when it was on standby. Suffice it to say, I am no longer using it as an alarm clock.

We have switched back to hard-wired Internet, as you suggested, and made the bedroom a low-electronic environment. Everyone seems to feel better – and sleep better. Thought it was just the stress.

## Kitchen

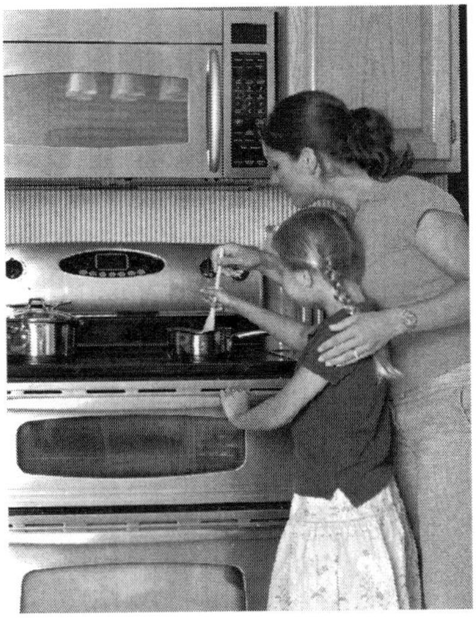

Adults without health problems are fine in most kitchens, as long as they stand far away from microwave ovens when they are on. Those who should use more caution include: pregnant women, children, people with poor immune systems or who suffer due to electro-sensitivity, convalescents, women with a history of breast cancer and men with a family history of testicular or prostate cancer.

When you're in the kitchen, you're often in the soup – of EMR. Test all plugged-in appliances with a Gauss meter (microwave ovens also need testing with the RF meter, as you may remember). If shopping for new appliances, take your testing equipment to choose the best options. Avoid induction ranges and cook tops as they emit very high magnetic fields. And steer clear of all 'Smart' Appliances as they waste energy and emit RF radiation, just like Smart Meters, and we know about them.

How many counter-top gadgets do you have? [When I use the kettle or blender I stand back, and I unplug them when I've finished].

[When my fridge expired I replaced it with a no-frills low energy consumption model. Each extra option that requires more power is going to add to the electro-magnetic fields.

I also removed the under-the-counter CD player/radio that was only a few feet from my head when I was in the kitchen. It was low intensity but high proximity and duration. The same player placed on the other side of the kitchen is less exposure].

The dishwasher, as you know, uses lots of energy and water, so being concerned about these, we don't run it more than we have to, always use the quick wash/air dry cycle, and don't stand against it when it's on.

In our kitchen there's no microwave oven, [reheating food on the stove only takes a few minutes]. What kind of stove do you have?

[Whenever possible I cook on the back burners on the stove as the electro-magnetic field from the front burners is much higher. The next time I buy a stove, I will get a gas stove and make sure it is well vented].

Gas stoves do not pose an EMR hazard as they don't use electricity. The sparks used to light the gas produce short bursts of high-voltage electricity, but these are insignificant. Some people with multiple chemical sensitivity need to avoid gas fumes.

Ovens, including fan-assisted convection ovens, electric fans/vents, even smaller toaster ovens are generating strong fields.

If you are standing close to the stove, with the front burners blasting, and the over-the-stove fan is on at your head, you are in a fairly strong field - test with a Gauss meter.

[Again the recommendation is stand back. Proximity is one of the best guidelines to keep in mind.]

## Laundry Room

The same is true in the laundry room. Washing machines and dryers create strong electro-magnetic fields so it is best not to stand directly beside them when they are on.

The other issue here is the toxic content of most laundry products unless they are non-toxic natural brands. I once felt like leaving a Pilates class because most women had either washed their clothes in standard detergent – chemically perfumed – or dried them with scented dryer sheets. I wanted to tell them that the chemicals from these products are absorbed through our skin. Ever walk past a house where people use these? You only need your nose to detect the dryer exhaust emissions.

## Vacuum Cleaners

Most vacuum cleaners have powerful motors and give off high EMR. Strap-to-your-back models are *not* recommended. If you are pregnant, upright models are also not recommended. [The canister kind is preferred as the motor is further away from your body than upright models. Use a plain mop or broom for non-carpeted floors. Best not to use chemically-treated floor cleaning pads.]

## Office

Whether we're talking about your home office, study, den or even your professional office, the same basic approach applies. We worked with the strongest exposures first – cordless and cell phones, other wireless devices, wireless Internet access and lighting. Then we tackled anything wired. Recently, I heard that there are problems with power bars that include surge protection – a fire hazard, evidently. See the Index. And it is crucial to test the electric, magnetic and RF fields.

## Your Cordless Phone Audit

How many cordless phones are in your home and office? Are they analog or digital? [We replaced all of ours with corded landlines that don't require electrical plugs, and use small batteries for the caller ID and speakerphone features.

You can also replace the handset cord with a 25 foot one, for long range wandering.]

## Wireless Routers

Proximity is a factor, even with a long-range device such as this. [Every EMR expert strongly recommends replacing wireless Internet with a hard-wired system.

You might check out the kind that connects your Ethernet through the house wiring; you can plug into an electrical outlet for your Internet access. Not inexpensive, but has its benefits in reducing significantly your EMR exposure by taking wireless Internet out of your home.

If you must have a wireless router, place it as far away from sentient beings as possible, only power it on when you use it, and turn it off after that; always have it powered off at night.]

The radiation range from the average router is about 175 metres, (575 feet). At night, and when you're away, be considerate of your neighbors and switch it off. Any bees and other migrating beings whose natural navigation systems are being thrown out of whack will also be grateful.

It is recommended to stand back from all office equipment, printers, copiers, fax machines etc, when they are working.

And I won't mention another word about the microwave oven.

## Experts' Action Plans

Many of these points have been touched on in previous sections, but it's interesting – and inspiring – to see how the leading authorities are putting their EMR-reduction advice into practice in their own homes and work places.

**Dr. Martin Blank** has no cell phone. His wife takes one in the car in case of an emergency. He has replaced his cordless phones with corded landlines. He's moved the electric clock away from the bed, got rid of circuits that have multiple electric switches on one line, as well as dimmer switches and instant-on devices.

He has also got rid of fluorescent bulbs in his house because they give off too much RF noise that has been linked to an increased risk of cancer.

Dr. Blank has meters and measures EMF levels at home from time to time. Instead of wireless Internet, Dr. Blank has a cable linkup between computers that are on opposite ends of the house. He and his wife do not own a microwave oven.

**Dr. Hans Scheiner** and his wife had to make changes to their house because of their exposure to EMF from the proliferation of antennas in their area.

Testing with meters found the levels were very high in Dr. Scheiner's main floor medical clinic and in the 3rd floor bedroom. He had the clinic walls coated with a special paint with small particles of carbon in it.

In the bedroom, the Scheiners had curtains made of shielding fabric, and on the outside wall have installed a thin metal plate that attracts electro-magnetic frequencies and grounds this energy into the earth. "The levels are much lower now."

**Dr. William Rea** offers his strategy for protecting his family from toxic exposures: "No cordless phones; no fluorescent lights, keep the chemical load down, consume organic food and safe water."

**Rob Metzinger** tells us:

"First, using special meters I evaluated exposure for Electric Fields, Magnetic Fields and RF (radio-frequency from microwaves – neighbors' cordless phones, wireless networks etc.) in all areas of the home, concentrating on the sleeping areas. Turned off power in all sleeping areas reducing electric field exposure by using demand switches.

- Removed all electronics from the sleeping areas.
- Installed shielded power cords on all computers and electronics.
- Moved computers and monitors as far away as possible from the users.
- Moved air conditioner away from children's sleeping area.
- Installed shielding curtains to deflect high levels of RF from entering the home.
- Replaced low voltage halogen, fluorescent and compact fluorescent lights with incandescent bulbs.
- Replaced dimmer switches with regular on/off switches

- Replaced spring mattresses with natural latex foam mattresses.
- Replaced electric alarm clocks with battery-operated units.
- Made a battery-operated night light for my children's rooms.
- Installed one analog 900 MHz cordless phone. All the other phones in our home are now land lines.
- Periodically retest exposure levels throughout the home.
- When purchasing any new electronic devices, I test them for EMF/ EMR emissions."

## Action Plan – Environmental Health Factors to Consider

Because we can't control everything around us, even the best action plan, up to this point, is reducing our chemical and electrical exposures, but not eliminating them entirely.

At the end of this section, you will see the detailed Action Plan to fill out, if this is what you want to do.

You or someone you know may already have some of the EMR-related symptoms and conditions listed in the questionnaire in Strategy 2. Even if you haven't, you'll benefit from the recommendations from some eminent complementary health practitioners on how to protect and improve your health in this hyper-tech world.

First, have you ever wondered how the health of people in our advantaged society got so far off course? Let's take a look at how this might happen. This analogy of a river gives us insights into our own health challenges, and wellbeing strategies.

## The River of Health – Pristine or Polluted?

### The River Runs Clear

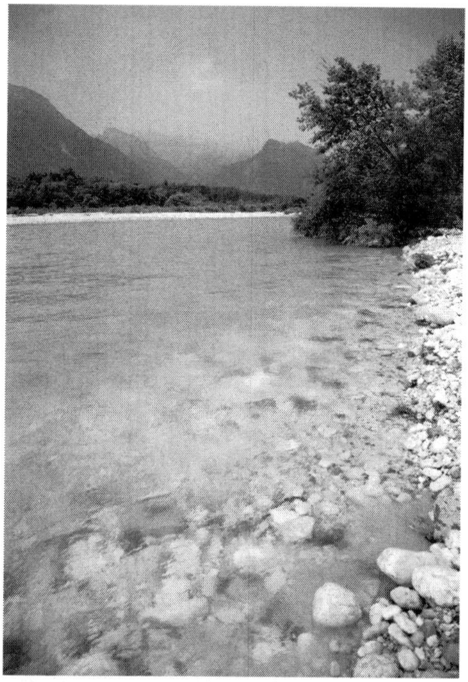

The clear mountain stream flows unhindered – translucent, its foundation bed of smooth river rocks can easily be seen. Light sparkles on its pristine surface and if you were to drink this pure, oxygen-rich water it would taste fresh and almost alive. It is mineral rich, being fed by pure mountain streams, so its acid alkaline balance is as nature intended. The rocks over which it travels are free of debris. There are no blockages in the river; it is not twisted and its flow is not blocked. The river banks are clean and free of clutter.

Then at some point toxic sludge enters the river – at first this is absorbed by the river, diluted and purified.

Then at another place downstream, more sludge is introduced and bit-by-bit the river's ability to absorb and detoxify these toxins becomes compromised.

The once-clear waters become clouded; the river bed covered with a dark slime. Debris builds up on the river bank and the river narrows. In places, the river slows to a congested trickle. Problems arise at that blockage.

The flow of energy, blood and lymphatic fluid that sustain our health, and our lives, is much the same. Its path, twists and turns are partly set by our genetic heritage and family health history, but everything that enters it has an effect.

Ideally, we want to start our lives with as clean and strong a river of health as possible, but this is an increasing challenge in the modern world.

The average North American diet contributes a great deal of sludge to the river of life, including highly acidic foods (disrupting the pH balance), pesticides and herbicides, assorted additives and trans fats.

And emotional and/or physical traumas early in life also take a long-term toll on the body's ability to heal itself.

## The River Reacts

Most children consume vast amounts of sugar and packaged foods – weakening the immune system and leaving them vulnerable to infection. Some children get recurring infections and lots of antibiotics. This can become a worrying cycle.

Antibiotics are truly wonder drugs and can save lives. Even if the family physician is careful only to prescribe antibiotics when strictly necessary, children may be ingesting antibiotics from foods such as industrially-raised chicken.

Antibiotics kill the bacteria we don't want, as well as wipe out the friendly bacteria – intestinal flora – that we need to maintain a healthy balance. A yeast overgrowth can result, overloading the immune system, leaving us vulnerable to more infections. If we are hit with a 'superbug' we may have nothing effective left in the arsenal.

Chemical sensitivities, asthma, and even childhood cancers can arise from a compromised immune system, many experts advise. Also, systems may be burdened by mercury in dental fillings or some vaccines.

The typical teenage diet of sugar, soda, fries, pizza, and other fast foods is highly acidic. And many young people don't get enough sleep.

We have now set the base for the potential of a lifetime of illness and disease. We can turn this around. Later on in this section we'll look at a number of factors that combine to support our overall health.

First, we'll start with electro-sensitivity, since to most people this is a new condition, and most people – even many doctors – are not aware of how this exposure affects every system in our bodies.

## Electro-hypersensitivity (EHS) – a new medical condition

We have a syndrome evolving called electro-sensitivity (ES), or electro-hypersensitivity (EHS). This is a phenomenon by which individuals experience recurring health effects that flare up during or after they are exposed to electro-magnetic radiation.

As Dr. Magda Havas points out, there are heavily-radiated parts of the world where an increasing number of people are so severely affected they have to live as far as possible from exposure. And she reports that as many as 35% have symptoms that significantly impair their quality of life. This impact on human health will rise until more of us wake up.

In Sweden, EHS is officially recognized as a functional impairment, and therefore employers and building owners are expected to try to rectify the problems and sufferers may be entitled to disability benefits. While EHS is not an accepted medical diagnosis yet, the Canadian Human Rights Commission recognizes it as an environmental sensitivity and classes it as a disability.

Dr. Scheiner treated thousands of people with EHS symptoms and warned the number of people affected was on the rise:

> Some people are electro-allergic – not only sensitive but hyper-sensitive. When they are exposed they have headaches, sleeping problems, exhaustion during the day, dizziness, vomiting, tachycardia, concentration and memory problems. They may faint or their vision might be impaired. It's likely these are signs of opening of the blood-brain barrier. Doctors often tell them their symptoms are psychological.

Dr. Scheiner said an electro-hypersensitive person can usually recover from the symptoms by avoiding the exposure. The next step along the continuum is what he calls an electro-allergic reaction, in which the body's response is a real illness. Some will feel no ill effects – then suddenly will be hit with something as serious as cancer, high blood pressure or a stroke.

Thomas M. Rau, MD, the Medical Director of the Paracelsus Clinic in Lustmühle, Switzerland, is convinced electro-magnetic loads lead to cancer, concentration problems, ADD, tinnitus, migraines, insomnia, arrhythmia, Parkinson's Disease and even back pain:

> At the Paracelsus Clinic (www.paracelsus.ch), cancer patients are now routinely educated in electromagnetic field remediation strategies, and inspectors from the Geopathological Institute of Switzerland are sent to patients' homes to assess electro-magnetic field exposures.

Source: www.electromagnetichealth.org, 'Electromagnetic Load a Hidden Factor in Many Illnesses' February 2009.

## Medical Help on the Horizon for People with ES

Dr. Heather McKinney attended a American Environmental Health Foundation (AEHF) and the University of North Texas Health Science Center conference in Dallas. The topic was The Chemical Mechanisms Leading to Electro-sensitivity. If you are dealing with chemical and/or electro-sensitivity, you will be heartened to hear about the progress in diagnosing and treating this, and related, conditions.

Dr. McKinney offers this to us:

> Physicians, researchers, scientists, nutritionists, counselors, and patients met to better understand and address the physiological signs and symptoms of electro-sensitivity. Their summary: the body is an electrical system that acts as an antenna – absorbing and receiving various information and sensations, including electro-magnetic fields from wired and wireless technologies. Health professionals from Australia, Brazil, Canada, Japan, the UK, and the USA discussed:
>
> **Testing strategies**: heart rate variability, blood sugar, live blood analysis, heavy metal test/hair analysis, mold/allergy testing, and lymphocyte sensitivity.
>
> **Triggers**: environmental and chemical stress, mold, thermal changes (exposure to heat/cold), sun spots, certain foods.
>
> **Signs and Symptoms**: poor circulation, skin changes, tremors, migraines, seizures, rapid heartbeat, diabetes, MS, chronic fatigue, asthma, allergies, food sensitivities/intolerance, memory fog, Alzheimer's and autism.

**Possible ES Treatments**: decreasing exposure, drinking lots of pure water, adrenal and immune support, vitamins/ supplements including magnesium and Vitamins B, C and D, hormone support, removing mercury fillings (with strict controls), acupuncture, chiropractic and other energy therapies, meditation, yoga, deep breathing techniques, homeopathy, Epsom salt baths, rotation diet, medically-supervised chelation and decreased exposure to metals.

## Refuges For People Suffering Due to ES – A Wake-up Call

Like polar bears on melting ice floes, an increasing number of people are finding the sphere they can safely inhabit is rapidly diminishing. While low-EMR places of refuge is good news for some, it may be a troubling sign of disastrous things to come. What will it be like when more and more people have to leave their homes, and their jobs, and retreat to remote hideaways? One such sanctuary is Green Bank, a small town in West Virginia in a 13,000 sq mile US National Radio Quiet Zone where there is no cell phone service and no public WiFi! These signals are strictly controlled in and around Green Bank as they would interfere with the nearby radio telescope. There are also refuges in Sweden, France, Italy, Spain, Canada and Japan. This back-to-the-land movement may be a life-saver for people with ES symptoms; it is also attracting people seeking a healthier lifestyle of reduced chemical and electro-magnetic contaminants in their bodies, food, air, and water. In our increasingly WiFi hot-spot world, these cool spots, quiet zones, may become examples of a saner way to live. No Google Glass here.

Please contact us through our website if you know of refuges developing, or if you are interested in finding one. Until this wireless world gives its head a shake and wakes up, we'll need these sanctuaries.

## No, EMR does not cause everything

At this stage you may well be wondering how electro-magnetic radiation can be blamed for such a lengthy and diverse list of symptoms and conditions. Research indicates there are about eighty immune system disorders that we didn't have twenty-five years ago before we really started microwaving the planet. Is there a connection, one wonders?

Whether a person develops symptoms, or not, can be influenced by the intensity and duration of the exposure, and by the individual's vulnerability – whether his or her overall health and immunity are strong enough to buffer the effects of EMR.

Reportedly, that is why ES/EHS is more common in people who already have chemical, or other environmental, sensitivities. Many may also be burdened by heavy metals in their systems and by food allergies.

Dr. Scheiner also said people who have had cancer are more susceptible to developing electro-hypersensitivity; their bodies are likely too busy fighting the cancer to be able to fend off this extra assault.

Even when exposure to EMR hasn't directly caused a disease, for instance diabetes, or a neurological condition such as MS, ALS or Parkinson's, the medical experts tell us that the symptoms may get worse as the person's body tries to cope with the additional burden of this exposure.

As you saw on page 215, our Tech-free Retreats are not only a way for the tech-obsessed to unplug, this is a refuge for people with electro-sensitivity whose ability to travel is increasingly restricted. And for those still without symptoms it is a useful wake-up call to meet those dealing with ES – the new health challenge in this digital age.

# EHS Symptoms and Related Conditions

(with the kind permission of Susan Parsons: www.weepinitiative.org)

| SYMPTOMS OF ELECTRO HYPERSENSITIVITY | | | | | | |
|---|---|---|---|---|---|---|
| Neurological | | Cardiac | Respiratory | Dermatological | Ophthalmologic | |
| headaches | depression | palpitations | sinusitis | skin rash | deteriorating vision |
| difficulty concentrating | anxiety | pain or pressure in the chest | asthma | facial flushing | pain or burning in the eyes |
| muscle and joint pain | confusion and spatial disorientation | low or high blood pressure | bronchitis | itching | pressure in/behind the eyes |
| memory loss | fatigue | shortness of breath | pneumonia | burning | floaters |
| dizziness | weakness | arrhythmia | | | cataracts |
| nausea | tremors | slow or fast heart rate | | swelling of face and neck | |
| irritability | muscle spasms | | | | |
| numbness | leg/foot pain | | | | |
| tingling | "Flu-like" symptoms | | | | |
| hyperactivity | fever | | | | |
| altered reflexes | insomnia | | | | |
| OTHER | | | | | |
| digestive problems | abdominal pain | testicular/ovarian pain/swelling | enlarged thyroid | great thirst | dehydration |
| nosebleeds | internal bleeding | hair loss | pain in the teeth | deteriorating fillings | Light sensitivity |
| swollen lymph nodes | loss of appetite | hypoxia | allergies | frequent urination and incontinence | night sweats |
| immune abnormalities | redistribution of metals within the body | ringing in the ears (tinnitus or similar chronic ear-noise) | impaired sense of smell | altered sugar metabolism | dryness of lips, tongue, mouth, eyes |
| **Severe reactions can include seizures, paralysis, psychosis, and stroke** | | | | | |

Doesn't it seem incredible that just about everything you've ever heard of is here? How could this be? Medical experts I've talked with explain this by saying that EMR affects every cell, organ and system in the body. So if you consider this, it doesn't seem as hard to believe that there are so many related symptoms and conditions.

If your house were flooded repeatedly, eventually everything within it would be affected.

How can you tell whether your symptoms are EMR related, or not? This is just what I asked Dr. Scheiner. He explained that each symptom might be unspecific (in other words not related to a particular illness):

> You can have a headache for a lot of reasons. It gets specific if you get lots of them, or sleeping problems. If you can't sleep at night this could be microwave syndrome from EMR exposure… not yet a sickness, it's a warning syndrome.
>
> The body is saying 'I am having trouble here'. It is a call for help. Allergies and food sensitivities could also be a test.

## More women than men? Not so.

Dr. Scheiner also made a gender observation:

> Women seem to have a finer sensitivity to their symptoms and to heed them more. Often men who attend our clinic will say 'I have *no* problem, but my wife really suffers.' Then we do some lab tests and discover both are being biologically affected equally.

A short wilderness retreat, if away from cell antennas, can give you useful information. Dr. Scheiner suggested removing yourself from some of the sources for a few days, and seeing what happens. If the headaches, insomnia, tingling and other symptoms improve when you're away, and return when you come back, this is probably a sign that you're electro-sensitive.

Cindy Sage of the BioInitiative Group, agreed:

> Symptoms quickly improve when away from EMF/EMR sources, particularly when the patient moves away from computers, fluorescent lighting, transformers, wireless antenna, cell and cordless phones, appliances and out of proximity to cell phone towers, electrical substations and power lines…
>
> Symptoms recur on returning to the irradiated environment. Over time, sensitivity is increased to smaller and smaller EMF/EMR exposures.

The renowned surgeon Dr. William Rea, offers the EHC-D protocol used at his Environmental Health Center – Dallas (www.ehcd.com). This facility is a complete testing and medical treatment clinic for environmentally-sensitive adults and children.

1. Eliminate exposure
2. Energy balancing
3. Mineral analysis
4. Skin test for minerals
5. IV nutrients twice weekly
6. Grounding at least 1 hour/day
7. Immune modulation
8. Sauna

Katharina Gustavs says, "Grounding and sauna, as mentioned above, are great therapeutic strategies for healing. However, if the grounding involves artificial grounding pads, the electric field exposure could increase during the grounding. Walking barefoot along the beach, of course, is always a winner. Infrared saunas are notorious for high magnetic and electric field exposures." One company that has been recommended has evidence that its low EMR emission infrared saunas are specifically designed for electro- and chemically-sensitive people.

Sarah Dacre, Trustee of ES-UK registered charity, was disabled in 2005 when she moved to a brand new house within close range of a mobile/cell phone mast in London. A myriad of symptoms forced Sarah to give up her London lifestyle and independent TV Production business. Sleeping within 200 meters of a phone mast (cell tower), excessive mobile phone use, a 24/7 activated WiFi internet connection and wireless burglar alarm, were all contributory factors to the development to a bad case of chronic fatigue syndrome, benign tumour, extreme environmental sensitivities, food allergies, eye sight disturbance, memory and balance problems. Sarah was forced to sell up on her urban lifestyle.

Her health has almost totally recovered and she now lives rurally. She has spent thousands of pounds on treatments and in building a shielded custom designed house. Some eight years on, she has re-established her consultancy business, helps out with local environmental campaigns and assists at ES-UK responding to enquiries about EHS. Sarah has featured in BBC, Channel 4 and ABC TV programmes, events and articles.

Sarah Dacre highly recommends the comprehensive new book by Michael Bevington MA (Oxon.), MEd. Chair of Trustees of ES-UK. *Electromagnetic Sensitivity and Electromagnetic Hypersensitivity* (Capability Books 2013.) It is available at: www.es-uk.info.

The WEEP Initiative has a section on living with EHS on its website, www.weepinitiative.org/livingwithEHS.html

Now, let's keep going and look at a few more conditions and explore how EMR exposure influences them. You may discover some connections with health issues in your family, and some useful medical advice.

Our library mum – a woman who has been reading parts of the book as they've been written – has noted some interesting inter-connections:

> It seems EMR is one of *various* environmental toxins that we are exposed to which are compromising our immune system. A couple of years back, I was exposing myself to a lot of bleach and when I stopped this, I recovered much of my health (slowly, over time).The challenge is that it is difficult to put our finger on *which* environmental toxin is the culprit because it is the overall load of toxins that get us. We need to abandon the search for a single cause.

## Immune System Impairment

## The Sweet Smell of Chemical Overload?

Why should you care about this? We only have one immune system, one lymphatic system, one liver, one set of kidneys etc, to deal with the daily onslaught of environmental toxins, EMR now included.

Your immune system, whether you know or not, is reacting to all of these environmental exposures. The more we can reduce the various chemical loads, the better it is for us, and for all life forms on this planet, including the birds in the air, and the fish in the rivers and oceans.

And most people who are electro-sensitive are also chemically sensitive, so this is vital information for them.

I asked Dr. William Rea what is of most concern to him these days. His answer: "Pesticide exposure plus wireless equipment. EMF sensitivity is a growing problem in the world. Everyone needs to be aware of its consequences."

Dr. Rea elucidates on the interplay of environmental influences:

> Various factors (heavy metals, inner terrain – yeasts, pH balance, emotional stress etc.) may combine to make us more vulnerable to a myriad of environmental toxins, including EMR. Dealing effectively with these factors can boost our ability to buffer the toxic effects. If the load is reduced, many times the patient can tolerate the EMR.

## Systems Overwhelmed?

A recent report on the rapid rise of serious food allergies in children (including life-threatening ones like peanuts) tells us that the experts cannot explain the nearly 20% increase in the last decade. Could it be the deluge of chemicals in our air, food and environment are overwhelming young immune systems?

Some companies were recently defending the several carcinogens found in their baby lotions and bath products, as just 'trace amounts'. I have also discovered one also needs to be vigilant for the wolf in sheep's clothing: chemically-laden products are labelled "natural" or "fresh," or some such disguise. A story comes to mind: when I had a counseling practice, a woman told me that she had used a plug-in air freshener for her son's bedroom to purify the air to help with his asthma. Like most of us, she was getting her health information from marketers.

You have probably heard that lead, tar and formaldehyde are used in most cosmetics and 'personal care products'. When they say 'perfume', unless they are using only essential oils, assume these are chemicals, as in most scented candles, cleaning products, air fresheners. Taking these things out of your home can ease everyone's immune and respiratory systems. Here's some more good information from Larry Gust:

> Fragrances commonly use phthalates, some of which are hormone disrupters. These, as well as synthetic musk compounds and other chemicals, accumulate in human tissue and are found in breast milk. Manufacturers don't necessarily test this stuff for neurological effects or respiratory effects – even though we know an increasing number of people have asthma attacks when exposed to scented products and two fragrance materials that had been used for decades were found to be neurotoxic.

Can we live in a pure, non-toxic environment? I don't think so. And, yes, our immune systems need a good workout – so we shouldn't swab down the decks too often with anti-bacterial soaps.

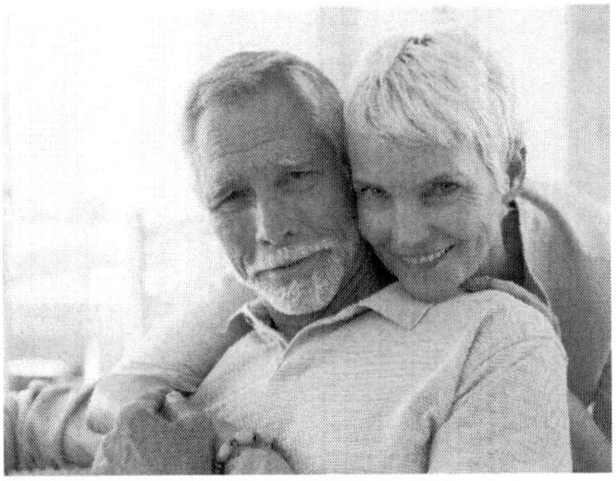

However, given the chemical pollutants in our environment it is wise to reduce all the exposures we can, and not agonize about the ones we cannot, and boost our ability to handle these – a serenity prayer for health. This will bring benefits as we age. Anti-aging experts advise a less polluted environment enhances health and longevity, as well as appearance. Reducing electro-pollution exposure is crucial. This new factor is missing in most anti-aging programs.

Dr. Mark Hyman is a physician who emphasizes the benefits of addressing environmental pollutants, including EMR:

> Clearly there are many environmental influences that can have a major impact on overall health, including your brain health. These toxins affect us all from our food, our water and air, medications, chemicals, metals, molds and electromagnetic radiation.
>
> Everyday choices we make to protect ourselves will have impact globally. The European Union, through new legislation (called REACH) designed to limit toxins in commercially produced goods, caused China to change its manufacturing practices.
>
> Buying organic food, refusing vaccines with mercury, or buying deodorant without aluminum will create a ripple effect throughout our economy and environment.
>
> You *can* heal yourself from brain damage by altering your diet, limiting your exposure to toxins, and changing the way you live. You can REVERSE the effects of depression, anxiety, bipolar disorder, autism, Alzheimer's, ADHD, and more if you know how to.
>
> From *The UltraMind Solution,* (Simon & Schuster 2009)

**Chronic Fatigue Syndrome (CFS)** In the UK, this condition is called myalgic encephalomyelitis (ME).

Several of our experts have advised us that EMR exposure weakens the immune system. An overwhelmed immune system cannot fend off environmental toxins, bacteria and viruses leaving us more open to colds, flu etc. Not only do we get sick more often, it can take us much longer to recover. And we feel more tired, more often.

A compromised immune system is also a contributing factor in, and a result of, Chronic Fatigue Syndrome, and many other conditions. (As you may know, emotional stress also weakens our immune systems.)

While CFS/ME is a complex illness with many possible causes, in October 2009 an American research team reported, in the journal *Science*, that a single retrovirus – a blood-borne pathogen – may play a major role. Retroviruses are known to cause neurological symptoms, cancer and immunological deficiencies, and many people with chronic fatigue report their symptoms emerged after a serious viral infection.

While it's too early to say whether this discovery will lead to better treatments, the news is heartening to the millions of people worldwide who suffer from this debilitating condition.

The reason I am including a section on this is that CFS and exposure to electro-magnetic radiation share many symptoms and are connected. And knowing about CFS can be a great boost to your overall health and your ability to heal from, or ward off, the effects of EMR.

In 1983, W. Grundler, in Germany, found even very low levels of EMR exposure affects the increased growth of yeast cells.

("Sharp Resonances in Yeast Growth Prove Nonthermal Sensitivity to Microwaves.")

Dr. Rau adds his recommendations for dealing with electro-sensitivity and fighting yeast conditions:

> Cultures have shown beneficial bacteria grow more slowly in the presence of electromagnetic fields allowing pathological (yeast – candida) organisms to dominate. Thus, a strategy with electrically sensitive patients, or with those facing chronic conditions, is the aggressive

> supplementation with probiotics and other Biological Medicine approaches to balance intestinal flora. Many people with chronic infections likely linked to EMR exposures, such as Lyme Disease, are symptom-free after an aggressive microorganism rebalancing program.

A proliferation of yeast cells (Candida albicans) in the bowel can be a contributing factor in many conditions, including Chronic Fatigue Syndrome, and will weaken the health of EHS people.

A physician specialising in complementary medicine, Carolyn Dean MD ND, author/coauthor of 17 books including *The Magnesium Miracle,* explained in a recent interview that it's not just fatigue:

> In brief, Candida albicans is a fungus living in our intestines that produces 180 chemical toxins capable of making you feel dizzy and fatigued, shutting down your thyroid, throwing your hormones off balance, and causing you to crave sugar and alcohol, and gain weight. It's associated with drowsiness, insomnia, numbness, tingling, PMS, loss of libido, painful intercourse, infertility, MS, Crohn's, colitis, IBS, acne, Lupus, white tongue, bad breath, body odor, sinusitis, bruising, sore throat, bronchitis, shortness of breath, heart palpitations, spots in front of eyes.
>
> The miracle of antibiotics has its downside as an underlying cause of yeast overgrowth. The refining of sugar and wheat has its downside by creating a simple food source for yeast.
>
> The tremendous levels of stress hormones that flood our bodies daily also make us prey to yeast. When yeast, bacterial, and food toxins hit the blood stream they

> trigger widespread inflammatory reactions by either directly attacking tissues or creating allergic reactions along with the production of histamine. It is mainly through diet and lifestyle change that you can overcome yeast overgrowth—but you *can* overcome it, and reduce the amount of inflammation in your life with some effort and support.

Original article: Total Health and Longevity Magazine Sept 2006 issue.

Dr. Dean also describes how magnesium can be useful in CFS and possibly EHS as these conditions share many symptoms, including insomnia and fatigue, as we have seen:

> Magnesium-deficient patients commonly experience fatigue because dozens of enzyme systems are under-functioning. An early symptom of magnesium deficiency is fatigue.

Dr. Dean is the medical director of the Nutritional Magnesium Association and has a wellness consulting practice in Hawaii.

The treatment suggested for CFS, and boosting one's immune system, includes cutting out sugar. Sadly, the more difficult this is, the more it may be needed, as craving sweets is one of the main symptoms. Physicians specializing in this also recommend supplementing with good quality probiotics – it's not enough to eat yogurt – and using an effective anti-fungal. There are more details at Dr. Dean's website: www.drcarolyndean.com

Another physician specializing in complementary medicine, and an expert in CFS, Dr. Jacob Teitelbaum has more information on the treatment of CFS on his site www.endfatigue.com. I asked Dr. Teitelbaum this question: "Many people, including those with EMR exposure, are tired and don't sleep well. So how do you know if you really have CFS?"

> Although many people are tired and have poor sleep, the fatigue usually goes away with rest and is not associated with the other symptoms. It is the mix of a common group of symptoms that define a syndrome. People who are tired, achy, 'brain foggy', can't sleep, have increased thirst and poor libido – even if these are not disabling – often have a milder form of CFS.

## Electro-sensitivity and CFS

Dr. Teitelbaum offers his responses to a patient experiencing sensitivity to electric fields and computers.

Q. "I had a relapse with CFS and have been out of work for a year. I notice that this time around a few months into the illness, that I am now sensitive to sitting in front of a computer screen. Symptoms: I feel hot and nauseated, and if I stay on the computer long enough, feel my heart racing. I notice that I'm really sensitive to it in the morning versus the evening. Any ideas?"

Dr. T. "There are those who get electro-sensitivity with CFS. In some cases, turning off the electric circuit to your bedroom before you go to bed (use a wind up alarm clock or a battery one kept away from your head) and leaving the electricity off at night (you would be amazed at some of the electromagnetic fields found in the bedroom ) can also help – especially since you report feeling worse in the morning.

In severe cases, there are specialists that can evaluate a home for electrical pollution and assist in remediation."

**Sleep, perchance to dream?**

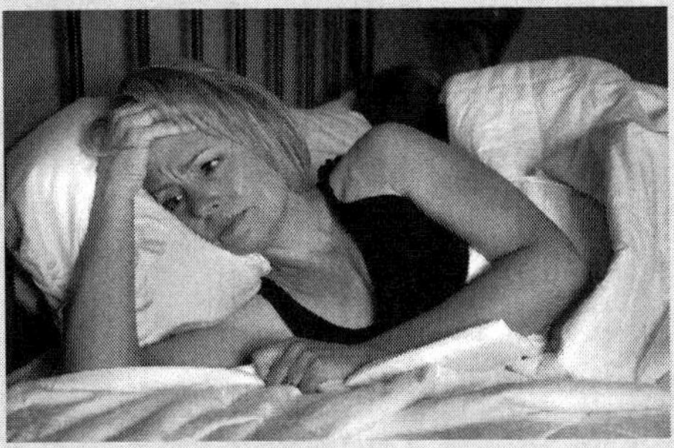

The curtains are drawn tightly. The spacious room is dark and seemingly conducive to sleep. The woman in the brass bed has one arm twisted around the sheets; her other arm is flung to the side and rests lightly on her wireless laptop. On the night table the digital clock marks the passing of another sleepless night.

Her trouble falling sleep, and then staying asleep, seems to be getting worse. "Stress, no doubt," the doctor advises and prescribes pharmaceuticals. Annoyingly, these seem to make her dozier during the day than they do at night. These pills perch on the table along with an arsenal of headache remedies. She read that room temperature is crucial, so, she either snuggles a heating pad or relies on an air conditioner.

She has surrounded herself with techno-delights to occupy her restless mind. In the middle of the night she often flicks on the light and taps away on her wireless tablet (the router is nearby) or calls a friend who lives in an earlier time zone.

Online, she can shop, plan vacations, watch a movie, and the alarm is so handy as she keeps her mobile phone on the bedside table. There's also a digital cordless phone right there – the powerful 6.0.

A Bluetooth sound system surrounds her with relaxing music. However, she can't get to sleep. Or stay there for long. She glares at the relentless clock and is sure that it's just stress keeping her awake.

## Insomnia, Stress, Mood

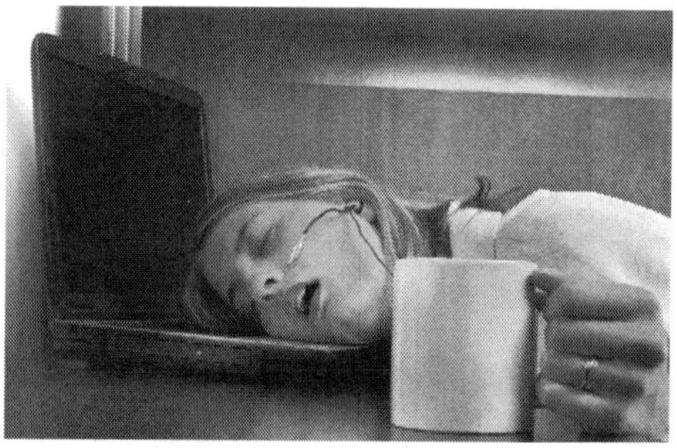

As you may know too well, not being able to sleep affects every facet of your life to the point where you can barely function. Specialists say it doesn't take long before sleep deprivation drives down your IQ (temporarily!), impairs reasoning and memory, makes adults more irritable and kids a little more "hyper."

As if that isn't enough, scientists also suspect that chronic sleep deprivation in children may also impair their growth and development. There are of course many factors that contribute to sleep disruption – caffeine, stress, hormones, a bedroom that faces a noisy street.

Not too long ago, our family was staying at a hotel when I attended a conference. I had chosen this hotel because it was one of the few that did not have wireless Internet access in the room.

My relief was short-lived, however, when I got into our room, looked out the window, and saw a nearby cell tower antenna. I had a small RF meter, which had a very sensitive audio signal. The levels were so high that this meter screamed as loud as it does next to a cell phone in use.

It wasn't easy explaining to the front desk why we wanted to change our room. I found a room on a lower floor, with less exposure, but when we left the hotel, I felt a pang of sadness for people seeking help in the sleep research centre that was on the top floor of this building. (Also I felt for the housekeeping staff with powerful vacuum cleaners strapped to their backs. Intensity. Proximity. Duration.)

In stress disorders and depression, EMR has been shown to affect levels of brain chemicals and hormones including norepinephrine, dopamine and serotonin, which are involved in regulating mood.

As you may know, these conditions are already epidemic so more research is needed here. Maybe this why we feel more calm, and our spirits are lifted, when we are out in nature and far removed from technology.

As Dr. Scheiner described, your ability to sleep can be a good indicator of your EMR exposure and sensitivity.

Many people who are not sleeping well may be unknowingly immersed in a high EMR environment. We know the agitating effect of EMR on the brain. Is it any wonder that difficulty sleeping is one of the primary and most prevalent symptoms?

Evidently, some people are using electric mattress pads to sleep better, and/or to enhance their health. You may remember reading about why this is a problem, in Strategy 3.

EMR exposure has been shown to make it more difficult to "wind down" and can also reduce the amount of melatonin in the brain. According to some research, using a cell phone for more than 25 minutes a day for two weeks can be enough to reduce melatonin levels. Katharina Gustavs adds, "According to J. Burch's research, the effect is exacerbated if you sit in a dimly lit office for most of the day."

As you may know, this hormone is necessary for deep, restful sleep, which also allows the body to recharge and heal itself.

(Many years ago, a remarkable immunologist told me that one of the primary functions of sleep was to recharge the immune system.)

A small study done by Sweden's Karolinska Institute and Uppsala University, with Wayne State University in Detroit, released in January 2008, revealed that people using a cellphone just before bedtime took longer to get into deep sleep, and spent less time in this deeper sleep phase.

(Published by the Massachusetts Institute of Technology's Progress in Electromagnetics Research Symposium.)

One of the researchers, Dr. Bengt Arnetz, said it appears that cell phones affect the areas of the brain responsible for activating and co-ordinating the stress system. It's also possible that radio waves disrupt production of melatonin, which controls the body's internal circadian rhythms.

Melatonin performs many crucial functions including regulating the timing of the onset of puberty.

Therefore it's no wonder sleep experts such as Dr. Jeffrey Lipsitz were especially disturbed by what this study implies for teenagers, who tend to use cell phones more in the evening, talk for long periods of time, and keep the phones on standby during the night.

As he told CTV News, a Canadian TV network:

> If they're using cell phones for long hours in the evening and then going to sleep and their sleep is disturbed this may have implications with regard to health and development and functioning in school and so on...

Insufficient sleep in young people is linked to mood and personality changes, ADHD-like symptoms, depression, lack of concentration and poor academic performance.

Dr. Lipsitz went on to say:

> You kind of wonder what else might be going on to the brain as a result of extended cell phone use, and what does that mean for all of us?... It certainly cries out for more research.

(Incidentally, the study was funded by the Mobile Manufacturers Forum, which called the results "inconclusive.")

Dr. Jacob Teitelbaum also writes about insomnia in *From Fatigued to Fantastic* and recommends: "magnesium 75 to 250 mg and calcium, 600 mg at bedtime and Hydroxy L-tryptophan (5-HTP) 200 to 400 mg at night. 5-HTP is what your body uses to make serotonin, a neurotransmitter that helps improve the quality of sleep." It may take four to six weeks to see the full effect of 5-HTP, though, so don't expect instant results.

Dr. Teitelbaum cautions that if you're taking anything else that raises your serotonin levels (including SSRI-type anti-depressants or even herbal remedies like St. John's Wort), "it is reasonable to limit the 5-HTP to 200 mg at night." In rare cases people may experience a reaction from excess serotonin.

As with all supplements that affect the body's natural production of hormones, for example, you should consult with a qualified clinician – physician or naturopathic doctor – before following any protocols. There may be contra-indications, conflicts with certain conditions and/or medications you need to know about.

Dr. Teitelbaum also has some useful insight:

> For most people with disordered sleep, supplementing melatonin to normal levels takes 3/10ths of a milligram. The usual dose is 3 milligrams, which is ten times the level I recommend.

I have found that sleeping in a dark room, and one that stays dark until you want to wake up, is very helpful. Try blackout curtains, or good eyeshades. Did you know that eyeshades keep the light out of your eyes and help in sleeping, but you need the whole room darkened to enhance the production of sleep-inducing melatonin? And, of course, make your bedroom a low EMR sanctuary.

## Sleeping Well Beyond the Electronic Cocoon

This once-sleepless mom heard our alert – loud and clear – and took action right away:

> I am a recovering breast cancer patient, and a life long skeptic, but after reading this book I found the information in the book so compelling, that I decided to make some immediate changes.
>
> To start, I replaced my cordless phones with land lines, moved my blackberry charger out of my bedroom, moved my bedside clock across the room, and stopped sleeping with the blackberry on my night table. We removed all of my daughter's electronics from her room, and got rid of her metal bed frame. As a family, we decided to try out a self-imposed one-hour-per-day-limit on how much time we would spend in front of the computer, television, DS and Wii for a month, and see what happened. We recognized

that there may have to be adjustments to computer time made to manage work and/or school obligations. To be honest, while it seemed like the right thing to do, I didn't expect to notice any immediate effect. However, I have been struggling with insomnia for the past three years, two years prior to my breast cancer diagnosis. The first night after clearing all of the electronics out of my room, I slept like a baby. Likewise for the next night.

While I am willing to consider a certain amount of placebo effect, I have now been sleeping well and deeply for a few weeks. I notice that I rarely wake in the night to use the washroom (before, I would get up several times in the night) and when I do wake up, I fall easily back to sleep.

My daughter, who at 13 has been complaining about not sleeping well for the last year, is also sleeping more deeply. Now that I think about it her sleeping difficulties began about the same time we put a cordless phone in her room, and mine began when I got my blackberry. Maybe just two coincidences. Or maybe not.

During my period of sleeplessness, I stopped drinking caffeine, and did everything I could to improve the quality of my sleep. I looked at all of the possible causes - new job, peri-menopause, caffeine intolerance, food allergies. I worked with a naturopath. While there was some small improvement, nothing was as dramatic as the effect of lowering the EMR levels in my bedroom and house.

My son has ADD and learning disabilities, and we wonder what other benefits our experiment in "unplugging" will reveal. Last night, we went to the park and played tennis after school, then had a rousing game of UNO after dinner. Playing cards and tennis are much preferable to the poor habits we had been slipping into, with each of us isolated in our individual electronic cocoons.

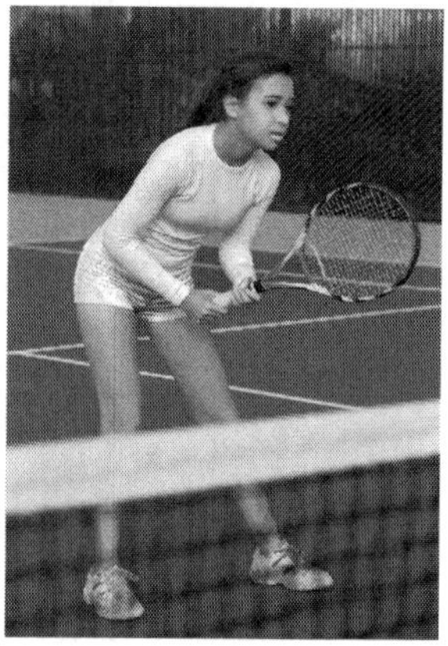

## Cardiovascular – Heart disease, TIA, Stroke

Cardiovascular disease is a major problem in industrialized countries, and it's not just because of the unhealthy western diet. Researchers explain that when EMR depletes the levels of antioxidants in the blood, high-density lipoproteins (HDL), the good cholesterol, will bind with free radicals (oxidants) turning the good cholesterol into bad cholesterol (LDL). This leads to thicker, "stickier" blood, which can form clots. (Emotional stress also thickens the blood, and constricts the arteries.)

And EMR has been shown to disturb our own sensitive electrical system – the brain and the heart, for example.

I have a friend who is a scientist at a leading university. Despite being fit, and in otherwise excellent health, she was rushed to emergency in cardiac distress. There's a claim by staff that a cluster of cancers is related to the high levels of EMR on her campus.

Could the cardiac symptoms also be related? Some electro-sensitive people can actually tell when there is a cell phone powered on nearby – they feel a change in their heart rate and rhythm, and/or a tightness in their chest.

Years ago I co-produced a program for Canadian network TV on heart health. I'd like to reconnect with the hundreds of patients I counseled when I worked in cardiac clinics, and encourage them to read this research and do an EMR audit of their homes and workplaces.

And I'd like to go back to all the cardiologists I once knew to ask if they're seeing an increase in "unexplained" cardiac symptoms.

In November 2009, Dr. Havas presented research demonstrating increased heart rate from wireless radiation exposure. Evidence included an increase in heart rate on exposure to a nearby cordless phone. The heart rate immediately returned to the baseline after that phone was unplugged (see www.magdahavas.com).

There is a concern that many patients today who are experiencing cardiac, and other electro-hypersensitivity, symptoms are turning to prescription drugs, instead of reducing their EMR exposure.

I welcomed this pioneering study and the opportunity to ask cardiologist Dr. Stephen Sinatra for his insight. He told me that he applauded Dr. Havas's research and offered this observation:

> We saw these cardiac effects ourselves in the middle of a study when a cordless phone was in use. If electro-pollution stresses the body like emotional stress then we already have mountains of evidence on how this affects our health including, of course, the cardiovascular system.

## Ophthalmological/Vision Problems

**Google Glass Alert!** Their SAR (radiation absorption) levels are reportedly higher than those of the iPhone 5. When asked for a comment Google evidently refused a sit down interview but did say in an email, "We've studied design comfort and safety very closely, and we haven't found cause for concern". Dr. Moskowitz warns of both WiFi and Bluetooth radiation and, "Just because these devices are legal does not mean they are safe". Exposure at a further distance has been shown to damage the eye's sensitive lens. Fifty years ago, in 1964 Dr. Milton Zaret was one of the first scientists to report dangers of microwave radiation and related ocular damage. According to Dr. Zaret, exposure to this radiation at either thermal, or non-thermal, levels can cause cataracts which sometimes remain latent for months or years. Zaret then had his research funds cut.

Metal eyeglass frames attract EMR, magnifying its effects. (A tip from an eye surgeon: blue-tinted lenses let in harmful rays.) Another expert has told me that our eyes are especially endangered by exposure to wireless radiation. Other vulnerable body parts are the testicles.

## Infertility, Miscarriages, Birth Defects

For couples longing to conceive, all this is deeply distressing. Some researchers in human reproduction are now telling us the more time men spend on cell phones, or carry powered-on phones in the pockets of their pants, the lower their sperm quality.

Occupational exposure may be a factor in men's reduced fertility. A study of 17 thousand military employees in the Norwegian navy, between 1950 and 2002, found men who worked within ten miles of high frequency aerials had a significantly higher risk of infertility than the ones who worked farther away. (Baste V et al *Eur J Epidemiol* 2008)

In Japan, with its massive concentration of electro-smog, an unusually high number of women are suffering miscarriages in their last trimester. (Nagaishi et. al., J.*Obstet Gynaecol Res.* 2004)

In August 2009, Dr. Louis Slesin of Microwave news reported:

> Martine Hours, the chief science advisor to the French RF research program, has called for serious studies on the effects of cell phones on male fertility. Now, Australia's John Aitken is saying the issue 'deserves our immediate attention.' In a new study, Aitken has reported that cell phone radiation damages human sperm – as well as DNA. Cell phone use and radiation has now been shown to harm sperm, in five different countries and including two different groups in the United States, one of which is at the Cleveland Clinic. Aitken's message is simple: Men who want to have children should not keep active mobile phones in their trouser pockets.

When couples trying to conceive know that EMR exposure decreases fertility they can now make informed decisions.

## More girls than boys in your play group?

There are also indications of a global prevalence of female births. Some researchers suspect this may be due to EMR. A Russian study in the 1950's found an altered sex ratio (more girls) in children born during the years of a radar station's operation in what was known as Latvia. That Norwegian navy study, which I mentioned above, showed similar results: a lower ratio of boys to girls were born to fathers who reported a higher degree of exposure to high-frequency antennas and communication equipment.

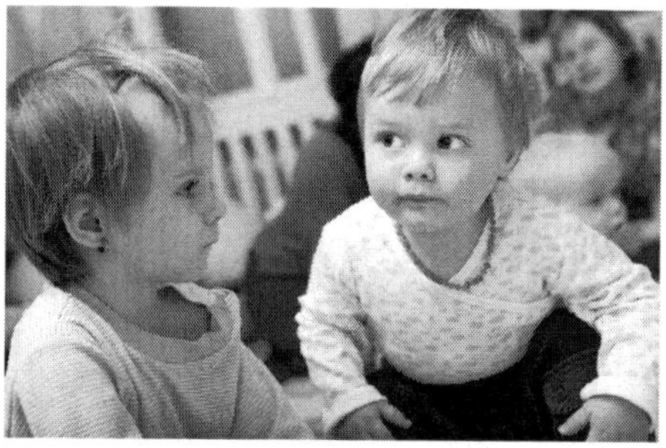

Evidently, the normal sex ratio is commonly 105 boys to 100 girls. But under adverse conditions – famine, for example - more girls are born. While this girl/boy imbalance may not seem troublesome, think of the ramifications over a few generations. And, perhaps we need to connect the dots with the growing signs of dysfunction throughout our ecosystem?

As I see it, information is the key to waking up, to getting ourselves out of this biological experiment, as Dr. Salford and Professor Johansson have cautioned us.

## Neurological Issues

Alzheimer's, dementia, Parkinson's Disease, ALS and MS may also be related to EMR, according to neuroscientists who explain this exposure can cause levels of neurotransmitters such as acetylcholine to drop abnormally. Low levels of acetylcholine are linked to a number of these neurological and neuromuscular symptoms and disorders.

(A side note: many people with these conditions improve dramatically when they deal with heavy metal toxicity and avoid artificial sweeteners such as those found in diet pop. Research the health effects of Aspartame, for example.)

You may not want to hear this; I know I didn't. While Alzheimer's Disease and dementia have generally been diseases of the elderly, based on the evidence of EMR biological harm, some experts are predicting these conditions will be afflicting people decades earlier.

## The Silent Epidemic

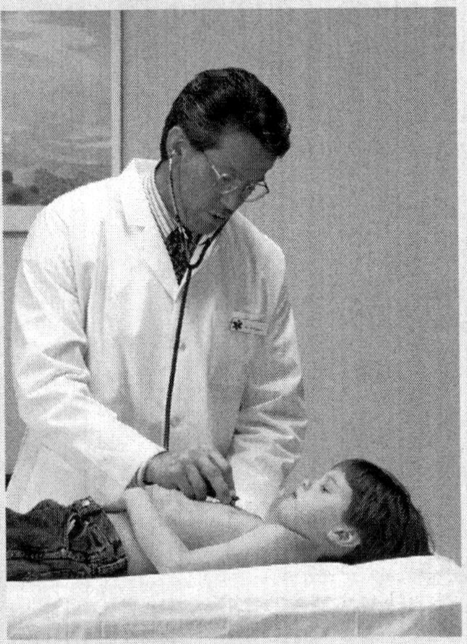

The young boy lies on the examining table banging his legs in an odd rhythm. He seems off in his own world. Standing close by, his parents look stunned: the pediatrician has just told them their child has autism.

They have known for a long time that something was not right, but nothing prepared them for the raw shock of the diagnosis they had feared.

He had been such a healthy baby and a normally developing toddler. Not long after his second birthday, however, they began to notice it was difficult to get him to focus, the development of his speech slowed, and he had occasional intense tantrums and hyperactivity.

They were taking extra steps to protect him, including a digital wireless baby monitor. They kept his environment as clean and germ-free as they could with highly effective cleaning products.

Now he spends a good part of the day on the iPad, which he loves, and screams if they try to take it away from him.

Then they hear about a possible connection with the microwave radiation from these wireless devices, including baby monitors. This possibility makes more sense when they read about children like their son improving in a WiFi-free environment. Why, they wonder, have they not heard about this before?

## ADD/ADHD and Autism Spectrum Disorders

If you are facing these challenges you don't need anyone to tell you how difficult this can be, especially in the initial stages.

However, many families, through their courage and determination to find out as much as they can, are improving other parents' success in helping their children. Truly dedicated parents who are leading support and advocacy networks are helping a great many families.

This section includes the research and recommendations of several leading experts in this field.

Here's what I've discovered: what most people call autism is a wide and varied range of neurological conditions with symptoms that may include difficulty communicating and functioning socially, various developmental disabilities, and cognitive challenges. Some people on the Autism Spectrum also have extraordinary musical or mathematical skills.

Not long ago I met a remarkable young boy who introduced himself right away, announcing, "My name is David and I have OCD (obsessive-compulsive disorder) and Asperger's."

His eyes were bright and alert; he was obviously highly intelligent, and he seemed agitated. David then became distressed when someone asked me about the book I was writing on the health effects of electromagnetic radiation.

"Radiation?" he squealed, "Oh no. I don't want to know about that. That's too scary."

Many well-controlled adults have had the same reaction, but this vulnerable boy was visibly distraught. I shifted gears immediately and sat down with him and his mother, to listen to his fears, and do what I could to calm him. He appeared to feel better when we talked about all the ways we can be safer.

Evidently, David's parents had recently installed a DECT 6.0 cordless phone in his bedroom; he told me that he loves to talk for hours with his friends. He is a talented musician who spends many hours on an electronic keyboard, as well as a wireless laptop. Being environmentally concerned, the parents had switched all the lights in the house to compact fluorescents.

David's mother had just got the new high-powered 'smart' cell phone, with wireless headset, and told me that she had it on most of the day, and that it was often charged on standby in their bedroom at night – "just in case there's an important call."

She had been considering getting her son a cell phone as "it would be helpful to know where he was, and so he could call us if he was in trouble."

Having read this far in the book, are you also concerned about this child, and many like him?

It seems a great deal of research still needs to be done into the ways EMR exposure, and heavy metal toxicity, may affect normal neurological development in children like David.

## What are some researchers and clinicians telling us now?

There seems to be no medical consensus on what causes autism and other seemingly brain-based disorders like ADHD, or how best to treat them. Many researchers say there are probably genetic factors that predispose a child to such conditions. But some are now piecing together a disturbing picture of how environmental toxins, heavy metals, molds, chemical/food sensitivities, infections, viruses, and EMR exposure can combine to create symptoms.

As you've seen in the symptoms chart a few pages back, concentration problems and hyperactivity are among the symptoms of electro-sensitivity, so it may well be that many thousands of children are being diagnosed and treated with drugs when removing them from EMR exposure could help them significantly.

Even children who don't have neurological problems can find it difficult to sit down, focus and succeed at school when there is a lot of EMR in the environment. (So why are so many schools installing wireless Internet?)

Some of the research that's coming in suggests a link: an American and Danish team of university researchers studied 13,000 young mothers who used cell phones during pregnancy. Their results, published in an epidemiology journal in 2008, found these women's children had a 50% higher than usual incidence of hyperactive behavior and emotional problems.

Having read this far, you are probably now aware that the radiation from the mothers' cell phones is likely only one factor.

A hospital in San Diego, California found that 14 out of a group of 18 autistic children studied had lesions in the brain identical to those in rats exposed to low electro-magnetic frequencies between one and six days after birth.

The medical pioneer, Dietrich Klinghardt, MD, PhD, is a physician who believes that the increase in autism is connected to the proliferation of EMR and our increasingly toxic environment.

In his ground-breaking work, Dr. Klinghardt is finding out how to recognize and treat the effects of toxic EMR on the genes of a developing fetus.

The hope is to prevent neurological and other problems from developing in the child.

In an interview, Dr. Klinghardt told me:

> In 10 of our autistic children we measured the EMR exposure of the mother in the location where she was sleeping before giving birth to the child – who later on would be diagnosed as autistic.
>
> We measured body voltage and microwave exposure from ambient background cell phone radiation.
>
> The results clearly showed significantly increased levels of EMF exposure in the affected mothers versus the control group.

Dr. Klinghardt has developed an approach to assessing exposure:

> We also take EMF/EMR measurements at the home (and whenever possible work location or school) of children

with ADHD, behavioral problems, developmental delay and in adults with severe neurologic disease (Parkinson's, ALS, etc.) and the results are similar: the higher the exposure at home and at work, the more therapy-resistant or severe the illness.

The promising news is that many children are showing significant improvement in their symptoms, thanks to treatments that include: detoxification; supplementation with vitamins, antioxidants, and cellular nutrients; dealing with food allergies and chemical sensitivities; infrared saunas; and a low EMF/EMR environment.

Katharina Gustavs adds, "As long as the infrared sauna being used is not a magnetic field hot spot."

Dr. Klinghardt's suggestions for reducing EMR exposure are not difficult and are affordable for most people. Here is the short list that is given to his patients, including those with ASD (autism):

a. no wireless technology and no cordless phones in the home (get wired broadband and corded phones)

b. switch off all fuses at night (unless you can measure body voltage and get specific)

c. use the sleep sanctuary principle: a silver-coated mosquito net over the bed as a Faraday cage (greatly decreases microwave exposure)

Gustavs says about shield/net fabric, "First, the electric fields in the room have to be measured – and reduced – to make sure they are not drawn into the Faraday cage increasing the radiation exposure. Be cautious of what RF shielding fabric you get. Cheaper varieties can become brittle and shed off tiny particles of the metals used in the fabric, which can find their way into food and bodies causing harm." I presented at an autism conference and was saddened to hear a speaker praise 'autism apps' and her well-intentioned (misguided, in my view) mission to put an iPad into the hands of all children with autism. Why would we risk their wellbeing when they can get the same educational and entertainment benefits on safely wired devices? While evidence of a link between EMR and autism is highly controversial, most experts extol the benefits of *all* children spending less time with electronic screens and more time discovering the simple wonders of nature.

## Screen Time, Children, and Nature

Is your son or daughter an 'inside' or 'outside' child? How often do you get them involved in activities that do not involve TV, gaming, or other mobile devices and screens? Child psychiatrist and Doctors For Safer Schools Board Member Victoria Dunckley, MD cautions that "screen-time can have profound and lasting negative effects on children's brain and body development, including effects on learning, mood regulation, behavior, and fitness level. Nature and time spent outdoors, on the other hand, are proven to enhance all of these aspects."

Check out the Campaign for a Commercial-Free Childhood's screen-free week and inspire your children. (More details on pages 313 to 319.) How many children these days play freely outside as we did?

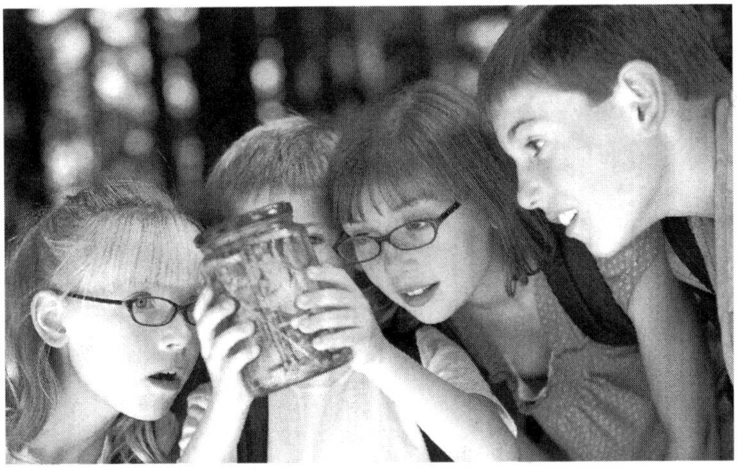

## Children With Autism Benefit in Low-EMR Environment

This 2008 case comes from Larry Gust, the electrical engineer and certified IBE environmental health consultant based in California. "A client had two children who were diagnosed with high heavy metals concentrations – particularly mercury. One was a 5-year-old boy with autism; his 3-year-old sister was behaviorally normal. Under medical supervision strategies were tried to remove this toxic load from the children's bodies, but the results (monitored via urine analysis) were poor. A full environmental assessment of the house showed the principal issues were electromagnetic pollution from:

- a wireless Internet connection.
- a 5.8 GigaHertz cordless phone system. (6.0 are even higher)
- AC Magnetic field level of more than 3 milliGauss in the girl's bedroom.
- AC electric field of more than 7 Volts/metre in all bedrooms.

**These changes were recommended:**

- Eliminate the wireless Internet and cordless phone, replace with hard-wired Internet connections and corded landline phone.
- Locate and repair wiring errors that cause high magnetic field.
- At bedtime, turn off the circuit breakers identified as causing the high electric field level in all the bedrooms.

Just before the above changes were implemented, the children had a urine test to determine if heavy metals were being eliminated from the body to the urine. There was little evidence of mercury dumping. One month after the changes another test was conducted. Mercury dumping doubled and uranium was showing up in the urine as well.

In a few months the son with autism was doing better than he had ever done in all aspects including behavior and his ability to learn."

A low-EMR environment may lead to an increase in heavy metal release resulting in a reduction in autism symptoms. This anecdotal evidence is not scientifically significant; it is, however, if it is your child who is getting better! Consider this theory: EMR compresses the cell membrane affecting the transport channels, and inhibiting the release of toxins, including heavy metals. Is this a factor?

Pediatrician Toril H. Jelter, MD, FAAP of MDI Wellness Center told me, "Some children with autism have significant improvements with a 2 week EMR remediation trial. After establishing a baseline of current function we do a 2 week EMR remediation trial i.e. turn off WiFi for 12 hours at night, unplug all cordless phones, use a land line only and turn off the electricity to the child's bedroom, IF this can be done safely. Then we repeat the functional evaluation 2 weeks later and if they have improved, we take EMR remediation to the next level.

A 4 year old with PDD-NOS who hadn't slept well for 2 years slept well within a few days - his cognitive level improved by 2 years in 2 months. A 10 year old boy with autism and aggressive behaviors said his first full sentence without prompting within a week of this trial and his aggressive behaviors vanished. His mother's seizure disorder improved. So the whole family's coping skills may benefit. Digestive problems like constipation also improved.

A 4 year old boy with autism stopped arm flapping when he visited grandma in a rural area without cell phone reception. When he returned to the San Francisco Bay Area his arm flapping restarted.

The cases I have mentioned showed dramatic changes in a short period of time. It is my professional opinion that all children with autism need a comprehensive EMR evaluation of their home and school early on, and yearly, by a trained individual. The ideal scenario would be a knowledgeable physician working closely with an individual that is certified to do EMR (electromagnetic radiation) measurements."

## EMR, Mercury, and Autism?

Words like 'detoxification' and 'mercury' come up in this discussion on autism. Some people view this as a plausible connection, others are highly skeptical. Clearly, more independent research is needed. The precautionary principle may apply here – better to err on the side of caution and avoid exposing pregnant women, infants, and children to toxicity. Holders of all views in this controversy would agree that those populations are most vulnerable to toxic exposures, as we have seen.

The still-forming picture of a possible mechanism is information that may benefit everyone who has issues with heavy metal toxicity, and may shed a new light on a range of immune and neurological conditions.

In his book, *From Fatigued to Fantastic,* Dr. Teitelbaum describes how the cell membrane works:

> All cells in the body are enclosed in a cell membrane, a balloon-like wall. Stiff cell walls can make it hard for cell membranes to perform their critical functions.

One theory is that when cells are exposed to EMR they go into a 'protective mode' to ward off a foreign invader. Part of the reaction may be compression of the cell membrane, making it rigid and impeding in-flow of nutrients and out-flow of toxins and waste products. This could make it difficult for compromised cells to clear heavy metals.

Boyd Haley, PhD is the former Chairman of the Department of Chemistry at the University of Kentucky and a National Institutes of Health post-doctoral scholar at Yale University Medical School. Dr. Haley's research into the biochemical abnormalities found in people with Alzheimer's disease led to his identifying mercury toxicity as a major factor. He was one of the first to suggest that Thimerosal, the mercury-based preservative often found in infant vaccines, was possibly involved in autism-related disorders. This is a highly controversial hypothesis. It seems mercury should be the focus, not safe mercury-free vaccinations that can be crucial in preventing disease.

Another theory is that a child can be exposed to mercury prenatally, through the mother's mercury amalgam dental fillings, or later if the child gets amalgam fillings. Heavy metal exposure could also come from the environment, as in the case of eating contaminated fish, particularly tuna, from polluted waters.

According to Dr. Klinghardt and others who treat ASD, it appears that people with a genetic predisposition to autism have trouble clearing heavy metals from their cells. This could be one of the genetic factors.

A possible explanation for this, offered by some scientists, is that when a child's blood-brain barrier is more fully formed – around the age of 18 months – it can make it extremely difficult for the mercury and other heavy metals to be excreted from the brain cells.

Pediatrician Jerry Kartzinel, MD explains his view on why some children seem able to detox themselves from metal exposures – and not develop symptoms of autism – while other children can't:

> We have natural pathways that are designed to clear toxic metals from our body. We are all born with different capacities to accomplish this. Some of our population is more easily poisoned than others.
>
> We know the very young and the very old are especially sensitive to poisonings and heavy metal…if they were never exposed to toxins in the womb, they might never have had a problem. If they were exposed to just 'regular' toxins of day-to-day living, they would be fine.

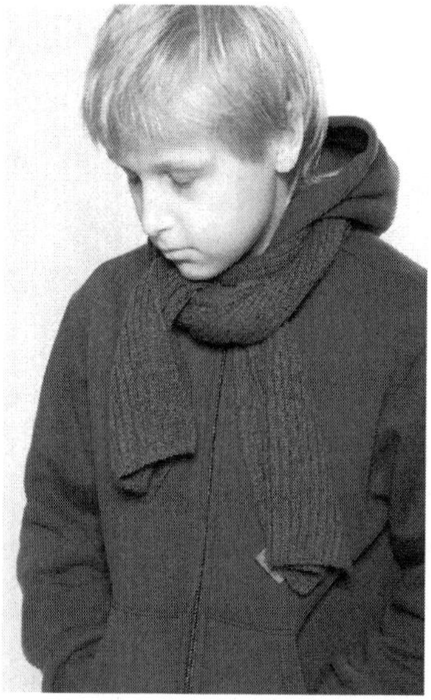

Remember, we are speaking of a total body burden of heavy metals and toxins. This burden starts soon after conception. By the time these babies take their first breath, their ability to mitigate the damage of toxic exposures is already taxed. Some children are barely taxed. Some children are almost maximally taxed. Those children born with a robust ability to detoxify sail right through. For the others, clinical signs and symptoms start becoming evident at a very young age.

Even if your family is not dealing with any challenge of hyperactivity/autism, don't you find the increasing incidence disturbing? I do. Even if the human side of this epidemic does not unsettle you, imagine the millions of dollars spent on assessment, treatment, and support services. Wouldn't it make sense to explore all avenues to seek the cause and cure of these conditions?

It seems to me that children with neurological symptoms/conditions should be at the forefront of our efforts to reduce the EMR and other toxic exposures in our homes, schools, health care facilities, and communities. And we should make it a priority to ensure they enjoy the benefits and advantages of technology in this digital age in the safest way possible.

Someone should develop a tablet that connects easily to the Internet safely using Ethernet, fibre optic, or other cable. *(See page 186 for one option.)* Until then, please teach all children how to place wirelessly-connected devices (including iPads, mobile phones, and iPods) in airplane mode and make sure they do.

## Detoxification

In *The Magnesium Miracle*, Dr. Carolyn Dean describes the many benefits of magnesium, including the process of detoxification and the ability of heavy metals to be released through the cell membrane:

> Magnesium is crucial for the removal of toxic substances and heavy metals such as aluminum and lead.

This is interesting in terms of the treatment of autism; I have also heard that magnesium is being used by some clinicians for EHS patients as it 'softens the cell membrane'.

Dr. Scheiner agreed detoxification is a key element in helping the body withstand even quite severe environmental assaults. He points out that while people in Finland were heavily exposed to radiation from the nuclear meltdown in Chernobyl, they had far lower levels of radiation sickness, and cancer, than you would expect. That's because, he says, the Finns' lifestyle includes saunas.

Sweating is one of the body's best mechanisms for clearing toxins. Some specialists recommend the far infrared sauna. Sit away from the electric element and look for a lower EMR model.

Dr. Teitelbaum also offers a key to detoxification and/or buffering the effects of EMR on the normal functioning of the cell membrane:

> This cell membrane is made up of fatty acids and a phosphorus molecule. Your body likes to use Omega-3 and -6 fatty acids when it makes cell membranes. When these are not available, your body has to use saturated fats and this results in rigid, poorly-functioning cellular walls. Essential fatty acids (EFAs) Omega-3 and -6 fatty

> acids play an important part here in keeping the cell membrane optimally functioning. This is particularly important when people are under severe physical stress or have increased sensitivities, including those sensitive to EMR. It is recommended to supplement even a healthy diet with good quality Omega-3 and -6 fatty acids."

A comprehensive protocol is evolving: magnesium from Dr. Dean, essential fatty acids from Dr. Teitelbaum, antioxidants from Dr. Scheiner and the therapeutic role of supervised detoxification from Dr. Klinghardt.

## Nutritional Supplementation

Not all supplements are created equal. Many are not absorbed by our cells. And if EMR compresses the cell membrane, it is an even greater challenge to absorb nutrients. Some supplements, including some forms of magnesium, may soften the cell membrane.

Dr. Scheiner also suggested several ways to strengthen and protect our immune system and overall health with supplements:

> First, avoid exposure of environmental pollutants, as much as possible. This will help get rid of excess free radicals. To combat these we need scavengers – antioxidant vitamins. It is not possible to get all the nutrients we need from even the healthiest diet. Our nourishment is losing antioxidants because of industrial agriculture. These days a strawberry has only 20% of its original amount of vitamin C. Therefore, it is necessary to use supplements including antioxidants, vitamins D and E, as well. All these water soluble vitamins don't enter the brain so we need scavengers that can pass the blood-brain barrier – melatonin, for example.

Salvestrols may be a much-needed supplement for this digital age. The British scientists who developed them report, "Cells in the body use Salvestrols to help correct themselves when things go wrong – like the cell's own police force helping to ensure the cell functions correctly. Salvestrols are useful when the body for some reason turns on itself and for inflammation. Antioxidants strive to protect our cells from DNA damage but are ineffective once the damage is done. Salvestrols work beyond antioxidants by eliminating the damaged cells, and only the damaged cells." There's some promising evidence that Salvestrols are effective in battling various cancers – without any adverse effects.

## Other Key Health Factors

We've heard the experts talk about all the factors working together in a negative way, harming our health. But we can also combine many factors to contribute positively to our family's wellbeing, by boosting our bodies' abilities to buffer the electro-magnetic load we experience every day. After you have reduced your EMR, and some chemical, exposures, here are effective ways to boost your overall wellness and ability to deal with the EMR load on your system that you cannot control. Some physicians offer recommendations that can enhance your family action plan; they have become central to ours. We begin with dental health.

## Dental Health

Dr. Klinghardt is only one of the physicians testing patients for heavy metal toxicity as one of the underlying causes of electro-sensitivity, Chronic Fatigue Syndrome, autism and many other conditions. Research the work of Dr. Boyd Haley, as well. This is the focus of many complementary medicine clinics, including that of Dr. Thomas Rau, the Swiss physician. Dr. Rau advises:

> A strategy to consider for those experiencing electrical sensitivity symptoms is to remove the electromagnetic 'hot spot' in the head created by the presence of metal fillings.
>
> Concern is thus not only for the neurotoxic aspect of mercury in fillings, an increasingly understood hazard, but because fillings themselves act as antennas in the presence of electromagnetic fields.

Dr. Rau says the removal of dental fillings can be an important early step in reducing electrical sensitivity, allowing some people to live in homes they otherwise could not tolerate.

(NOTE: removal of mercury fillings must be done by a dentist using a strict protocol, otherwise you, and the dentist, will be exposed to the mercury during the removal process. You must receive supplemental air during the procedure, I am told.)

Dr. Myron Wentz, a medical research scientist with a doctorate in microbiology and immunology, is also an internationally recognized virologist and cell biologist. Dr. Wentz is the founder of the comprehensive medical clinic, Sanoviv. Dr. Wentz has written a book detailing his concerns, *A Mouth Full of Poison*, (Medicis, S.C. 2004):

> Today we know that mercury is the most toxic, non-radioactive heavy metal on the planet. Despite its toxicity, mercury is still used in manufacturing including the production of: batteries, thermometers, barometers, semi-conductors, electronic instruments, lighting and chemicals.

> Mercury exposure, even at very low levels, diminishes the ability of the immune system to meet the slightest challenge.
>
> The number of T cells in the blood declines markedly when mercury amalgam is placed in the teeth, and the cells have now been programmed to undergo apoptosis – cellular death – in the presence of this mercury.
>
> If you have personally decided to get vaccinated, or are required to do so, I urge you to opt for one that is free of mercury-containing thimerosal.

## Biological Dentistry

John Snively, DDS, practised 25 years as a Biological Dentist incorporating complementary modalities of homeopathy, detoxification, supplementation and energetic medicine. Dr. Snively explains this approach:

> Toxic metals and other materials often become implanted in our teeth resulting in a long term burden to our immune system and root canals can also have devastating effects. The teeth and jaw joint provide us with a valuable sense of proprioception and discrepancies here can manifest throughout the body.
>
> Dissimilar metals in the mouth can create not only an electrical current but can also act as an antenna for other invisible Electromagnetic and Microwave forces.

In seeking a Biological Dentist one must first be certain that the office is "mercury free" and provides protection not only for you as a patient but that the dental team is wearing appropriate masks when removing toxic metals.

Some sort of biocompatibility testing should be offered to determine which materials are most tolerable for your immune system. Clifford Consulting & Research, of Colorado Springs, offers this testing – a dental materials screening. (www.ccrlab.com)

## Safeguarding Your Family's Health the Holistic Way

As you may know, the complementary medicine approach has a lot to offer those of us who want to protect our families' health in this increasingly irradiated world.

Complementary health practitioners tend to focus more on prevention and natural remedies such as those advocated by Dr. Andrew Weil and the others mentioned in this book, whereas the conventional medical model uses more pharmaceuticals to treat disease.

In this emerging field of electro-sensitivity it seems crucial to understand the complementary approach, as there are no drugs to treat this condition, and many conventional tests and treatments may exacerbate symptoms and conditions rather than improve them.

Dr. Scheiner described the electro-sensitive person who's experiencing a range of symptoms when exposed to these frequencies. Unfortunately, this percentage of the population is growing dramatically in virtually every corner of the world. Few people, and few of their doctors, recognize these symptoms and their potential cause.

Therefore, after many medical or non-medical tests and therapies, patients' symptoms may remain and over the long term even worsen, as they have not been able to identify and treat the source. For some, the source is the invisible waves of radiation that surrounds us all.

The best possibility here is that people have recognized their body's wireless wake-up call, are hearing the body's alarm, and taking steps to avoid the exposure.

While many people are suffering, with their daily activities severely limited, feeling overwhelmed and victimized by the electro-pollution, in some ways these canaries in the coal mine may be doing better than the miners, who are also being exposed and affected, but do not hear and/or heed the symptoms.

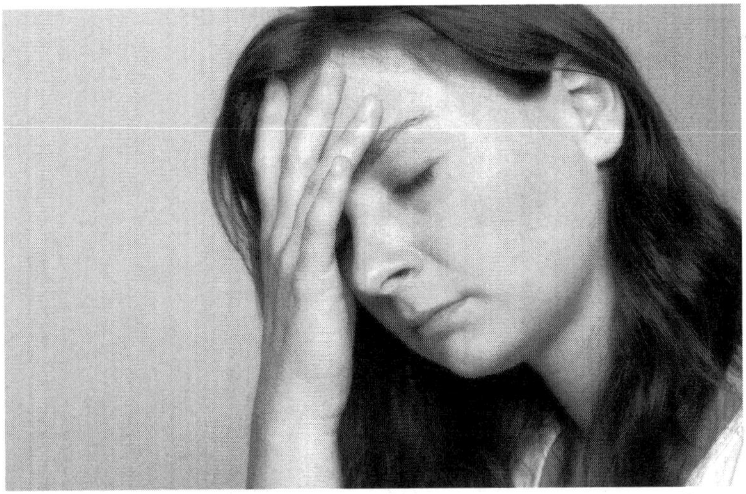

One of the main objectives of this book, and my new health advocacy, is to get the word out that if you're having a lot of trouble sleeping, if you're fatigued, having skin tingling, burning sensations, difficulty focusing, any light-headedness or dizziness, this collection of symptoms may well be your body's attempt to let you know that this exposure is harmful.

Dr. Scheiner's observation:

> Each symptom, like the headaches, sleep disruption, dizziness etc. can be unspecific – caused by a lot of different reasons. It gets specific, however, when you experience several of these – this could be what we're calling microwave syndrome – this is not a sickness, it is a warning system.
>
> Your body is trying to alert you, saying, 'I'm having trouble here, get me out of this situation'. These symptoms are a call for help. As you may know, in our conventional medical system, it is often our approach to deal with these symptoms, in a sense trying to shut the body up, masking the calls for help and giving relief of the symptoms.
>
> The cause of the distress, however, may not be addressed and therefore continues the harm. What we see, clinically, is that this can progress to more serious conditions.

I had the good fortune to have several very long conversations with Dr. Scheiner, and the more I heard from him of how EMR affects the cells and stresses the body, the more it reminded me of much of the work I had been doing in emotional and physical stress.

In my previous book, *The Healthy Type A*, I developed an Early Stress Warning cue to help people tune into this stress reaction sooner, giving themselves greater success at reducing this potentially harmful response.

With Dr. Scheiner's inspiration, I began to develop an exercise to recognize the early symptoms of EMR exposure.

## Your Early Warning Cue

This is an exercise where you take note of the first signs – the slight tingling, the slight light-headedness, etc. It is much easier to deal with these symptoms when they are just beginning, as you would assume.

This early indicator can serve as a cue, an alert to wake you up that you need to do something about where you are right now.

When you recognize this cue, the first obvious step is to reduce the exposure. For example, are you in a wireless hot spot? Has your neighbor installed a new router; have you up-graded the cordless phone model?

You might go back to the questionnaire in Strategy 2 and look at the symptoms you checked off. Then note the ones that seem to occur first. These can become your early warning cues.

When you recognize this cue, you know it is time to get away from what you are doing, and where you are, if you can. This is where an EMR detector is so helpful. It can alert you to high EMR areas, and also to lower ones you can seek when you recognize your cue.

Getting outside, away from electronics, is often good, unless you are close to power lines, masts or cell tower antennas.

Having a cool, or warm, shower can be helpful. And being beside a waterfall, fountain, stream, river, or ocean can be restorative.

Now let's take a look at a variety of ways we can protect and restore our health – our greatest treasure, as you know.

## Wellbeing Strategies

### Grounding Exercises

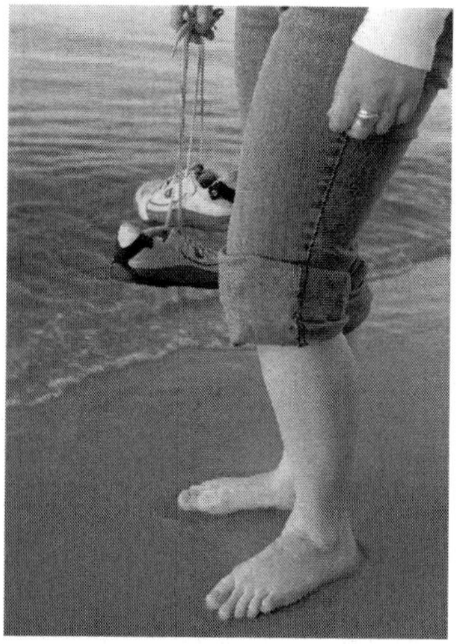

A physician who specializes in energy medicine told me that he advises his electro-sensitive patients to remember the healing, restorative power of nature. This is not as far-out as you might imagine. Remember what Dr. Becker told us about the natural electro-magnetic fields of the earth. This doctor recommends going outside and standing barefoot on the actual earth, if at all possible (sand, dirt, grass are best, but pavement is ok).

Lean or crouch over so that all your fingers touch the ground. If you're feeling light-headed or dizzy, you might need support. He suggests doing some relaxed deep-breathing, and feel as much as you can that you are reconnecting with the earth and the natural energies around you. The surgeon Dr. Rea also recommends this grounding practice.

There are explanations for this grounding – it might be that with hands and feet both on the ground you're completing a circuit and allowing the buildup of artificial electro-magnetic energy in your body to be discharged into the earth. Dr. Sinatra contributed to *Earthing* (Basic Health Publications, 2010 with Clinton Ober and Martin Zucker) on the physiological benefits of grounding. As you may know, what Dr. Sinatra calls "good vibes" can heal and balance us when we connect with the harmonious forces of the natural world – walking barefoot on the earth is the best way, or leather-lined moccasins (no rubber sole).

There are earthing, grounding pads to sleep on, or have under your feet at the computer. Not sure why but these help some people and not others. Probably something to do with the surrounding EMR/RF.

Dr. Sinatra talks about natural grounding:

> Our research has shown that these grounding exercises can calm and balance our systems and produce a physiological shift from the sympathetic nervous system (stress mode) to the parasympathetic (relaxation mode). The results of this shift have a positive effect on many cardiovascular risk factors: thickened blood was normalized, heart function was balanced, there was a reduction in oxidative stress from free radicals easing the disruption of blood vessels, inflammation was reduced, and there was an easing of anxiety. These are significant health benefits.

Another good way to ground: pause and take a few deep breaths, letting go as you exhale. Not heavy breathing and hyperventilating; it's more changing the way you breathe – lower and deeper with the abdomen moving. With each inhalation, focus on breathing in energizing oxygen, and with each exhalation, expelling stale air, and some of your stress. More on this coming up in a few pages.

## Anti-aging – Healthy Aging – Important New Discoveries

No other generation has faced our health challenges; we need to adapt. This is one focus of Dr. Sinatra, who is a founding member of the American Academy of Anti-Aging Medicine (A4M). Both of us speak at the annual conference. As we've said, EMR has been shown to: impair DNA repair and other cellular and organ functions; decrease memory; suppress immunity; diminish melatonin and cause sleep problems; affect eyesight, and increase inflammation – primary aging factors. As Dr. Blank's research shows, living amidst the increasing smog of electro-pollution also produces unhealthy stress on our cells.

And remember the German study that found EMR exposure impaired our neurotransmitters – the electric impulses in the brain. Not good! So each step you take in this plan brings a wealth of anti-aging benefits.

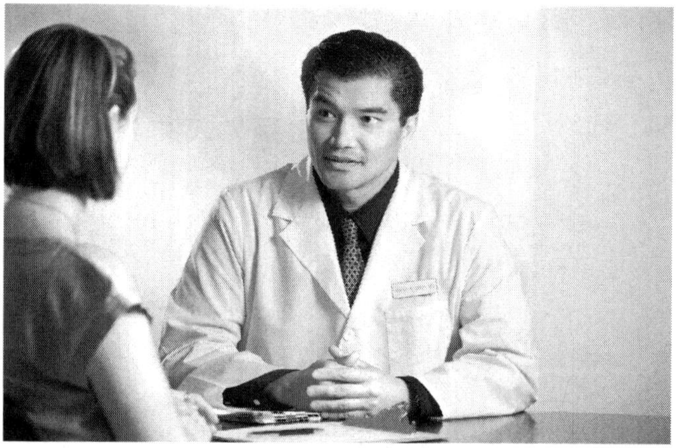

I hope this book inspires you to take better care of your body's electrical system – your heart and nervous system. This is critical as we age. I highly recommend tai chi and qi gong. These practices have been used for thousands of years to balance and ground our life force energy, and promote longevity and lifelong wellness. These ancient spiritual and health belief systems completely understood "the body electric" – hence the development of acupuncture and other forms of energy medicine.

## Acupuncture

Traditional Chinese Medicine (TCM) has its roots in Taoism. Its practitioners have known for at least five thousand years that the life energy of humans and other living creatures is connected with, and influenced by, the energies in our environment, whether these are natural or artificial. TCM practitioners see the human body in terms of a system of pathways, or meridians, through which our life force energy (called qi, or chi) travels. Our health depends on the balanced and unhindered flow of this energy.

Dr. Hong Zhen Zhu, author of *Building a Jade Screen: Better Health with Chinese Medicine* (Penguin Canada 2001), has treated a number of patients with EMR-related symptoms. Although EMR is a relatively new kind of assault on our bodies' natural electro-magnetic energies, Dr. Zhu applies classical TCM theory to what he's observed in his patients' symptoms.

Dr. Zhu explains:

> EMR disrupts the normal direction of energy flow along the meridians, affecting many body systems and functions. It also disturbs mental functioning, mood and spirit. Acupuncture is helpful in treating the brain fog, insomnia, and other EMR-related conditions such as Chronic Fatigue Syndrome and sensitivity to noise and light.

Dr. Zhu also recommends such mind-body balancing practices as tai chi, qi gong and meditation.

Dr. Carrie Hyman, LAc, OMD, a Doctor of Chinese Medicine, recommended specific herbs and antioxidants:

> A TCM practitioner can recommend Chinese Tonic herbs. These are a unique class of herbs that are preventative and restorative. The numerous benefits include adaptogenic properties. Many of these longevity enhancing "superior herbs," have been valued by the Chinese for thousands of years. Modern science reveals that they are high in polyphenols (green tea), flavonoids (berries...anti-inflammatory), polysaccharides and antioxidants. Moreover, they support the body's ability to manufacture endogenous antioxidants like SOD and glutathione peroxidase. This is important as EMFs increase free-radical – oxidative stress, thereby increasing our need for antioxidants.

## NeuroModulation Technique, NMT

This is another treatment that works on the principles of energy medicine. NeuroModulation Technique (NMT) was developed by a chiropractor/complementary health practitioner, Dr. Leslie S. Feinberg, DC, in 2002. His website www.nmt.md describes this approach:

> The informational basis of illness and disease may be the most common, yet the most overlooked, roadblock to healing. NMT is best described as 'informational medicine,' because it works to identify and correct the informational source of illness – the confusion that can interrupt our innate healing mechanisms.
>
> Many people believe that illness results from some external affliction that viciously attacks the mind-body. The NMT position is that illness is the inevitable result of informational confusion and faults in the systems responsible for regulating body functions, making them unable to produce the balanced internal-body state that wellness requires.
>
> A good example of this is food allergy, where the immune system is so confused that the body damages itself by its misguided reaction to a food that it should see as beneficial nutrition. Seen in this light, illness or "dis-ease" in the body happens by default when the mind-body is not sufficiently aware of its internal conditions and the requirements for healing.
>
> The mind-body is a self-correcting system that always seeks to find and maintain the balanced internal state in which optimal health and vitality thrive.

I asked Dr. Feinberg how this system might benefit people with EMR exposure symptoms and conditions:

> With thermal exposure there is obvious harm – heating of the tissue. As you have told me, most of the concern in the scientific community is with non-thermal levels from cordless and cell phones, WiFi etc., where the radiation is not strong enough to heat tissue, but is causing harm nonetheless. We could use the analogy of allergy and toxicity. Mercury is highly toxic – harmful to everyone. This could be compared to thermal EMR exposure. An allergy, however, happens when the immune system is provoked to react in an 'inappropriate' way, causing reaction symptoms – inflammation etc. This could be compared to what happens on the cellular level with non-thermal EMR exposure. Perhaps it is not so much that this level of radiation is harmful to the body, as it is confusing.

Confusing? I remembered what I had heard about the mechanism of harm – the cell membrane going into 'lockdown' mode as it does not recognize these new artificial frequencies – and that it was this reaction (misinterpretation) that affected the normal functioning of the cell.

I found this conversation with Dr. Feinberg illuminating and encouraging. You can imagine what it has been like for me to be immersed in this issue for the past four years, reading more and more research that presents increasingly troubling results. I asked Dr. Feinberg how this 'confusion' might explain electro-sensitive people. He said that some people are very reactive and have symptoms. With electro-sensitive people it might be tingling of the skin, headaches, difficulty sleeping etc.

Remember what Dr. Scheiner told us about people becoming "allergic" to electricity?

But what about something like leakage of the blood-brain barrier? I asked Dr. Feinberg. Although this specific area has not been the main focus of Dr. Feinberg's work, and he was not familiar with Dr. Salford's research, he replied that this could be explained by inflammation – one of the body's primary reactions.

I wanted to three-way Professor Salford into the conversation right away, and to bring in all our other experts. Hopefully, one day we can get these researchers and clinicians together to provide a more complete picture of how this all works, and how best to diagnose and treat EMR exposure. Not only for the millions of electro-sensitive people, but for all those with high EMR exposure who have not yet developed symptoms.

## NMT and Autism

Dr. Feinberg told me that NMT was used recently in a research study with children with autism, led by Dr. Robert Weiner, a Clinical Psychologist in Dallas, Texas. The trial was stopped after 18 children completed the study.

The results were so positive that Dr. Weiner wanted to report the findings as soon as possible rather than waiting another 6-12 months to collect more data before he announced the findings and published the study. Dr. Weiner designed the study to determine the effectiveness of NMT in improving the functioning of children with autism. The study ran for 12 sessions over 6 weeks. Statistically significant improvement was noted by the end of 6 sessions, with continued improvement occurring through the end of the study.

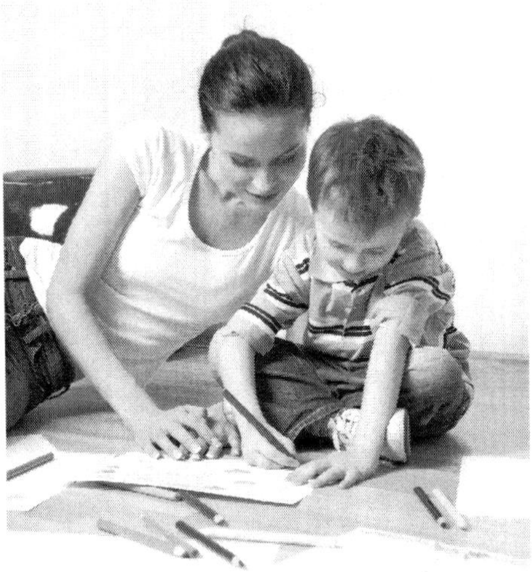

Parents whose children were in the study were amazed at the changes they saw in their children during the course of the study. Each session averaged 45 minutes, so the study demonstrated that NMT was able to produce profound changes in these children in a total of only 9 hours of NMT treatment.

This is a small study, with encouraging results. We need to help these families get their children back so they can all thrive.

I wanted to call Dr. Klinghardt right away to tell him this news. Then Dr. Feinberg told me that Dr. Klinghardt knows his work, so is probably already aware of this study and its promising results.

I was "connecting the dots" during this conversation and saw a comparison, not only with allergies, but with the "miscommunication" of the fight or flight response – the source of our emotional stress. This is when the body gets all geared up – muscles tighten, blood pressure goes up, etc. – with our basic instincts to fight that tiger, when the only threat is slow traffic.

## Another Key Factor – Your Acid-Alkaline (pH) Balance

There is a Swiss naturopathic doctor who specializes in this area. Dr. Christopher Vasey ND, in his book, *The Acid-Alkaline Diet*, explains why this balance is so important to overall health, and why most of us are overly acidic. Not good news: most of the foods in our Western diet are highly acidic – meats, starchy foods (white-floured pasta), sugars (most fruits, all cakes, cookies, sodas etc.) alcohol and, of course, vinegar. Dr. Vasey reports that fatigue is a primary symptom of being overly acidic.

Other symptoms include: irritability, depression, headaches, inflamed gums, skin inflammation, red blotches, itching, heartburn and other stomach and digestive problems, excessive urination, fungal diseases (yeasts thrive in the acidic environment), joint and muscle pain and our old friend insomnia.

This list reminds me of the Chronic Fatigue and the EMR checklists. It may seem puzzling; however, everything is interconnected in our body. And when the natural balance of this vital pH is thrown off, it affects all the fluids and systems in the body, producing many symptoms.

Briefly: Dr. Vasey describes effective ways to test urine and saliva – good indicators – and how to bring the pH back into healthy balance. All green and colored vegetables – without any sweet or sour sauces – are the primary alkalizing foods and should be included in every main meal, he recommends. This doesn't mean we give up acidic foods like meat, sugar and many grains; it does mean that we balance with alkalizing foods: vegetables, green drinks, soft cheeses, almonds and avocados.

## Keeping Hydrated

This is vital. Virtually every complementary medicine practitioner highly recommends that we drink lots of pure water. Sorry, this does not include coffee, tea, juice, soda or alcohol. This means good, filtered $H_2O$. Every cell and system in the body must have sufficient toxin-free water to maintain healthy functions.

And this is crucial for any kind of detoxification. It is also helpful in terms of our EMR exposure, as much of our cells' composition, and our cell membranes, are lipids and liquid and need to stay permeable, as Dr. Teitelbaum explained.

Here's a good tip: drink your large glass of water, with alkalizing greens, between meals. There are also mineral drops and powders that you can add to alkalize your system. It is best to hydrate and alkalize *between* meals, not with them, as you don't want to dilute your digestive enzymes. It is also good *not* to drink ice water with meals, as this hampers digestion.

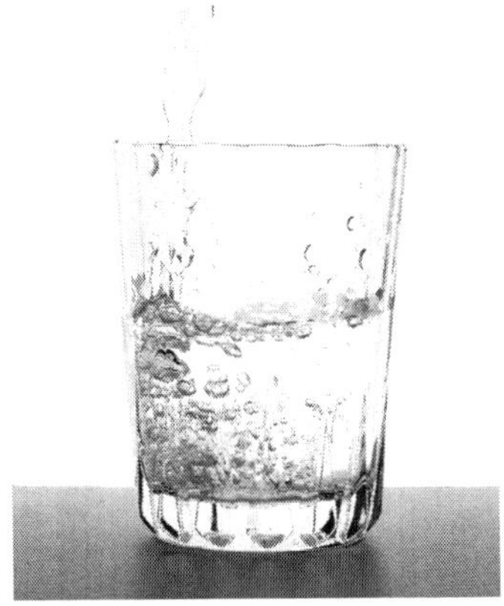

## Techno Speed, Stress and Everyday Frenzy

Are you discovering there are many facets to this discussion, not just health concerns? In this digital age of distraction, electro-seductions can grab our attention by the throat and not let go. I read that when we are staring at a computer screen, we blink a fraction of the times we should. Ever felt dizzy at the keyboard when you realize you have been so ramrod focused that you forgot to breathe? (Even at your yoga class?)

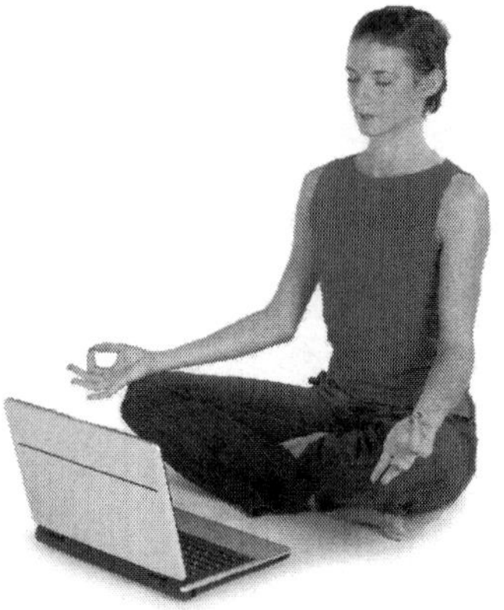

We may tell ourselves, "take breaks, breathe, stretch," yet the hours go by and we're hunched up, tightened up and bleary-eyed, still staring at the screen. It's as though we've lost touch with the fact that we have a body, until we notice the aching low back, sore neck and shoulders and wrist pain. Some people even think computering can be good down time. The hyper-speed that all this technology affords us is a two-edged convenience. People used to have to wait for you to return messages; now, they demand instant access.

And there used to be quiet moments in our day – waiting for the kids after school, waiting for a bus, or just hanging out. Now, we never have to be alone. There never has to be a gap. We can fill every bit of space with texting, if we can't be talking or shopping online. This can lead to a very speedy mind. Our dazzling display of technology feeds right into, we could almost say enables, unhealthy stress.

Remember Toad of Toad Hall, in *The Wind In The Willows?* How he would have loved instant messaging and video gaming. Zooming from one call to the next can feel so exhilarating. We hardly need to take a breath in between.

All this speed can make us feel so alive; it is, however, hard on the system. When the body responds with a surge of adrenaline, heart rate and rhythm are disrupted, blood pressure goes up, the blood thickens – not a good combination – muscles tighten, the normal functioning of immune and gastro-intestinal systems is suppressed, and more.

Foolishly, the body thinks these responses are going to save us from that saber-toothed tiger, when in fact, these 'adaptations' work against us. (Reminds me of the theory of the cell membrane's misunderstanding of non-thermal EMR exposure.)

This misplaced stress response disturbs our sleep, makes us tense, ages us more rapidly and can lead to a wide range of symptoms and conditions. You know this feeling – you're restless, edgy and impatient. It's not only the jet-fuel java accelerating your heart, it is also the stress response.

Our high-tech toys feed our Type A need for speed. I know this from my research, and personal experience: high-energy go-getters can be a tad impatient. I realize that this personality style plays a role here.

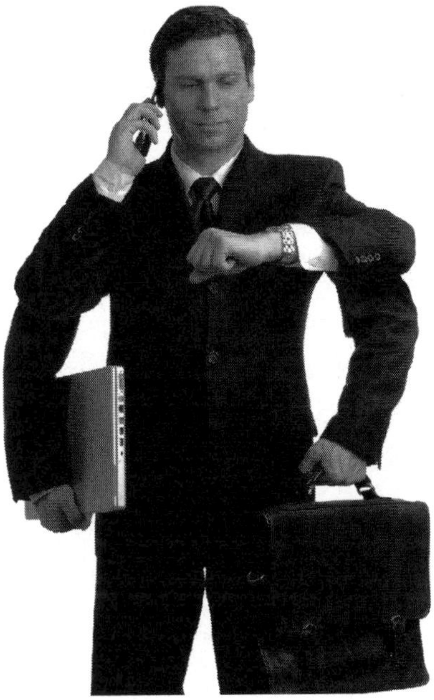

If we are going to reduce our EMR exposure, unhook ourselves from our tech obsession, it seems we need to cut this cycle of urgency, speed and stress. A challenge: do you know anyone who is not stressed these days?

Even vacations don't seem to provide much of a gap. Here's a good space-filler I saw recently: a luxury resort is now offering your own wireless television set, complete with wireless headsets, poolside. (No, I don't remember the name of it.) We can quite literally, go into withdrawal when someone, some thing attempts to take away our 'drug'. Try taking your child off computer games 'cold turkey', or forgoing texting, emailing, YouTubing, Facebooking and web-surfing for a day. We may need to come off slowly.

Whatever you can do to reduce the adrenaline will help. In fact, cutting back on caffeine – gradually, to avoid a withdrawal headache – is a very helpful way to slow you down and will make it easier to cut back on your tech time, assuming this is what you want to do.

Before you got caught up in this swirl, do you remember what more slow-paced pastimes you enjoyed? Reading? Walking in the park? Sitting on a log at the beach? Without headphones. Maybe visit a friend. Yes, actually, go and *see* them. And sit and chat. Reconnect. When we allow our mind to slow down, our body will follow. This is a good approach for digital detox.

There are some ways that we can enjoy these together. Meditation, for example. Just plain sitting. Being with your breath. Being with your mind. Being where you are. Unplugged. An outrageous thought, perhaps? To sit quietly. To tune in. To just take some down time to be with ourselves, to be with this moment, somehow goes against the grain in our modern world.

### SIMPLICITY: Mindfulness Meditation Made Easy

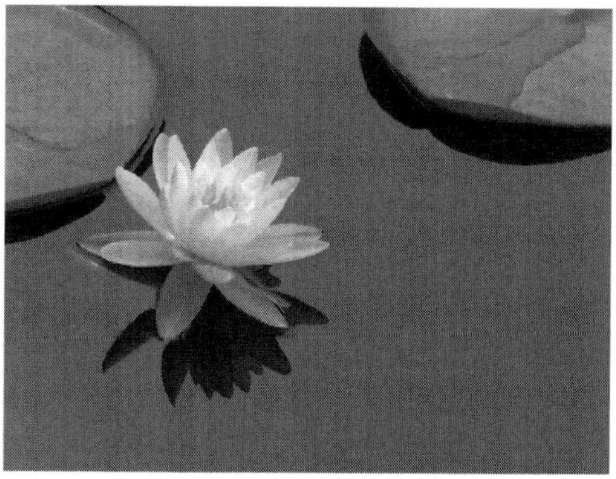

Interestingly, in Japan, one of the most frenetic cultures on this planet, many people still seek out the quiet contemplative environment of Zen meditation. Nothing religious, just taking time to slow down, and tune in.

I have studied meditation, flower arranging and Tea Ceremony for many years – an accomplishment for a go-getter. When I had a clinical practice and taught people progressive relaxation, I used to combine this with simple breath meditation. This was before we were so crazed and dazed by technology, so it is even more useful now to pull ourselves away from the screen, power off, and sit quietly for a few moments.

Dr. Jon Kabat-Zinn is the author of *Wherever You Go, There You Are: Mindfulness Meditation In Everyday Life* and founder of the Stress Reduction Clinic at the University of Massachusetts Medical Centre.

Dr. Kabat-Zinn describes what it is like to have a meditation practice:

> ... by making some time for this each day doesn't mean that you won't be able to think any more, or get things done. It means that you are more likely to know what you are doing because you have stopped for awhile.

### Simplicity 5-Min Meditation: Quick Calm and Focus

**Posture**: Sit comfortably on a straight-backed chair or on a cushion on the floor. Let your shoulders relax and let your arms hang straight down by your sides. Rest your hands, palms down, comfortably on your legs.

**Eyes**: Your eyes are open – helpful in keeping from dozing off. Your gaze is soft and relaxed; you look out and down slightly.

**Breath**: try to refrain from fancy breathing. You are not trying to bliss out, or get caught up in any other entertainment. Just sit quietly and breathe normally. Once you settle a bit your breathing will become more natural. Just breathe in through your nose, and out through your nose. Let your jaw relax. Slowing down you feel your body, feel your breath, feel yourself just being here.

**Attention**: The more you need to do this, the more difficult it may be. Some of us haven't sat quietly with ourselves for a long time. It's hard to grasp but the action here is to just be. Just let your attention rest on your breathing. Enjoy the space.

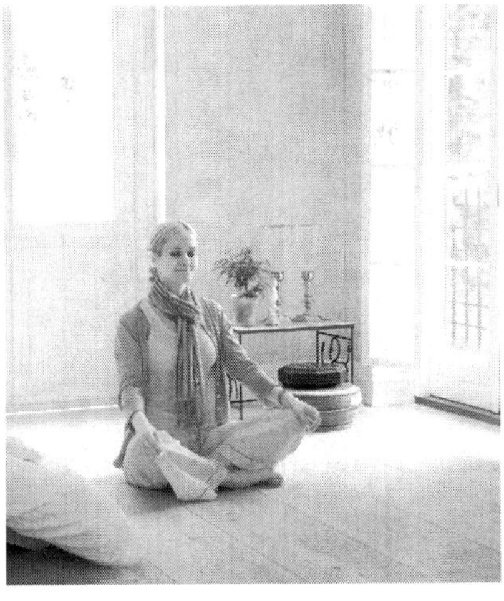

**Unplug. Breathe. Exhale.** Try just five minutes; see how you feel. If three is all you can do, that's a start.

**YOU ARE NOT TRYING TO STOP YOUR THOUGHTS!**

This only creates more. Let the thoughts – and all those colorful emotions – come and go. When you wake up and realize that you have been carried away by them; come back. Come back to the gentle movement of the breath. This helps to train, focus and calm the mind.

**The Benefit**: What has this got to do with our Safer-Tech Challenge? When we are no longer uneasy in the space of things as they are; no longer edgy when alone, or frantic when nothing is 'happening', we find ourselves spending more time away from the computer and our other diversions. And every moment we are unplugged reduces our EMR exposure.

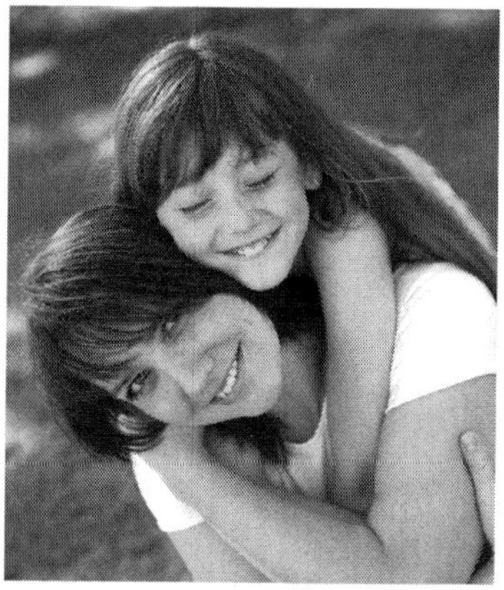

When we get outside, just being in nature, our energy soars. And when we walk barefoot on the earth (or wearing unlined leather moccasins without rubber soles) we are grounding and enjoying many benefits. May I suggest you try this and see.

## Yoga, Tai Chi, Qi Gong and Other Body/Mind Practices

The benefits with these practices are numerous, in this context they help us reconnect with ourselves, ease the stress in our bodies, clear the clutter from our minds and release the stale breath from our lungs, as well as focus the mind. I'm sure you can find a good class at your local recreation center, if you want to try out these body/mind exercises. My husband Charles Blackhall and I teach these disciplines and also a contemplative photography workshop and webinar, The Mindful EYE. This Zen art of seeing practice is to slow down and see our world with fresh eyes. It's fun! Visit us at www.TheMindfulEYE.org.

These body/mind activities, particularly when done out in the fresh air, and when we breathe deeply, helps to recharge our life force energy and helps us to reconnect with the natural energy fields of the earth.

## Walk, Stretch, Swim, Enjoy

Remember the River of Health, and how it can be flowing or stagnant?

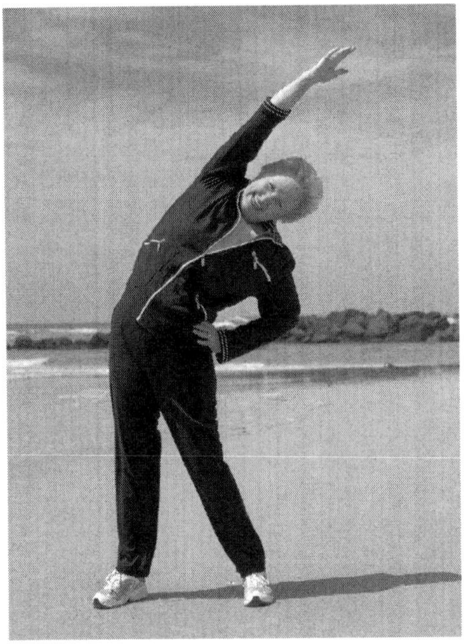

An easy way to diagnose your own inner river is: if you feel tired and low energy, the flow is sluggish, toxins are building up, and you're lacking oxygen.

One of the best ways to recharge our EMR-overloaded systems is to get this river moving again; our blood moving, lymph flowing and chi circulating. Stretching at the computer keyboard is good for crunched muscles, but it's even better to get away from it.

You may have built up resistance; exercise being a way to lose weight. You may have come to resent feeling pressured into being fit. But let's look at being more active from a different perspective, one that is pivotal to staying healthy amidst environmental pollutants.

You don't have to walk, cycle or run for miles; just get a stagnant system moving. Flowing. The vitality of our lymph system is a key element in dealing with almost all of the symptoms and conditions we've been discussing.

If this clearing house is not functioning well there is a build-up of toxins, the immune system becomes overwhelmed and we are more likely to be sensitive to chemical and electro-pollution, have allergies and food sensitivities, among other problems. Being more physically active helps the lymphatic fluid clear toxins and this improves so many conditions.

A spry 90 year-old woman at our rec center coached me on her swim routine: warm up your muscles in the hot tub, take a brief cool shower, then swim. She does ten slow and steady laps, while I splash around in the aqua-fit class. After you get out of the pool, she suggests, have a steam to help the body flush out any toxins from the pool water. Some gentle stretching and re-hydrating with lots of pure water completes her routine. Try it.

When you recognize the Early Warning Cue which tells you that your stress, or EMR exposure, levels are rising, get up and get outside. Lie on the grass. Look off into the distance.

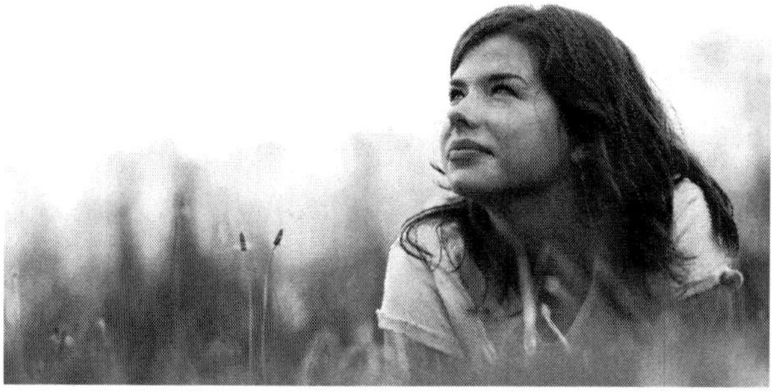

Watch birds in the sky.

This is good for eyes that spend long hours staring at various electronic screens. Swing your arms. Breathe deeply. Move.

This, and staying hydrated, are the best ways to keep the river flowing. Swim. Play tag with your children at the park. Put on your era's favorite music and dance just like you used to do. That will make them smile. I encourage you to add to your action plan twenty minutes daily of being outside in the fresh air. Feel too tired? All the more reason to get moving. You may find it more effective, and more fun, than the usual ways we try to deal with fatigue – the sugary carb, or the caffeine kick. (Isn't it annoying that many of the things that taste good aren't good for us?)

## The Communication Challenge

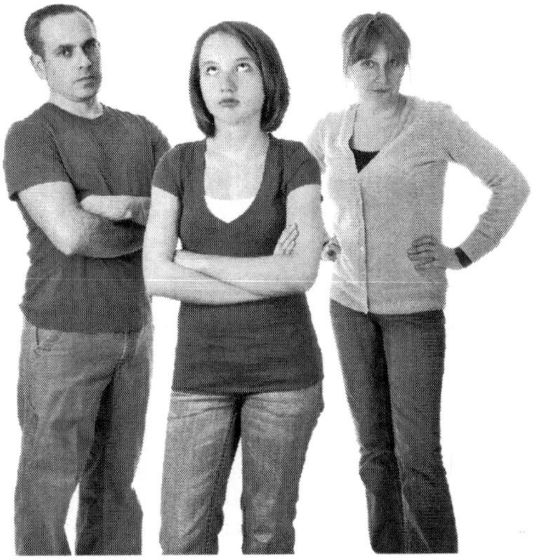

Recognize this eye roll? Persuading supposedly rational adults to adopt a safer-tech lifestyle is one thing. How do you get your teens to understand that their beloved cell phone, so central to their social life, is as much of a safety issue as sex, drug use, wearing a helmet, driving safely and so on?

I spoke with Dr. Allison Rees, a counsellor and parenting expert, who agrees that dealing with this hyper-tech generation can be a real challenge:

> Teens need and want to make their own decisions, just at a time when they aren't good at doing that! So we attempt to educate, state our concerns and negotiate, as best we can. I suggest not indulging children with the technology, and not seeing these devices as a privilege. I'm concerned with the sense of entitlement kids have around getting this 'stuff'.

Dr. Rees offers some ideas for communicating more effectively with your children, which may be helpful whether you're talking about technology, or any other issues.

Here are some of her key points:

- Say what you want to say; don't just react to the child's statements or behavior;
- Stay on one topic, be brief and to the point, and don't bring up issues from the past;
- Do respect the teen's need for independence and request a positive change;
- Don't lecture or try to control by making demands, commands, threats, or guilt-inducing statements, or fear-inducing warnings.

Dr. Rees adds:

> People, including children, tend to resist being pushed, coerced, or otherwise forced into changing their behavior. When a parent forces a child to change his or her behavior, the child reacts like someone whose head is held under water by a bigger, more powerful person. He/she does anything possible to resist. If the parent succeeds, the child feels resentful and wants revenge.

> It is therefore important for us as parents to make requests rather than give orders. We should recognize that it's up to our children to control and change their behavior, rather than trying to impose such changes on them. Only in situations where there is actual physical danger should we try to control our children.

I would suggest that in the case of radiation exposure, as with other health and safety issues such as alcohol consumption and driving, you engage your teens in a problem-solving discussion around solutions that will keep them safer while still respecting their need for autonomy and some privacy. For instance, can they agree to abide by some of the safer use guidelines for cell phones – limiting use, keeping them powered off and away from their heads at night, and using the speakerphone or wired headset? As with so many issues that come up as our children grow into young adults, we have to be clear about our reasons and give them the information they need. As Dr. Rees reminds us, lecturing breeds resistance.

## Other Technology Issues:

A Good Morning America segment interviewed five top texting teens – one boy sent up to 35,000 messages a month. I was amazed that his parents did not seem horrified with this saying, "Well, it doesn't seem to be affecting his school work."

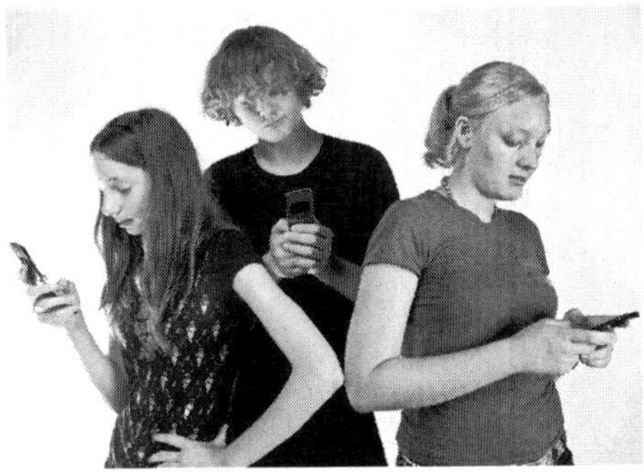

Let's consider the radiation exposure. However, there are also concerns with teens and technology that go beyond physical health effects and distractions at school. For instance, vicious attacks of cyber-bullying, where a young teen is targeted with abusive emails or instant messages.

Or the obsession with texting, which has developed a sideline where young people send each other nude photos of themselves by cell phone. Check in with your children and teens about their communications. Check the bill to see how often the phone is being used.

## Internet Safety, Privacy, Social Media in this Digital Age

The health hazards are not the only concern. Ever notice that kids suddenly switch screens when you walk in? Look at the window tabs.

Jesse Miller, founder of Miller Consulting Services warns:

> Social networking websites can provide your personal information to other companies, with your approval based on agreement of the prescribed terms of use.
>
> Not knowing, and/or not caring, about any consequences, our youth see Facebook, for example, as a place where they can be who they are, communicate with friends openly without adult judgement.
>
> The consequences to this behaviour when un-monitored, or unaddressed by parents can be detrimental to their endeavours in the future – permanent traces are left behind. It is common for potential employers, school and university admissions to use Facebook, and other sites, in the screening process. The people I talk with assure me that their profile is secure. I show them how easy it is to access and retain their personal information, pictures etc.
>
> Less common, but potentially tragic, police investigations track home invasions, abductions, sexual assaults and homicides that have resulted from seemingly innocent online encounters. Parents should explain that passwords should be available (maybe in a sealed envelope) if access

to these accounts is needed in a police investigation. Today our personal information – pictures, home addresses, when you are home alone, away on holiday, and telephone numbers – is digitized into public view.

Renowned singer and children's advocate Raffi Cavoukian's new book *Lightweb Darkweb* (Homeland Press, 2013) is a much-needed guide for parents and educators with concerns about how social media affects young people. Raffi asks probing questions and offers three excellent reasons for social media reform: safety, intelligence, and sustainability – "B4 It Re-forms Us". It's a call for sanity in this digital age and for acting in the best interests of our children, and theirs.

Raffi is founder of the Centre for Child Honouring – Respecting Earth and Child, "honouring children is the best way to create sustainable, peacemaking societies". He is an eloquent spokesperson for living with heart, and with respect for each other and the world in which we live. Raffi is an inspiration to me and to all who hear his message.

I know social media is supposed to connect people, but it can also increase isolation and a loss of privacy. A Silicon Valley expert told me, "I don't do social networking. I know what they do with the data".

## Disconnect from the Internet to Reconnect

In 2014, someone in Vancouver, Canada opened the Faraday Cafe – a metal mesh enclosure blocks WiFi and cell phone signals – as a gathering place to enhance social interaction. The owner's inspiration was to encourage people to unplug from their digital gadgets and reconnect with each other. There will be more such places.

One day we'll see WiFi-free zones in airports, hotels, schools etc. until WiFi is banned in public places due to health concerns – like smoking.

## The Safer-Tech Family Challenge and Digital Detox

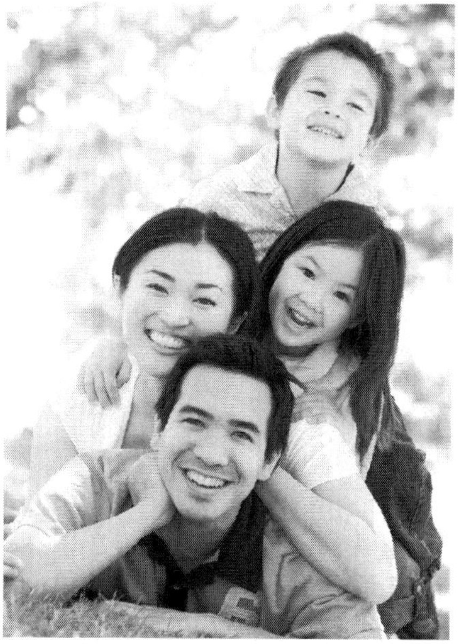

Roberto Salti and colleagues at the University of Florence in Italy found that when 74 children, aged 6 to 12, were deprived of their TVs and computers for a week, and other sources of artificial light were reduced in their homes, there was a beneficial outcome: the production of melatonin increased by an average of 30 per cent. The increases were highest in the youngest children.

And as you may know, being outside in the sunshine triggers the internal production of Vitamin D, which is also essential to our health.

Ever wondered what might happen if your family were to unplug from the virtual world and reconnect? This is for families wired on wireless who want to reconnect with each other, and the natural world around us. If you've had children in primary schools, you might have participated in "turn off the TV week," when families are encouraged to spend time reading, playing games, listening to music, going outside – any activity that doesn't require a television or computer monitor.

There was a TV challenge some time ago for families to go without for a month. I remember one young teen complaining it "was like a death in the family." Interestingly, there were similar stages – irritation, boredom, anger and eventually, if they could hang in there, some times of once-lost fun and jokes. Some parents reported that it was really refreshing not to have to drag the kids away from the TV show or the "next level" in the video game when it's time for dinner.

I'd like to propose a safer-tech family life and digital detox. Rediscover each other, and maybe the joy of reading, books, the printed page?

Don't panic – you don't have to toss out all things electronic. I'm hoping this process will give you the time and mental space to see how much of the technology is really necessary in helping you function and stay connected, and how much is just a habit and mental clutter.

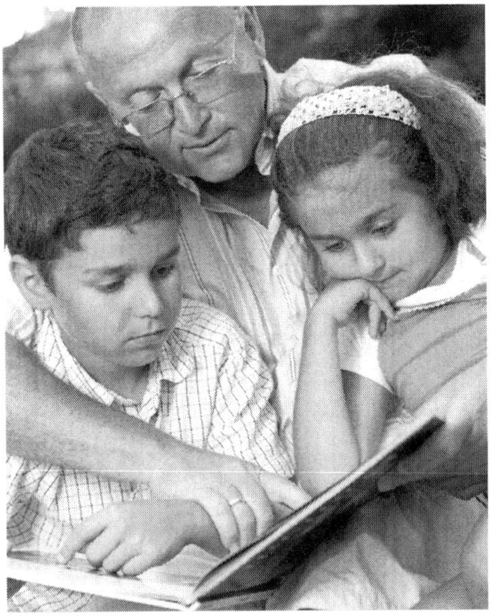

Take another look at the questionnaire to see how central technology is to your family's activities. In the evening is everyone in their own space texting, emailing, watching TV, playing video games? Isn't every family, you might ask?

There are many families, ours is one, who enjoy some "no-screen" evenings listening to music and reading, or playing cards, board games. Sharing laughs. Last Spring Break we went to a family resort that offers lots of outdoor activities. We were surprised that the nature trails were empty, while the parking lot was full. We had a wonderful time exploring the woodsy wonders below the forest's canopy, digging in the inter-tidal zone, splashing at the water's edge and sitting on logs watching birds.

We have given our children hand-me-down digital cameras; this is a great way for them to develop an appreciation of nature, and have fun taking pictures and sharing them with friends. (Yes, most of the time on Facebook.) Reconnecting with each other doesn't have to be rare family holiday time, it could be part of your weekly life.

## One Family's Safer-Tech Challenge and Digital Detox:

Here's a follow-up with our 'library mum':

1. Thought about nature deprivation. We don't live near any woods but I unplugged the kids and went to the park the other day. Played and had a wonderful time.

2. Today, took the kids to the ocean, bypassed children's playground and went straight to tide pools and rocky shore. Had a great time with them exploring barnacles, shells and watching the tide, thought about nature deprivation and how wonderful it felt to be with them in this unscripted environment.

3. Thinking about how to redesign life in ways that aren't just about restricting or taking away toys/ conveniences, but finding creative ways to do things that contribute to overall wellbeing. This is in response to my son who is concerned that our discussions will lead to the restriction of things that he loves (and it probably will, but he may end up happier as we spend more time outdoors in nature!)

It could make a powerful difference if more women were as quick to re-think their families' balance between nature and technology, as our library mum and her neighbour have. There was a recent article from BBC news in the UK, reporting on a surging number of "geek mums." It seems many women are using their emails, cell phones, texting, Twittering, blogging, to counter the loneliness and social isolation of being at home with children.

Consider the fact that more than 60% of electronic devices are evidently purchased by women; you see the potential impact mothers, grandmothers, sisters, aunts can have on this issue, if they choose. It's quite amazing that a small shift in the family focus can bring great benefits. We haven't made any major changes – just less time on the computer – all of us that is, as I was spending a lot of time there myself writing this book. We are making an effort to get outside more, even in less than brilliant weather.

## Our Children's Connection With Nature?

The latest Oxford Junior Dictionary (Oxford University Press) has deleted nature words like: beaver, dandelion, heron, magpie, otter,

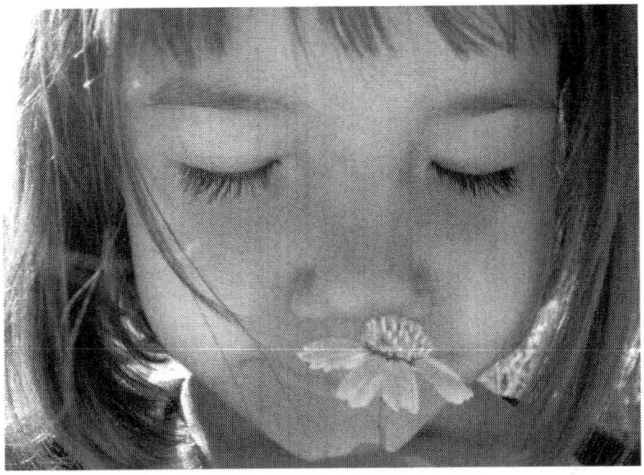

acorn, clover, ivy, sycamore, willow and blackberry? In their place, they have substituted more popular terms, like the electronic "Blackberry," "blog," "MP3 player," and "broadband."

Canadian wildlife artist and conservationist Robert Bateman, whose "Get to Know Program" has been inspiring children to go outdoors and "get to know" their wildlife neighbors for more than a decade commented on this disconnection with nature:

> If you can't name things, how can you love them? And if you don't love them, then you're not going to care a hoot about protecting them or voting for issues that would protect them.
>
> And I have to add, much of what young people see on their screens is just junk food for the soul.

If you are feeling inspired about changing direction with the focus of your family so they will have a greater appreciation of nature, and unplug now and then, I encourage you to approach this with tact.

As you know, it is not easy to guide your children in the direction you want them to grow. And it can be irritating, even heartbreaking, that they seem to insist on moving in the opposite direction – you want them to be playing outside in the fresh air, and they prefer being inside, glued to video games in darkened rooms.

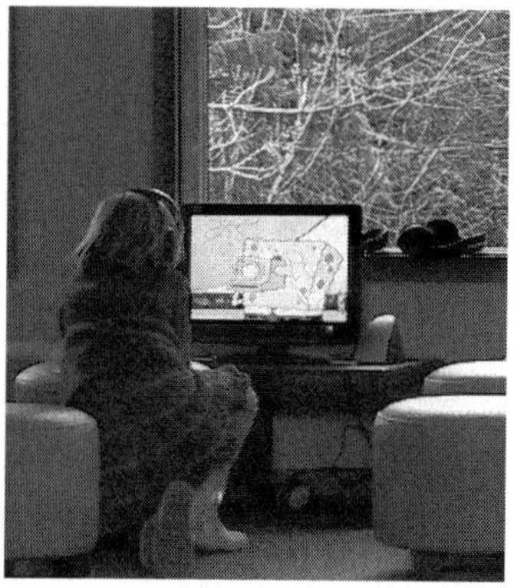

Richard Louv, author of *Last Child In The Woods*, has a great quote in his book from a child who declared, with one of those looks, "Of course, I prefer to play inside. That's where all the electrical outlets are." This is funny, in a way. And tragic, in another. Richard shares his insights on saving our children from what he calls nature-deficit disorder:

> People around my age enjoyed a kind of free, natural play that seems, in the era of kid pagers, instant messaging, and Nintendo, like a quaint artifact.
>
> Within the space of a few decades, the way children understand and experience nature has changed radically. Today, kids are aware of the global threats to the environment – but their physical contact, their intimacy with nature, is fading. Yet, at the very moment that the bond is breaking between the young and the natural world, a growing body of research links our mental, physical and spiritual health directly to our association with nature – The health of our earth is at stake.

Richard Louv goes on to inspire us about the possibility of a "new frontier – a better way to live with nature." His work has evolved into the Children & Nature Network (www.childrenandnature.org) and the Leave No Child Inside program. It's tempting to keep including quotes here from his wonderfully thought-provoking *Last Child in the Woods.* This book offers so much great information that it is pivotal to our Safer-Tech Family and our Tech-free Retreat. (See page 215.)

*Contemplative photography by Charles Blackhall*

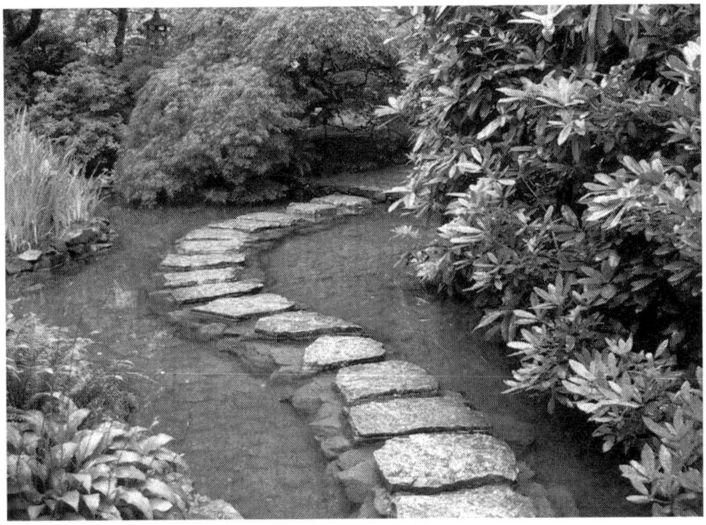

The Mindful EYE program that my husband Charles and I offer, that I just mentioned, is a good way to reconnect with the natural world. And it's great family fun – tech-free (we use non-WiFi digital cameras).

We have led this workshop in Hawaii and Mexico. It's wonderful to be in such luscious tropical destinations, but this practice also shows us how to tune into being present, in the moment, and appreciate our daily lives. When your mind is clear and calm, have you ever noticed colors are much brighter? Has the simple beauty of the morning light streaming in the window ever caught your eye? Tuning into the visual world can wake us up, and bring us joy – with or without a camera.

Here's a story of a dad who became so electro-sensitive that he sought not only to regain his own health, but to prevent such a situation with his young family:

> When I was younger we were outside most of the time, except for those long hours in school. My friends and I used to make up games where we would roar around and using our imaginations in all sorts of scenarios. We discovered how things worked by putting things together; well, mostly taking things apart in all sorts of places – in the garage, the back yard and down by the river.
>
> Some days we would just sit there and watch insects. But mostly we were climbing trees, challenging ourselves. I remember working with the fast flowing river discovering how to have fun without drowning. I didn't know it at the time, but we were developing social skills – working with each other, getting along and sorting out our differences – who was going to lead the next game.
>
> We used to make up a lot of games. We began to see other people's skills – Joey was very good at seeing things intuitively, and Billy could fix things in his dad's tool shed – we relied on him for many engineering projects. We developed trust in each other; we were in real situations where you had to count on people. We were looking at birds squawking at each other, all the life in the wetlands, watching the fish and their cycles. You learn a lot about life cycles watching salmon – see them spawning, and watching them die. Without making a big deal of it, we were connecting with the impermanence of life, the changing of the seasons, and how things are.

My wife and I both work hard. We put in long hours – virtually all inside – and it is a struggle just to keep the kids fed, dressed and schooled. But I see that there are so many times in the day where we are making choices that involve sitting in front of a computer, TV or video screen.

Inspired by the book *Safer-Tech Solutions,* we decided to make an effort to wean ourselves off of these entertainments. It seemed daunting at first. The kids rebelled. Then my wife and I sat down and had a family discussion about how all these technology things had been part of making me sick. They, of course, shot back that was because I was 'old' and they were just kids so it was okay for them. I didn't subject them to all the evidence, but my wife and I did our best to explain why spending too much time around these electronics was not a good idea for kids.

We found that rather than trying to tackle this head-on, that we would plan some outings. As I unplugged more myself, I got better – I was sleeping much better and had more energy. So instead of collapsing in front of the TV when I got home, I'd say 'let's go outside and kick a ball around'.

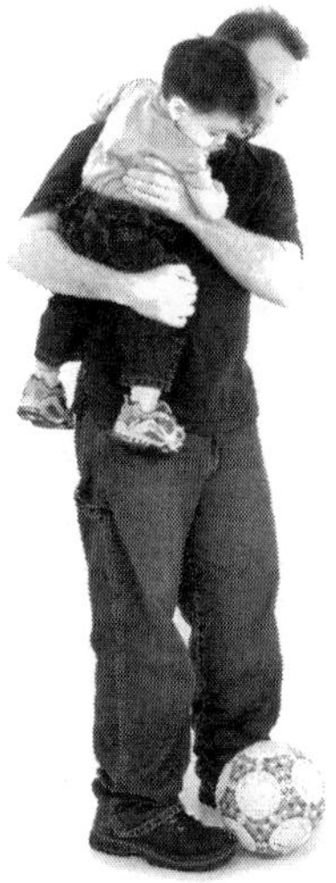

Once we were outside more, I noticed the kids were really into it and even took themselves outside now and then. Our somewhat pasty-looking kids began to look healthier. Sometimes we just go outside and sit on the ground and chat. And listen to each other.

## What Was It Like When You Were Young?

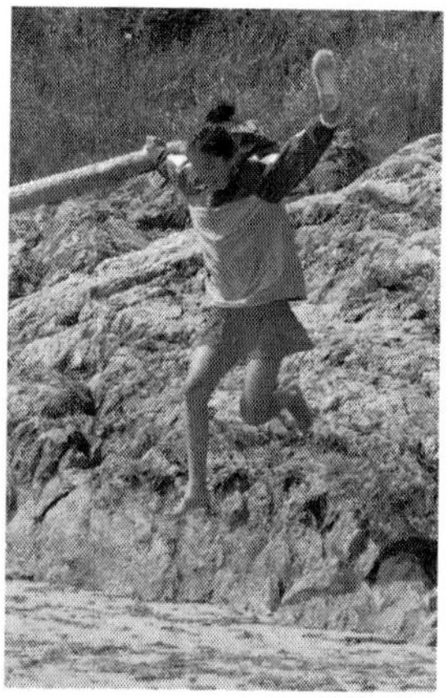

What kind of stories are the children you know going to tell? What stories, and values, are they going to pass along to their children, and grandchildren? If the rate of technology continues at the current supersonic speed what kind of lives are all of us going to have in ten years? In twenty? It's not too late. We can take better care of the health of our families, and our home – this blue planet is our only home.

## From Good Intentions to Effective Changes

This is a lot of information; important things for us to consider to safeguard our families. The challenge: not to get overwhelmed and give up into hopelessness. After you waded through Strategy 3, I included an intention plan to help focus on what you wanted to deal with first – your priorities. Here is that list again. Just skip over it, if you want.

### Reviewing Our Safer-Tech Challenge Intentions

Top Priorities – what I want to tackle first:

________________________________________

Secondary priorities – what I want to deal with after that:

________________________________________

I should consult a professional to assess the following:

________________________________________

Other environmental exposures I want to address:

________________________________________

Now that you have been through Strategy 4, which has enough aspirations to last a lifetime, let's look again at winnowing this down into bite size chunks.

## Our Safer-Tech Challenge Action Plan

| Area | Action intended | Action completed |
|---|---|---|
| Front Porch | | |
| Master Bedroom | | |
| Children's Rooms | | |
| Bathroom | | |
| Kitchen | | |
| Laundry Room | | |
| Vacuum Cleaner | | |
| Office | | |
| Cordless Phones | | |

| Area | Action intended | Action completed |
|---|---|---|
| Internet Access | | |
| Other Environmental Exposures | | |
| Your Physical Health | | |
| Nutritional Supplementation | | |
| Dental Health | | |
| Other Well Being/Lifestyle Factors | | |
| Safer Tech Family Communication Challenge | | |
| Safer-Tech Family Challenge | | |
| Other Personal Goals | | |

WE CAN MEET THIS CHALLENGE but please don't imagine that you are going to reduce the risks all at once. We have been developing this unsafe-tech environment for a long time and many people are deeply hooked. Detoxing from a digital addiction has become the latest trend, as some of us predicted a few years ago.

*2 Minute Quick Read Summary*

## Hope For the Future

Let's take this one step at a time and feel good about each one. By this stage in our plan, you've accomplished a lot: how to be tech-savvy *and* healthy, and more mindful of your digital environment. And you know more about this issue than most of the regulators and legislators responsible for public health and EMR safety standards.

Hopefully, you have made a few positive changes – simple steps like putting your mobile device in airplane mode whenever possible; keeping it away from your head and your body; using the speakerphone; and limiting the number and duration of calls. These habits can make all the difference to your health.

For more benefits, replace your WiFi with a safe, wired Internet connection. If that doesn't seem possible, have you thought of putting the WiFi router on a good quality power bar – maybe a timed one – to limit your exposure, and place the router far away from everyone? Wired is safer than wireless (your mouse, keyboard, laptop, TV).

Replacing your cordless phone with a corded landline may be the best strategy in dealing with vertigo, heart rate and rhythm problems, headaches, or insomnia. Enjoying an EMR-quiet sleep zone?

I hope you will continue through this last section to hear from some of our experts about their hopes for the future, while you contemplate yours. You have our support in taking better care of each other and this planet which is our only home.

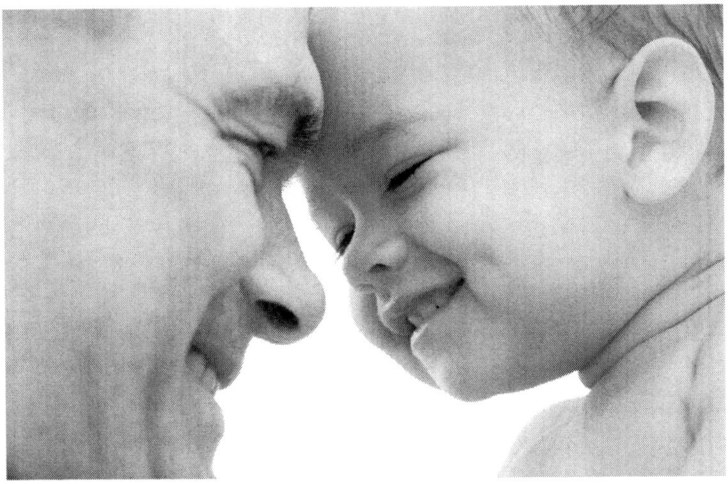

# Hope For the Future

## Moving from Knowledge to Action

It may surprise you to know (or maybe by now it won't surprise you) that some American scientists have been telling their government about EMR biological effects for more than 35 years!

Robert O. Becker, MD, was one of the researchers looking into the U.S. navy's plans to install a 6,000 mile underwater messaging system to communicate with submarines.

Dr. Becker said:

> As far as I know, our testimony (in 1975) was the first ever openly given by American scientists stating that electromagnetic energy had health effects in doses below those needed to heat tissue, and that power lines might therefore be hazardous to human health.

> We criticized the White House Office of Telecommunications Policy for failing to follow up a tentative 1971 warning that harmful effects from electro-pollution were proven.

There are hopes that the US administration will take a courageous stand on this issue.

As I mentioned early on, one of the leading lights in fighting the installation of cell towers is Eileen O'Connor, the founder of EM Radiation Research in the UK. She was one of the presenters to the 2010 President's Cancer Panel that studied the possible links between radiation (nuclear and electro-magnetic) and cancer.

Ms. O'Connor was pleased the issue is being taken seriously:

> President Obama has said science is about ensuring that facts and evidence are never twisted or obscured by politics or ideology. It's about listening to what our scientists have to say, even when it's inconvenient and I welcome this approach.

Many of us have the "audacity of hope" that this administration, and the next one, will show true leadership in this other inconvenient truth. Steps taken to protect people's health are likely to be echoed around the world.

As you may know, most politicians take their lead from the majority of the electorate's demands; it's not the other way around. Yes, there's industry lobbying, but when enough of us unite to demand safer limits for this technology for the health of all of us, especially our children, then things will change.

## What Your Town Can Do

Have some shiny new palm trees, pine trees or church spires sprung up in your neighborhood? Near your child's school? You can do something about these cell tower antennas.

There is an excellent book edited by B. Blake Levitt: *Cell Towers: Wireless Convenience? or Environmental Hazard?* This is a quote from Blake Levitt:

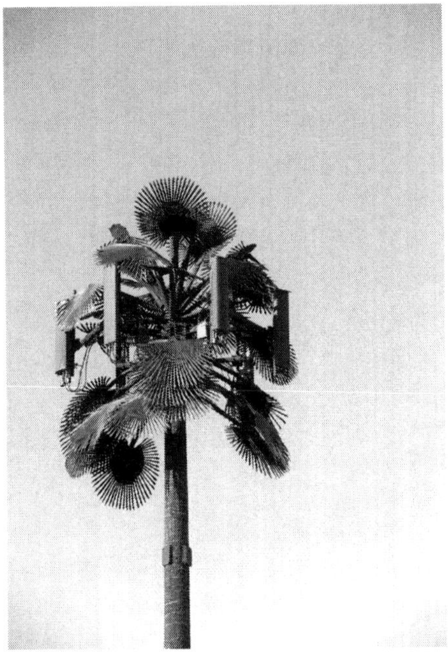

> Something municipalities fail to keep in mind is the basic legal fact that it is up to the providers of a service or product to prove that their wares are safe. It is not up to us to prove that they are unsafe. The tele-communications industry has largely failed to do that. Just because they are within the FCC guidelines for RF emission, does not prove safety. No town today should allow itself to be intimidated by telecom service providers or adjunct industries like tower companies...
>
> Those in decision-making positions need to understand that this form of land use regulation is very different than traditional forms. This is NOT just an aesthetic issue. It is a medical one.

This could be used at a public meeting. Most likely, no official would sign. Their reluctance, however, should be of interest to those residents, parents, and others who will be directly affected.

**Statement of Accountability**

My stated position is that the (cell tower antenna, WiFi router, Smart Meter) that has been proposed or approved in or near (______________________) should go ahead or remain as it does not present significant health risks within _________ *(feet or meters.)*

I am aware that the World Health Organization has reclassified this radiation and cautioned "it is possibly carcinogenic to human health," and that adverse biological effects have been linked with the levels of radiation emitted by this technology, including increased cancer and leukemia with proximity to cell tower antennas, and of other health risks with wireless exposures. I am aware of the research indicating children and pregnant women are most vulnerable; that many countries have set limits on the placement of this technology; and that cancer and other related diseases can take years to develop.

I acknowledge that public health official David Carpenter, MD called government regulators, "Just plain wrong" and their standards are challenged by many other experts as not accurate, and not protecting us. I am aware these regulations did *not* consider adverse effects on children, nor long-term exposure. I have heard this statement to the wireless industry by Dr. David Gee, of the BioInitiative Report:

> They are forewarned now, and saying 'but we were in compliance with ICNIRP (the international regulatory agency) safety limits' will not be sufficient reason for ignoring the growing evidence.

And I have read the remarks by electrical engineer Alasdair Philips:

> Many people living near masts (cell tower antennas), and other RF exposures, experience ill health: sleep disruption, headaches, dizziness, behaviour changes in children, nosebleeds, epilepsy, and increased rates of cancer. (See www.powerwatch.org.uk)

I have heard the quote by cardiologist Stephen Sinatra, MD that "Electro-pollution is the greatest medical threat of our time. As the heart is electrical in nature and vulnerable to this radiation, there can be cardiac, as well as cancer, risks from these exposures. Pregnant women, children, and those with heart disease are most at risk."

If you have been assured by another expert in this field that this system does not present health risks, please list his or her name and credentials: ___________________________________________

The reason I believe this installation be implemented or remain is:

________________________________________________

I believe that those responsible for this installation ________________________ do not have any past or present health-related disputes regarding this technology.

Please note exceptions: ____________________________

I believe that any adverse health effects, or medical conditions, attributed to this short and long-term exposure are covered by the insurance policy provided by ______________________________

Your name: (*Please print*)_____________________________

Your title and official position:

________________________________________________

Today's date: ______________________________________

Your signature: ____________________________________

Witnessed by: ______________________________________

*For your information, a list of the individuals who have been sent this letter has been forwarded to ______________________________ (media names). As there is strong community interest in this issue, they have been sent a copy of this letter and asked to follow up with you.*

This form is available, contact us at: SaferTechSolutions.org.

Professor Johansson is widely regarded as one of the leading experts. When officials, at all levels, heed his words we will all be more hopeful for the future:

> I strongly advise all governments to take the issue of electromagnetic health hazards seriously and to take action while there is still time.
>
> Governments should act decisively to protect public health by changing the exposure standards to be biologically-based, communicating the results of the independent science on this topic and aggressively researching links with a multitude of associated medical conditions.

As you know, there are many things we aspire to in this life. Fundamentally, is there anything more truly worthwhile than safeguarding our family and the future of our children?

That's why I have spent more than four years researching and writing this book. For you, and for your family.

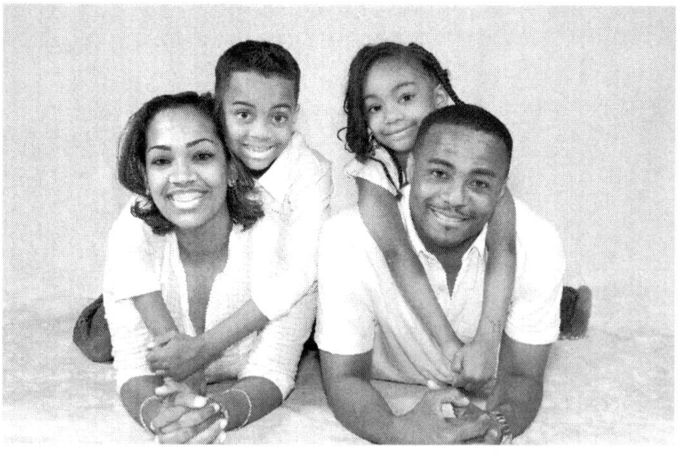

## Promising Signs On the Horizon

Are you old enough to remember the movie The Graduate? A young man is given a tip for success by one of his parents' friends, "The future, Benjamin, is plastics." The advice now might be: fiber optics. Why? Several of our experts have mentioned this as the wave of the future.

## Progress In Technology

### Fiber Optics – Safe and Secure

Many telecom technical experts also prefer this system. One told me that, "Fiber optic lines are thin strands of optically pure glass. This is the best way to move large amounts of data – digital information – over long distances. Security is a big factor, (as we mentioned before). Fiber optics is a secure, closed system (the shot-gun approach of satellites and wireless radiation firing through space is not). And fiber optics do not have the same radiation issues."

Evidently, there are plans in some places to bring fiber optic connections to homes and businesses, instead of wireless, for Internet access.

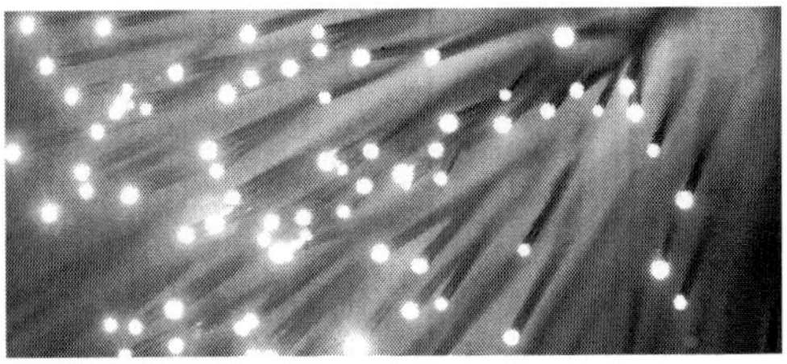

Let's promote this! The safest communities will provide online access with fiber optics to buildings that provide cable/wired access.

Not everyone in the wireless industry is onside with this alternative. Not yet. As you know, things change. In a few years we will see a shift.

Researchers at the University of Edinburgh are developing light-based wireless communication – without microwave/radio waves. This LED light technology may be more secure, and safer.

## Breaking Out of the Cyber Cocoon

If you have read through most of this book – glanced at a few pages? – you know this message is piercing.

It cuts to the heart of our techno-addictions: have we become too attached to the convenience and to those scintillating 'pings' and downloaded rings of cyber-connections? Are we immersing ourselves in clouds of radiation in the process? Are we closeting ourselves, and our children, inside and filling space with hyper-speed entertainment, the instant gratification of texting and Twittering?

Acknowledging any addiction is a tough message to take in. And that's without all of the "too scary" stuff about cancer and brain damage.

I have tried my best, without sugar-coating anything, to focus on the ways we can turn around this potentially perilous situation, and reduce the health risks, without losing the conveniences of this never-ending stream of technology.

Now, let's rouse our energies and look on the bright side of possibilities and prevention. Working together, let's do what we can to rescue our families. I am hopeful.

As a whole generation of baby boomers age – many who are already self-proclaimed 'crackberry' addicts – there is concern about health effects after so many years of sitting in front of computers and being hooked on electronics.

It is encouraging that there are treatments evolving to deal with these effects.

## Clinical Progress

There is hope on the clinical horizon. Innovative doctors are using effective ways to heal and prevent EMR symptoms and conditions. There is also hope for the millions of people already suffering due to electro-sensitivity (ES), and for those with autism symptoms and related neurological conditions.

Physicians with specialties in pediatrics and environmental medicine have recently joined our advisory board, Doctors for Safer Schools, and we are collaborating with a group of physicians in the UK. Each year when we present to doctors, and to the general public, we see a greater awareness of this issue.

Our next project is a handbook for doctors and their patients on ES and medical care in this digital age: how to recognize and reduce related symptoms and conditions.

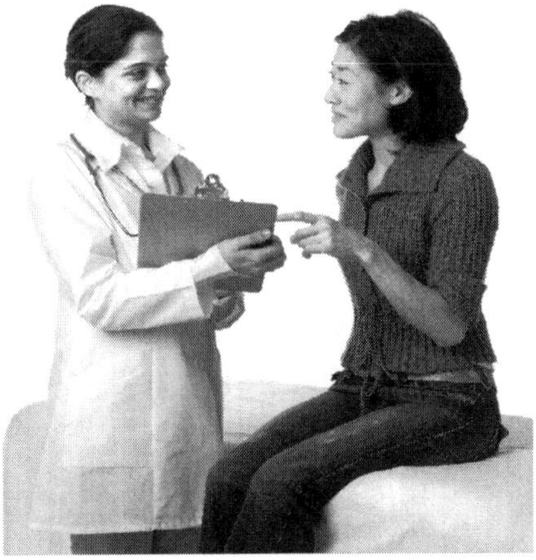

Join us in demanding more research in this area as the conventional medical approach of relying mainly on X-ray diagnostic tests, pharmaceuticals and/or surgery does not seem the best approach when dealing with environmental assaults. We need a multi-disciplinary approach focusing on holistic, non-invasive ways to heal and prevent environmental conditions. And, as the electro-magnetic fields affect us on a frequency level, we should be looking at energy medicine for some clinical clues.

We call upon clinical and technical experts to provide the information and tools we need to safeguard our health and develop safer technology.

## Parents and Grandparents Demanding Safer Products

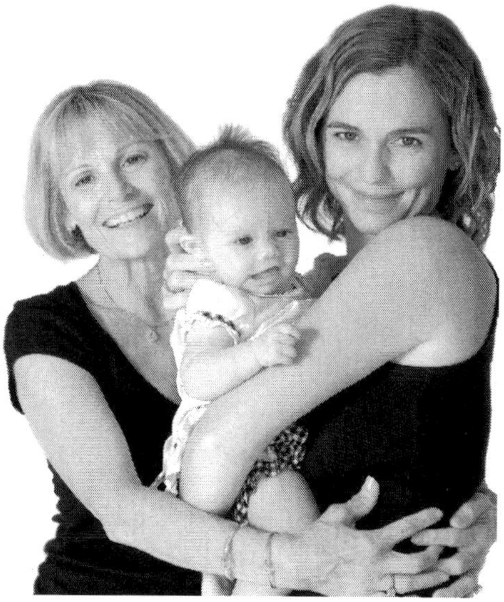

I am confident that most people will follow the lead of our library mum and make an effort to cut back on cell phone use and get our families unplugged and outside whenever we can, and that informed parents, grandparents and educators will limit our children's exposure in the ways we have discussed.

As we have seen in Europe, some legislators are listening to the independent scientists and inching forward to bring regulations within recommended safe limits, and safer products, including a less hazardous baby monitor, are being developed.

All are encouraging steps. Will all of this be in time to prevent the global EMR-related pandemic that some fear? Can we rescue this hyper-tech generation? Yes, if we act now.

## Progress With Our Families' Safer-Tech Challenge

### Library Mum

> Basically, this program has made me more aware of the addiction that my family and I have nurtured around technology. I will be increasingly more wary of gadgets which promise to increase my well being by providing me with efficiency tools.

In his video series, John Bradshaw uses the metaphor of a hanging mobile to show that when one part of the mobile moves and changes, it sends reverberations and changes throughout the whole system. I feel that this book has done a similar thing with our family. It seems that the changes that I am attempting to implement are leading to profound changes in our family interactions in general. It hasn't all been easy.

On one hand, these changes have been bringing tensions to the surface (for example, my son's Internet and technology savvy seem to be in direct conflict with my desire for a low radiation home and a de-emphasis on 'screen culture').

So, through these changes, we are learning how to navigate each other's needs and respect each other; whereas without this particular technology challenge, we have had very little conflict to work through (I found myself at the height of frustration yesterday when I thought that my son was reconnecting the WiFi and I pulled the computer power cord out of the outlet and banned the computer from use!)

The changes that I've been making have also had an impact on my relationship with myself. The cell phone, in particular, makes me feel important and necessary; efficient, productive and connected.

This is a heady mixture in a society that places such value on these qualities. The cell phone is a transformative wand which takes me from being a 'housewife' and ‘mother’ (negative terms in today’s society) and magically transforms me into a ‘modern, West Coast, work-at-home executive.’

Is this true? Is it what I really feel and think about – or is it the effective machinations of savvy marketers?

Because every change invokes a challenge to a personal relationship, my attempts to cut down the electromagnetic radiation in our lives are not simply a matter of just making simple technology changes.

For this reason, I have experienced profound shifts. All this navigating takes personal energy.

And so, I have not been able to implement all of the book’s suggestions in a straightforward, progressive way.

Instead, the process looks messy – it has turnarounds and circle-backs. This will likely continue. Yet, as I reflect on this today, I believe that this is natural.

Even blame, self-doubt, perfectionism and discouragement can be seen as part of a larger spiritual process of growth and renewal (as long as they don’t lead to an abandonment of the whole project!).

We begin to exercise our right to make choices and to create an environment rather than accepting one that is pre-packaged. This, in itself, is sufficient reason to begin the journey!

## Neighbor Dad

Changing gears is not as easy as it may sound. Some days, I feel we have failed hopelessly with our good intentions to live a more simple life, and to rely less on all this technology. The least bit of rain keeps the kids inside and begging for their gaming.

My wife still goes right to the computer in her jammies, bleary-eyed and clutching her coffee mug, to check her email. We have made some progress since reading this book. We should feel good about that, but this is going to take some time. I'm determined, though, to ease us gently away from this fixation, and focus on the successes, and more family fun, which we are enjoying these days.

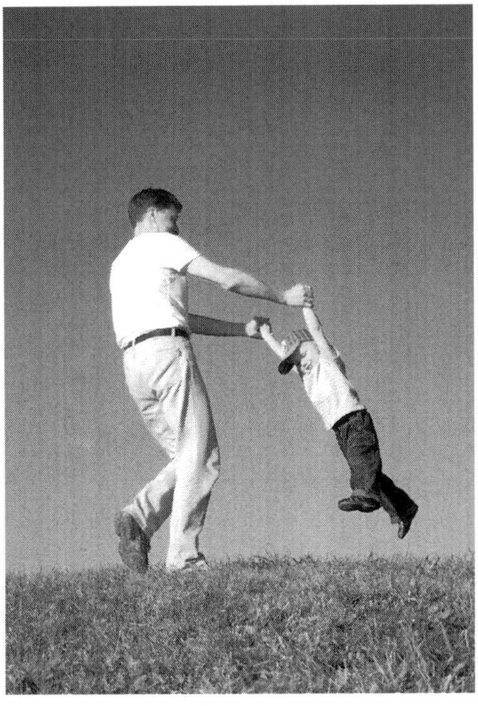

## Your Action Plan

As you can see, this is a process with "turnarounds and circle-backs." As these families have described, we are not only dealing with our own households, we are dealing with a culture that has evolved around instant gratification. Please take it step by step, feel good about every exposure you reduce, and don't give up.

## Your Safer-Tech Family Challenge?

When you are ready, see if you can get everyone on board and make this a sporting event. Try a positive approach: add more of the outdoor activities that your family enjoys, rather than ripping the gaming stations out of the kids' hands. Please be patient, with your family, and yourself.

Each week, spend one evening away from the computers and the TV's, and get outside for a walk in your neighborhood, or a nearby park. Try "no-screens" for a day. Or a week? – as inspired by the Campaign for a Commercial-free Childhood.

Check out garage sales for good deals on bikes, balls, badminton racquets, playing cards and board games. Ask everyone in your family, depending on his or her age, to come up with a non-electronic activity for that week. Maybe it's a rousing game of cards, or charades?

I know we are really busy, and many of our children have back-to-back lessons, sports and other after-school activities. These too can contribute to limiting EMR exposure, particularly if we watch the soccer game instead of texting on the sidelines.

I read one local hockey arena went wireless so the parents could work on their laptops during those long games and practices. How often do you see families at a park, or on the beach, and instead of being together, instead of really being there, they are immersed in the virtual world? What does this teach our children about how to interact in the real world?

Once you go through the withdrawal and your texting, gaming, Twittering fingers stop shaking, you may find you feel greatly invigorated by safer-tech activities.

This technology, and the world-wide Internet, have brought our global village many benefits. We can continue to enjoy and expand upon those. As with most powerful influences, we just need to use them more wisely.

## Progress In Consumer Awareness

The message is getting out. People are waking up. Remember that great line from the film Network? "We're mad as hell and we aren't going to take it anymore."

Dr. McKinney has offered to work with me to develop awareness and education and programs to get this message out:

> As results surface from scientists, researchers and clinicians it becomes important to share this information with citizens around the globe.

We will keep this updated on our website: SaferTechSolutions.org. And will continue to bring you the latest research and technical advice.

We owe a debt of gratitude to the many people who helped with this book and to the thousands more working tirelessly in this field.

Recently, I wrote to one of our contributors:

> Thanks to the dedication of pioneers like yourself, I predict we are reaching a tipping point where consumers, particularly parents and grandparents, are waking up. Soon the industry is not going to be able to hold back the tide of public demand for the truth, for truly safe products. And governments will be pressured into action for accurate safe standards.

I have asked some of our contributors for their hopes for the future.

Dr. William Rea, and several others, offered that they were optimistic. This is encouraging as Dr. Rea, for example, is treating people every day who are already suffering from EMR exposure.

**Dr. Stephen Sinatra:**

> I am hopeful as each year I see more doctors, and the public, becoming aware of this issue. Educating them is key to meeting the health challenges of electro-pollution.
>
> First, increased medical awareness will assist in the diagnosis and treatment of those presenting with related symptoms – dizziness, sleep disruption, tinnitus, and heart rate and rhythm disturbances. People will get the treatment they need, and may avoid tests (often involving diagnostic radiation exposure) and pharmacologic intervention (often involving side effects.) Second, education will raise public awareness about the need to use wired and wireless electronic devices with more caution and could encourage legislators to bring the safety standards in line with the science.

**Alasdair Philips:**

My hope for the future is that politicians and business leaders start acting with integrity regarding sustainable living and deal with problems like EMF/RF exposure now instead of ignoring them in order to make short-term financial gains.

**Dr. Magda Havas:**

I hope that those individuals who are in positions of authority, and this includes parents, teachers, employers, as well as government officials, will make the necessary changes required to minimize our exposure to electromagnetic pollution. I hope that it will not take decades, as it did with tobacco, to do the right thing. May those who are sensitive, who are the 'early warning indicators', not suffer in vain. May their experience alert us to the problem and give us the courage to resolve it. May we have the wisdom to live up to our name Homo sapien sapien and not have to change it to Homo greedicus ignoramus.

**Dr. Sarah Starkey:**

My hope for the future is that people will come to accept that creating a sustainable future for our planet involves reducing artificial electromagnetic fields. I would like children to grow up knowing that to protect their own health, that of future generations and their environment they need to limit their use of microwave-emitting technologies.

**Dr. Heather McKinney:**

My hope is that consumers around the world will raise their voices to encourage scientists, politicians, and corporate executives to be proactive, and look at this situation as an opportunity for research and long term restructuring. I am optimistic that this can happen.

**Dr. Carrie Hyman:**

We need more private citizens asking questions about the safety of these products. We all need to work hand in hand with clinicians, environmentalists and politicians to address this health issue quickly and responsibly.

**Dr. Louis Slesin:**

My hope is some breaking down of the research roadblocks. This is a challenge as there are so many vested interests on the hazards side; so much money involved. To be honest, I am not optimistic. I am encouraged, however, on the clinical side; there's progress with biomedical applications – this may be the key.

**Dr. Devra Davis:**

The government should work with phone companies to protect our children and to provide data to Professor Gandhi, and to other independent researchers, so that we can find the safest way to use this revolutionary technology which has also brought many benefits. In an ideal world, the profitable companies would compete to design the safest and sleekest phones.

## Now You've Heard The Whole Story

How are you feeling about all this now? Not too overwhelmed? I am confident in speaking for our contributors: our hope for you is the ability to make more informed decisions, and to use wired and wireless technology more safely.

We are also working to increase medical awareness so you can have more support from your doctor and others charged with the public wellbeing. And we're fighting hard to make our schools safer for all.

To summarize, let's take a look at these **Best Practices** strategies again.

**7 Key Reminders – wired over wireless and corded over cordless.**

1. Switch your cordless phones to corded ones. Please don't give up your landline phone (and they are also health-savvy gifts);
2. Seek wired solutions for all things wireless, including your Internet access, keep laptops, iPads and all wireless devices off your lap, and please do not use digital baby monitors, or wireless sensor pads;
3. Keep your cell phone simple (basic, low SAR), and away from your head, your heart, pregnant women and the young. Limit its use;
4. Use your mobile's speakerphone, rather than wireless, or wired headsets, and remember the most hazardous option of all is holding a mobile device against your head;
5. Avoid using a cell phone for an alarm clock, or sleeping near it;
6. Tell your airline and hotel that you want a wireless-free environment;
7. Talk to your local legislators, calmly and clearly. Provide some information (not overwhelming them) and ask for a response.

Please take this slowly and don't lose heart about the future. We can meet this challenge. We just need to keep focused and keep going. It's a journey that will bring many benefits. Ready to give it a try?

May you rediscover the delights of unplugging and stepping outside of your electronic cocoon, and reconnecting with the natural world.

May you have the courage to face the inconvenient truths, for yourself and your family, and this blue planet – our only home.

May you, and all of our children, and grandchildren, thrive.

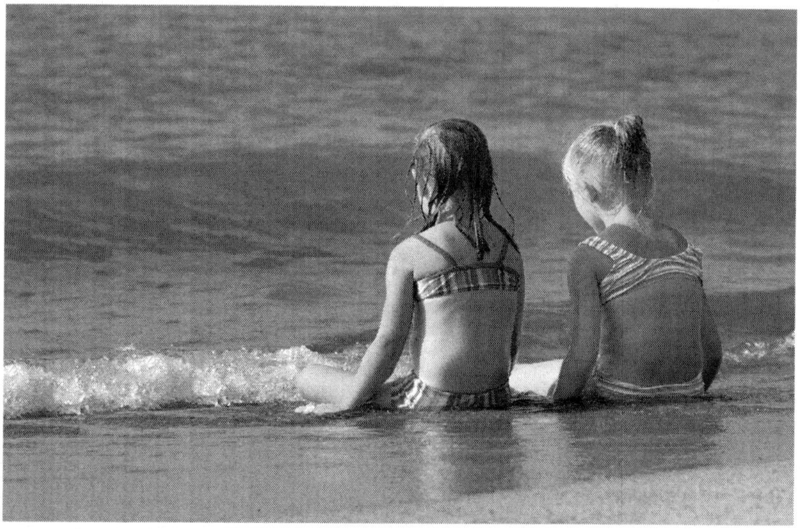

And, after reading (skimming?) this book, I hope you are inspired by our risk reduction plan for optimal health. This whole book, and our strategies, can also be a vital part of your anti-aging program, addressing the key factors that most other approaches are missing. Longevity is not only living longer, but living well – healthy aging in this new digital age.

> *You will succeed if you persevere; and you will find a joy in overcoming obstacles. I have confidence in the human spirit.*
>
> Helen Keller

> *Never doubt the ability of a small group of thoughtful people to change the world. Indeed, it is the only thing that ever has.*
>
> Margaret Mead

# Resources

## Research, Advocacy and Electro-Sensitivity Support Groups

### USA

- **www.antennafreeunion.org**

The San Francisco Neighborhood Antenna-Free Union (SNAFU) is a grass-roots, city-wide coalition of individual residents and neighborhood organizations.

- **www.bioinitiative.org**

In 2007, an international working group of scientists, researchers and public health policy professionals (The BioInitiative Working Group) released its report on electromagnetic fields (EMF) and health.

- **www.electromagnetichealth.org**

One of the most effective voices is that of Camilla Rees. She is the founder of ElectromagneticHealth.org and co-author with Dr. Magda Havas of the book, *Public Health SOS: The Shadow Side of the Wireless Revolution.*

- **www.emrpolicy.org**

The mission of The EMR Policy Institute is to foster a better understanding of the environmental and human biological effects from such exposures.

- **www.energyfields.org**

The Council on Wireless Technology Impacts is concerned about the safe use of technologies which use electromagnetic radiation.

- **www.ewg.org**

Environmental Working Group (EWG), a Washington, DC-based nonprofit organization, is dedicated to protecting children, babies, and infants in the womb from health problems attributed to a wide array of toxic contaminants. Their other mission is the relevant federal policies.

**• www.guineapigsrus.org**

Joanne Mueller's pamphlet, *Are You A Guinea Pig?* tells how to sleep better and feel better by reducing EMR exposure.

**• www.microwavenews.com**

*Microwave News* is meticulously researched and documented, making it one of the world's most authoritative sources of information on EMR/EMF health risks. Its founder and editor for more than 30 years is Dr. Louis Slesin.

**• www.centerforsaferwireless.org**

Christine Hoch founded Center For Safer Wireless, a national non-profit organization dedicated to enhancing the public's understanding of wireless product safety. The group engages in educational activities aimed at increasing awareness of EMR and the potential health implications of wireless products.

## CANADA

**• www.c4st.org**

Canadians For Safe Technology, led by Frank Clegg, former President of Microsoft Canada, is a not-for-profit volunteer-based coalition whose mission is to educate and inform Canadians and their policy makers about EMR, and to work with all levels of government to create healthier communities for children and families.

**• www.causetm.ca**

Citizens Against Un-safe Emissions (CAUSE) was founded by Sharon Noble. Her group has made great strides forward in educating the public.

**• www.citizensforsafetechnology.org**

Citizens For Safe Technology was founded by Una St Clair-Moniz. CST's goal is to raise awareness about this issue so that the public is empowered to protect themselves, their children, and their environment.

**• www.hans.org**

The Health Action Network is a charitable natural health resource. HANS provides information through its website and regular events.

• **www.weepinitiative.org**

The Canadian Initiative to Stop Wireless, Electric, and Electromagnetic Pollution (WEEP) has a mission to inform the public about the potential environmental effects associated with electromagnetic immersions.

**IRELAND**

• **www.ideaireland.org**

The Irish Doctors' Environmental Association (IDEA) was established by health professionals to promote the right to health worldwide.

**UK**

• **www.es-uk.info**

Sarah Dacre is a trustee of ES-UK, a registered charity in the UK advising and educating about electro-sensitivity and ways to lessen symptoms.

• **www.ssita.org.uk**

Safe Schools Information Technology Alliance works to identify issues and concerns regarding WiFi and other wireless technologies in schools, nurseries, day care environments and colleges.

• **www.mastsanity.org**

Mast Sanity is a national group of community members who campaign against the unsafe placement of mobile communications towers.

• **www.mast-victims.org**

This is an international community website for people suffering adverse health effects from mobile phone masts in the vicinity of their homes.

• **www.powerwatch.org.uk**

Powerwatch is a non-profit independent organization that has been studying the health effects of electro-magnetic fields for the last 20 years.

• **www.radiationresearch.org**

EM Radiation Research Trust researches EMR and related health effects and lobbies the U.K. Government and the EU. for policy change.

**• www.wifiinschools.org.uk**

WiFi In Schools has been set up by Dr. Sarah Starkey and a small group of other scientists concerned about the rapid spread of wireless technologies in schools. The group recommends application of the precautionary principle.

**• www.wiredchild.org**

WiredChild is a charity run by a group of concerned parents, raising awareness of the potential risks to children of exposure to radiation from mobile phones and other wireless technology.

**EUROPE:**

**• www.hese-project.org (German)**
**• www.hese-project.org/hese-uk (English)**

HESE (Human Ecological Social Economical project) is an international, interdisciplinary collaboration of scientists, institutions and informed lay people, which brings together research and advocacy information in several languages. Many of its contributors have suffered health effects from EMR.

**• www.next-up.org**

This France-based organization brings together the latest research, regulations and European news on lobbying efforts and public action.

**• www.priartem.fr**

PRIARTéM (Pour une réglementation des Implantations d'Antennes Relais de Téléphonie Mobile) is a citizens' group created in 2000 to monitor the installation of mobile phone antennas.

**AUSTRALIA:**

**• www.emfacts.com**

EMFacts was established in 1997 by Don Maisch, PhD as an independent source of information on the health and safety issues arising from EMR.

**• www.emraustralia.com.au**

EMR Australia is a consumer advocacy group which is working to alert people about the growing concerns in that country.

## NEW ZEALAND:

- **www.neilcherry.com**

Dr. Neil Cherry (1946-2003) was Associate Professor of Environmental Health at Lincoln University. He had discussions with many of the researchers.

- **www.canterbury.cyberplace.co.nz/ouruhia**

Oururah NZ is a group providing information on its website about cell tower antennas - masts - and mobile phone health hazards.

- **www.banthetower.co.nz**

Ban The Tower is working hard to alert people to the risks of wireless radiation and where cell towers are located, and planned.

## INTERNATIONAL:

- **www.doctorsforsaferschools.org**

This international advisory board is an association of professionals, and others, concerned about the health risks of EMR, especially wireless radiation exposure, in schools. The mission is to give parents, educators, doctors and others accurate information on health concerns and the safer-tech solutions.

- **www.iemfa.org**

The International Electro-Magnetic Fields Alliance is an independent global body of empirically-based scientific experts, with a multidisciplinary health focus. Founding members: Alex Swinkels, Netherlands; Brian Stein, Eileen O'Connor, United Kingdom; Camilla Rees, Diana Warren, Elizabeth Barris, Elizabeth Kelley, Janet Newton, United States; Daniel Oberhausen, France; Don Maisch, Australia; Sissel Halmøy, Norway

- **www.icems.eu**

The International Commission for Electromagnetic Safety (ICEMS) is a non-profit organization registered in Italy that promotes research and develops strategies for assessment, prevention, management and communication.

- **EMF Refugees: The International Coalition for an Electromagnetic Safe Planet (IC-ESP)** This group brings people together to form their own EMF-free communities in natural environments where they can heal and create healing environments for the Earth and others.

**Autism Related Issues**

• **www.autismcanada.org**

Autism Canada Foundation is a registered Canadian Charitable organization committed to improving the lives of Canadians affected by autism. Having firsthand experience with autism, our board of directors were more than aware of the lack of representation in Canada for all effective treatments and therapies.

• **www.GlobalAutismAlliance.com**

The Global Autism Alliance (GAA) is a network of autism organizations who are actively partnering on specific projects and programs on a global scale. Some of the plans include sponsoring international conferences, creating professional training webinars, establishing networked treatment clinics, translating important articles, and much more.

**Children & Nature**

• **www.childrenandnature.org**

The Children & Nature Network (C&NN) was created to encourage and support the people and organizations working to reconnect children with nature. C&NN provides access to the latest news and research in the field and a peer-to-peer network of researchers and individuals, educators and organizations dedicated to children's health and wellbeing.

• **www.childnature.ca**

In North America there is a growing movement to reconnect children and families to nature for improved health and wellbeing. The Child and Nature Alliance is a non-profit organization in British Columbia that is formalizing the movement provincially, and eventually across Canada.

## Medical Clinics/Professional Practices

**Robert Abell, ND, LAc** is a naturopathic physician who uses auricular medicine, homeopathy, acupuncture and Biotherapeutic Drainage as his primary therapeutic tools. He lectures on the assessment and treatments of neurological disorders including ADHD and autism. Dr. Abell treats children with ADHD and autism in his clinics and does phone consultations.

**Be Well Acupuncture & Natural Medicine Clinic**
Laguna Hills, California & Austin, Texas
Website: **www.bewellhealthclinic.com**

**Nancy A. Didriksen, PhD** has a private practice in health psychology/ behavior medicine and neuropsychology. She specializes in evaluation and treatment, including for EMF sensitivities. She is an adjunct professor of psychology at the University of North Texas.

Richardson, TX
Email: **drnancy@airmail.net**

**Leslie S. Feinberg, DC** developed NeuroModulation Technique as a result of his many years of studying energetic medicine and the principles of western science and Traditional Chinese Medicine. Dr. Feinberg teaches this technique to other health professionals from many disciplines.

**Columbia Chiropractic Clinic**
NeuroModulation Technique NMT Seminars,
Hermiston, Oregon USA
Website: **www.nmt.md**

**Mark Hyman, MD and Elizabeth Boham, MD** practice at the UltraWellness Center where they focus on identifying and treating the underlying causes of illness, starting with extensive diagnostic testing. Dr. Mark Hyman is the author of several books on wellness issues including: environmental influences, supplementation, metabolism, detoxification and the conditions ADHD and autism. Dr. Hyman also offers training programs for health professionals through the Institute for Functional Medicine.

Lenox, MA
Email: office@ultrawellnesscenter.com
Website: **www.drhyman.com**

**Dietrich Klinghardt, MD, PhD** was one of the first practitioners in the U.S. to include comprehensive detoxification in his medical treatment strategies. Dr. Klinghardt has pioneered many diagnostic and detoxification strategies and is considered one of the world's leading authorities in this rapidly advancing field. He is one of the Contributing Experts for this book.

For an appointment with Dr. Klinghardt's team at the Sophia Health Institute, 18106 140th Ave NE, Woodinville, WA 98072, phone: 425-402-4401.

There is an extensive list on the following website, under 'Find a Certified Practitioner', of doctors and other health professionals who have trained with Dr. Klinghardt.

The Klinghardt Academy is the official resource for Dr. Klinghardt's information, protocols, articles, educational materials, audio and video files and training.

**Klinghardt Academy of Neurobiology**
Website: **www.klinghardtacademy.com**

**Stephanie McCarter, MD** is an internal medicine/environmental medicine physician who works alongside Dr. Rea, treating those with EMF sensitivities. She is also active in bringing together physicians, healthcare professionals, researchers, and scientists to explore this biochemical phenomenon.

Website: **www.ehcd.com**

**Jean Monro, MD** is the Medical Director at the Breakspear Medical Group in England, and is a London Hospital Medical School trained physician. She is internationally active in educating other physicians, colleagues, patients, and the public about physiological mechanisms behind EMF sensitivity, and possible treatments.

**Breakspear Medical Group**
Herts, UK
Website: **www.breakspearmedical.com**

**Ron Overberg, PhD, CCN, RD, LD** is a nutritionist at the EHC-D. One of his specialties at the clinic is working with EMF sensitive patients. He is also active in helping to educate physicians and the public about EMF sensitivity, and corresponding nutrition considerations.

Website: **www.ehcd.com**

**Thomas Rau, MD** is the medical director of the Paracelsus Klinik in Switzerland which is the core of the international network of Paracelsus Biological Medicine. It was established in 1958 and is widely recognized as a center of excellence for natural medicine.

Website: **www.drrau.com**

**William J. Rea, MD** is a thoracic and cardiovascular surgeon with a strong passion for the environmental aspects of health and disease. Dr. Rea is founder of The Environmental Health Center - Dallas, Texas, which offers comprehensive medical tests and treats human health problems including sensitivities to pollens, molds, dust, foods, chemicals, air (indoor/outdoor), water, electrical sensitivity (electromagnetic- EMF) and many more.

Website: **www.ehcd.com**

**Gay Riley, MS, RD, CCN, NASM-CPT** is a licensed and registered dietitian able to provide Medical Nutrition Therapy (MNT), and a Certified Clinical Nutritionist, which includes training in complementary alternative modalities, therapeutic supplementation, diagnostic testing and functional nutrition, and education in vitamin and mineral supplementation.

Website: **www.netnutritionist.com**

**Sanoviv Medical Institute,** founded by Dr. Myron Wentz, is a cutting edge medical and healing center, located south of San Diego, in Baja California. Sanoviv offers integrative, patient-centered medical treatments complemented by individualized personal care programs.

Website: **www.sanoviv.com**

**Stephen T. Sinatra, MD, FACC, FACN, CNS** is a board-certified cardiologist, certified bioenergetic psychotherapist and certified nutrition and anti-aging specialist. He is a fellow in the American College of Cardiology and the American College of Nutrition, former chief of cardiology at Manchester Memorial Hospital, and an assistant clinical professor of medicine at the University of Connecticut School of Medicine. He writes a monthly national newsletter entitled Heart, Health and Nutrition (Healthy Directions, L.L.C.), lectures world-wide, and facilitates health-related workshops.

Website: **www.heartmdinstitute.com**

**Dr. Briana Sinatra ND, LAc, MSA and Dr. Drew Sinatra ND, LAc, MSA** utilize a holistic approach to reduce the detrimental effects radiation can have on a cellular, biochemical and physiologic level. This includes education on ways to identify and reduce EMR exposure, along with ways to help the body cope with unavoidable EMR. Dr. Briana Sinatra uses Traditional Chinese Medicine and Dr. Drew Sinatra practices 5-Element Acupuncture to help connect people to the cycles of nature, which are disrupted with EMR exposure.

Living Wellness Center, South Surrey, British Columbia
Website: **www.livingwellness.ca**

**Martha Stark, MD** is a Harvard trained physician. She has a private practice in psychoanalysis, and is on faculty at Harvard Medical School in the Center for Psychoanalytic Studies. She works with environmental physicians and scientists to explore the impact of physiological EMFs on the body, including oxidative stress, excitotoxicity, and mitochondrial disruption.

Harvard Medical School
Email: **MarthaStarkMD@HMS.harvard.edu**

**Jacob Teitelbaum, MD** is a board-certified internist and Medical Director of the national Fibromyalgia and Fatigue Centers, Inc., in the U.S. He focuses on expanding the understanding of hypothalamic dysfunction in Fibromyalgia (FMS) and Chronic Fatigue Syndrome (CFIDS). His work has led to the development of an effective treatment protocol for these diseases.

Website: **www.endfatigue.com**

### To Find a Practitioner of Holistic/Complementary Medicine

Website: **www.holisticmedicine.org**

### Research and Education

**Magda Havas, PhD** is an associate professor at Trent University. She focuses on teaching and leading research on the health and environmental effects of chemical contaminants on electromagnetic pollution.

Environmental & Resource Studies, Trent University
Peterborough, ON Canada

**Heather McKinney, PhD** is a researcher who specializes in strategic planning for effective change and health improvement within individuals, organizations and communities. She is working with the author in developing the Safer-Tech Challenge education program.

Email: **DrHeatherMcKinney@gmail.com**

**Cyril W. Smith, PhD** is a physicist and author. He has a special interest in the scientific mechanism of EHS and aims to help healthcare professionals understand the quantum science behind this phenomenon.

Eccles, Manchester UK

### Biological Dentists

**International Association of Mercury Free Dentists**
Website: **www.dentalwellness4u.com**

**International Association of Biological Dentistry and Medicine**
Website: **www.iabdm.org**

**Holistic Dental Association**
Website: **www.holisticdental.org**

## Professional Services

### Healthy Buildings:

International Institute for Bau-Biologie (IBE)
Website: **www.buildingbiology.net**

### IBE/IBN Certified Consultants:

### CANADA

**Guelph**, Ontario – Servicing South Western Ontario and the Greater Toronto Area, Associates throughout North America
Safe Living Technologies Inc. Rob Metzinger, President
Testing equipment and protective/solution products: shielding fabrics, protective bed canopies, shielding paint, demand switches and more.
Email: rob@slt.co
Website: **www.slt.co**

**Montreal**, Quebec
3E Electro-magnetic Environmental Expertise Inc.
Stéphane Belainsky
Website: **www.em3e.com**

**Victoria**, British Columbia
Rainbow Consulting
Katharina Gustavs, Building Biology Environmental Consultant (IBN)
Website: **www.buildingbiology.ca**

### USA

**Carlsbad**, California
Environmental Testing & Technology, Inc.(ET&T)
ET&T was founded in 1986 by Peter Sierck to provide an indoor environmental testing and consulting service for patients, physicians, home owners, corporations, institutions and builders.
Website: **www.emfrf.com**

**Ventura**, California
Gust Environmental. Lawrence J Gust
Email: lgust@GustEnviro.com
Website: **www.GustEnviro.com**

**New York City, Long Island, Eastern NJ, CT, lower and upper state NY**
Matt Waletzke, BBEC
Healthy Dwellings Tel: 612.242.4558
Email: matt@healthydwellings.com
Website: **www.healthydwellings.com**

**Clearwater**, Florida
Indoor Environmental Technologies, Inc.
William H. Spates, III – BBEI
Website: **www.ietbuildinghealth.com**

**Lyles**, Tennessee
Wings of Eagles Healthy Living, Inc.
Vicki Warren, BBEC
Website: **www.wehliving.org**

**Baltimore**, Maryland
Healthy Home Arts, LLC
Jennifer Michalack, BBEC
Website: **www.healthyhomearts.com**

**Battle Creek**, Michigan
Mike Weston
Email: **westonmf@comcast.net**

**St. Paul**, Minnesota
Damon Coyne
E-Mail:damon@intentionalenvironment.com
Website: **intentionalenvironment.com**

## Other EMF/EMR Consultants

## CANADA

**South Western British Columbia**
ElectroSmogSolutions
Chris Anderson & Associates,
EMR consultant following the Building Biology principles since 1999.
Website: **www.ElectroSmogSolutions.ca**

**USA**

**Boulder,** Colorado
Radsafe
Stan Hartman
Environmental health testing specializing in electro-magnetic fields and radiation.
Email: stan@radsafe.net
Website: **www.radsafe.net**

**UK / NATIONWIDE**

**Offices in: Surrey, Yorkshire & Powys**
Electric Forester Investigations Ltd.
Roger H Moller BSc.Ind.Eng. - Principal Investigator
T: (44+) 1591 610167
On-Site and Remote Electromagnetic Surveys & Investigations
Homes, offices, factories and other built environments
Email: surveys@electricforester.co.uk
Website: **www.electricforester.co.uk**

**EUROPE**

**Esslingen,** Switzerland
Peter Schlegel
EMF/EMR testing of buildings; consulting in shielding; publicity & presentations in the field of EMF/EMR protection
Email: info@buergerwelle-schweiz.org
Website: **www.buergerwelle-schweiz.org**

**AUSTRALIA**

**EMF/EMR Testing:**

**Tasmania/Melbourne**:
EMFacts Consultancy
Don Maisch, PhD
Email: dmaisch@emfacts.com
Website: **www.emfacts.com**

**Sydney**:
EMR Surveys
John Lincoln
Email: emrsurveys@optusnet.com.au
Website: **www.emrsurveys.com.au**

**Sydney**:
EMR Australia
Lyn McLean
Email: contact@emraustralia.com.au
Website: **www.emrandhealth.com.au**

**Melbourne,** Victoria
Magshield Products, Intl.
Garry Melik
Email: **gmelik@magshield.com.au**

**Melbourne**, Victoria (Australia-wide)
Brookes EMS Pty Ltd.
Ken Brookes
Email: ken@brookes.com.au
Website: **www.brookesems.com.au**

### Testing and Shielding Equipment

First, here is a brief description of each item; followed by sources listed by country.

### Frequency Detection:

**RF meters** detect radio and microwave frequencies from mobile phones, wireless devices etc.

**Electric Field meters** detect lower frequencies from plugged-in devices, wiring etc.

**Protective Shielding:**

**Air Tube, RF-Reducing Cell Phone** – The sound travels up the plastic air tube, limiting the amount of radiation to your brain from either cell phones or portable phones. If you must use a cell phone, using this headset will reduce radiation to the brain significantly.

**Bed Canopies** – People who are electrically sensitive find shielding bed canopies essential, as do high performance athletes and, increasingly, business executives bathed in frequencies all day. Must be done properly; the material cannot rest on you and/or the bed.

**Shielding Fabrics** – Shielding fabric by the foot can be used to line curtains, walls and can even be put under carpets or desk chair pads to shield from the wireless radiation of neighbors downstairs.

**Shielding Films** – Placing plastic shielding film on glass windows can significantly block out ambient radio-frequency radiation-from where it comes into the building most easily.

**Shielding Paints** – Metallic water-based paint can be placed under latex paints or wallpapers. Suitable for many types of exterior surfaces as well. Caution: The surface of this paint is highly conductive. It does need to be grounded and should <u>not</u> be installed without the services of an electrician.

Also, do <u>not</u> put shielding paint on the walls if the room will contain RF emitting devices, such as computers, cell phones, wireless routers, compact fluorescent bulbs, etc.

**CANADA**

**Safe Living Technologies**

Website: **www.SLT.co**

**RF Meters:**
RF Detector
A broadband detector allows you to hear and assess all the invisible microwave emissions around you.

**Electric Field Meters:**
eME3030B Dual Function Gauss/Tesla Meter and Electric Field

*Safe Living Technologies continued:*

**Shielding Materials** – A full line of bed canopies, fabrics, window foil and paint.

**Air tube, RF-Reducing Cell Phone Headsets** – Avoid the health hazards of traditional headsets. This headset allows for safer cell phone use.

**Demand Switches** – eliminate Electric and Magnetic fields in living spaces by automatically shutting off the power when it is not being used.

**Shielded Power Cord** – Help reduce electric fields by replacing your existing power cords with shielded power cords.

**USA**

**Less EMF Inc**
Website: **www.lessemf.com**

776B Watervliet Shaker Rd
Latham NY 12110 USA
Tel: 1-888-537-7363
lessemf@lessemf.com
Specializing in Electromagnetic Field Safety Products for the home and office since 1996. EMF Meters, shielding, appliances, books and more. They have a good selection of cell phone shield holders.

**EMF Safety Store**
Website: **www.emfsafetystore.com**

**RF & Other Meters:**

ELECTROSMOG METER (RF Fields)
Very Sensitive, Affordable RF/MW Meter

4180 ELF GAUSS METER (Magnetic Fields)

BUDGET BUZZ STICK (Magnetic Fields). This little unit won't actually measure anything numerically, but detects magnetic fields, letting you 'listen' to them.

ELFLX DETECTOR (Electric Fields)

AC Electric Field Finder

This inexpensive little unit has no numerical readout, but will detect AC electric fields from 100 to 600 volts (50-60 Hz), displaying them with a red LED and an audio output.

Air tube RF-Reducing Cell Phone Headsets.

**UK/EUROPE:**

**Sensory Perspective**

Website: **www.detect-protect.com**

**RF Meters**

The Acoustimeter (MW-AM10) features an extraordinarily wide Frequency Range (200MHz-8000MHz... 8GHz!), and with the sound of the iconic Electrosmog Detector and state-of-the-art measurement circuitry, it tells you what you need to know, including both the average reading in microWatts per square metre, and the peak/highest reading detected (in Volts per metre) since you turned it on.

HF32D – Digital Microwave Analyser for 800-2500 MHz - For a quick and competent digital assessment of microwave exposure between 800 MHz and 2.5 GHz. This range includes mobile/cellular phones, cordless phones, Wi-MAX, Bluetooth, and computer/broadband wLANs.

**Electric Field Meters**

ELF-3030B - Digital ELF Meter for E & H Fields 16Hz-2kHz

Sensitive and informative, with digital display and sounder, it allows you to check electromagnetic radiation from the delivery and use of electricity around you.

**Shielding Materials** – a full line of bed canopies, fabrics, wallpaper and paint, clothing and demand switches.

**Publications**. *The Powerwatch Handbook* – Simple Ways to Make Your (EMF) Environment Safer (this is highly recommended.)

Please visit our website: SaferTechSolutions.org. for the following:

**Evidence of Harm – Reference Material, including these documents:**

- ***Summarizing the Science***– by Dr. Henry Lai. For those who argue there's not enough science to link electro-magnetic radiation exposure and health effects, here is a summary from one the most qualified scientists in this field. Dr. Lai details studies conducted over the past twenty years. Many of these show that EMR can affect cancers, immunology, genetics, cellular & molecular biology, behavior, reproduction and growth, hormones, the nervous system, the blood-brain barrier and metabolism.

- ***Key Studies*** cited by Dr. Sarah Starkey. This neuroscientist offers an extensive list of published studies detailing adverse health effects from EMR exposure. Dr. Starkey is a strong advocate of safer-tech solutions for schools and encourages them to replace harmful WiFi networks with wired and/or fiber optics. Website: www.wifiinschools.org.uk

- ***Cellphones and Brain Tumors – 15 Reasons for Concern***, August 2009, Lead Author: L. Lloyd Morgan, USA, Bioelectromagnetics Society, Electronics Engineer (retired) The full BioInitiative Report can be found at: www.bioinitiative.org/report index.htm

- ***Symptoms of Electro-Magnetic Hypersensitivity – a Detailed List with References*** From Larry Gust Environmental. This is a comprehensive document and very informative. Website: www.healbuildings.com

- ***Breast Cancer Risks and EMR Exposure*** – a list of published studies. This potential cause of breast cancer is not well known, but should be. (A woman should never carry a mobile phone in her bra, or anywhere on her body, when the mobile is in its sending/receiving mode.)

- ***Scientists' Concerns About Wireless in Schools*** An Open Letter to Parents, Teachers, School Boards. Regarding WiFi Networks in Schools - May 5, 2009 by Dr. Magda Havas, Associate Professor, Trent University. Websites: www.magdahavas.com and www.doctorsforsaferschools.org

- ***Wireless in the Air - Health and Safety Concerns*** The full letter written to airline executives by Dr. Hans Scheiner and the German Environmental Physician Initiative. (When booking, please ask for WiFi free flights.)

# Index

## F



## G



## H



## I

## N



## O



## P



## Q

## R



## S

29653232R00214

Made in the USA
Middletown, DE
26 February 2016